Evidence-Based Protocols for Managing Wandering Behaviors

Audrey L. Nelson, PhD, RN, FAAN, is Director, Veterans Administration Patient Safety Research Center and has over 28 years of experience in nursing. She currently serves as the Associate Chief of Nursing Service for Research at the Tampa VA and Director of the Tampa Patient Safety Center of Inquiry. Dr. Nelson is Associate Director of Clinical Research at the University of South Florida College of Nursing and is a Research Professor in the Colleges of Public Health and Engineering. She is a national leader in patient safety and has established and chairs the International Research Consortium on Wandering. In 2005, Dr. Nelson was awarded the John Eisenberg Award for Lifetime Achievements in Patient Safety and Quality. Dr. Nelson has expertise in research methods, wandering/elopement, safe patient handling and movement, wheelchair-related falls, and patient safety technology. She has had studies funded from Veterans Health Administration, VA Health Services Research & Development and VA Rehabilitation Research and Development, and the Agency for Healthcare Research Quality (AHRQ).

Donna L. Algase, PhD, RN, FAAN, FGSA, is the Josephine M. Sana Collegiate Professor of Nursing at the School of Nursing, University of Michigan, founding Director of the Center of Frail and Vulnerable Elders, and Director of the Intervention Development and Measurement Core of the Michigan Center for Health Interventions. Her research program focuses on dementia-related behaviors with specific emphasis on the phenomenon of wandering and models to quantify and explain it. Dr. Algase has been awarded over $6.5M in research grants from the Alzheimer's Association, the National Institutes of Aging and Nursing Research, and other foundations. Her research has resulted in numerous publications, national and international presentations and consultations, and leadership of the Need-driven Dementia-compromised Behavior Collaborative Research Group. Her accomplishments also include development of multiple research instruments to measure wandering and other dementia-related behaviors and concepts including the Algase Wandering Scale, the Wayfinding Effectiveness Scale, the Ambiance Scale, and others.

Evidence-Based Protocols for Managing Wandering Behaviors

Audrey L. Nelson, PhD, RN, FAAN
and
Donna L. Algase, PhD, RN, FAAN, FGSA
Editors

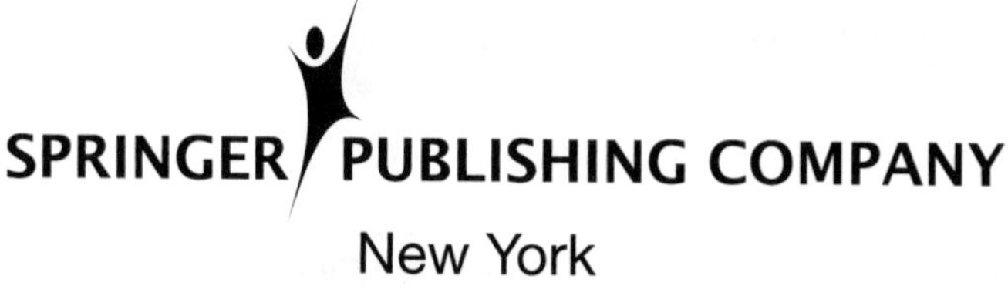

New York

Springer Publishing Company, LLC
11 West 42nd Street
New York, NY 10036
www.springerpub.com

Acquisitions Editor: Sally J. Barhydt
Production Editor: Carol Cain
Cover design: Joanne E. Honigman
Cover Photo Artist: Alana Papernik Stein
Composition: Apex Publishing, LLC

07 08 09 10/ 5 4 3 2 1

Library of Congress Cataloging-in-Publication Data

Evidence-based protocols for managing wandering behaviors / Audrey L. Nelson, Donna L. Algase [editors].
p. ; cm.
Includes bibliographical references and index.
ISBN-13: 978-0-8261-6365-3 (alk. paper)
ISBN-10: 0-8261-6365-3 (alk. paper)
1. Dementia—Complications. 2. Evidence-based medicine. 3. Walking. 4. Agitation (Psychology). I. Nelson, Audrey L., PhD. II. Algase, Donna L. [DNLM: 1. Dementia—complications. 2. Dementia—therapy. 3. Walking. 4. Aged. 80 and over. 5. Aged. 6. Clinical Protocols. 7. Evidence-Based Medicine—methods. 8. Psychomotor Agitation. 9. Safety Management—methods. WT 155 E93 2007]
RC521.E955 2007
362.196'83—dc22 2007012051

Printed in the United States of America by Bang Printing

Contents

PART III. SPECIAL ISSUES ASSOCIATED WITH WANDERING

PART IV. INTERVENTIONS

Preface

Wandering is among the most frequent, problematic, and dangerous of dementia-related behaviors, and, arguably, the one that brings the greatest risk, highest volume, and most burdensome cost of them all. Associated with high potential for negative consequences such as weight loss, falls, elopements and getting lost, injury, fractures, and even death, wandering is a challenging behavior in both home and health care settings. For lay and professional caregivers alike, caring for those who wander raises difficult questions in balancing autonomy, choice, privacy, dignity, comfort, and safety for people already confronting the impact of cognitive loss. The projected growth and important impact of the population with dementia is undeniable. Together with current and anticipated realities of restricted health care budgets and shortages of health care providers, expansion of available and tested methods for wandering management are especially critical.

For nearly three decades, the complexity of wandering has intrigued gerontologists from multiple disciplines. Steadily, methodological and theoretical challenges associated with the study of wandering are being overcome, and consequently, much has been learned about this perplexing behavior. However, gains in synthesizing this learning into a comprehensible body of knowledge have been slower to evolve.

This book is addressed to gerontologists and to nurses who face the day-to-day challenges of caring for persons who wander in nursing homes, assisted living facilities, home health agencies, and hospitals. Our purpose in developing this book is to aid them in advancing the science of wandering and improving the care of wanderers. This book presents a comprehensive analysis and synthesis of a large body of work drawn from the research, clinical, health care management, and policy literature on wandering into concise meaningful summaries and practical tools. It is our hope that this book will help standardize the language and measurement of wandering, shape theory to guide intervention, reduce variations in practice, and improve quality of care. The book has a special emphasis on addressing the difficult and stressful problems of daily patient care, improving safety of those with cognitive impairments, and enabling those with dementia to remain independent longer.

This book is the product of a large group of interdisciplinary collaborators collectively identified as the International Consortium for Research on Wandering. Launched in 2003, under the umbrella of the Patient Safety Center of Inquiry at the James A. Haley Veterans Hospital in Tampa, Florida, the Consortium has rapidly expanded to include over two dozen nurses, gerontologists, psychologists, social workers, geriatricians, dieticians, social scientists, anthropologists, engineers, health economists, architects, and statisticians whose efforts are escalating both the quality and quantity of wandering science and disseminating it to advance practice and improve care for wanderers and their families.

The book is organized in five parts: (I) the construct of wandering, (II) assessment, (III) special issues associated with wandering, (IV) interventions, and (V) future directions.

The first part, *Construct of Wandering,* provides an introduction to the complexity of wandering. Chapter 1, "Wandering Definitions and Terms" includes the terminology that is a necessary first step to standardizing language in practice and research. This chapter includes two useful tools: discussion of the Compendium of Wandering-Related Terms and Definitions (found in Appendix A) and a conceptual map of wandering (Fig. 1.1). In Chapter 2, "Theoretical Models of Wandering," new and emerging theoretical models of wandering are presented. These models, derived from research, can be used to guide clinical practice as well as to contribute to the science of wandering. The scope of the problem of wandering is elucidated in Chapter 3, "Epidemiology of Wandering," which includes data on the incidence and prevalence of wandering, as well as characteristics of wanderers and consequences of wandering behaviors. Lastly, Chapter 4, "Neuropsychological Correlates of Wanderers," reviews findings of neuropsychological testing in persons who wander.

The second part, *Assessment,* includes Chapter 5, "Assessment of Wandering Behaviors," which describes the WING-AP, a wandering assessment protocol based on the Need-driven Dementia-compromised Behavior Model and the Model of Risky Wandering and on validated tools for assessing wandering. The WING-AP also includes an assessment guide and approaches to compiling and organizing assessment data for identifying and prioritizing treatment goals.

Caring for wandering patients requires far more than knowledge of disease processes and treatment modalities alone. The third part, *Special Issues Associated With Wandering,* includes five chapters focusing on biopsychosocial issues likely to affect wandering behaviors and responses to interventions. In Chapter 6, "Impact of Wandering on Functional

Status," functional outcomes of wandering are described in the context of seven functional domains most affected: mobility; elimination; eating; bathing, dressing, and grooming; communication; nutrition and eating; and resting. In Chapter 7, "Caregiver Issues Associated With Wandering," the authors explain how wandering affects family caregivers and describe issues in the implementation of wandering interventions that can be used by family caregivers. In Chapter 8, "Cultural Issues Associated With Wandering," issues related to wandering behavior are examined to promote culturally competent assessments and interventions for persons who wander. Given the cultural diversity in the United States, health care professionals need skills for successfully negotiating cultural differences. In Chapter 9, "Root Cause Analysis Reported of Wandering Adverse Events in the Veterans Health Administration," provides information on missing patient events contained in the VHA Patient Safety Information Database, including when and where patients are reported missing, as well as the root cause/contributing factors and actions identified to address system vulnerabilities. Lastly, in Chapter 10, "Getting Lost: Antecedents, Wandering Behavior, and Search Strategies," the devastating experience of getting lost is described. In addition to summarizing real life situations in which individuals become lost and what happens after they are lost in the community, methods and successful search strategies that law enforcement agencies can use to find them are presented.

In the fourth part, *Interventions,* practical solutions are described for enhancing the safety for persons who wander. In Chapter 11, "Behavior Management of Wandering Behavior: Staff Training Issues," the authors focus on training relative to implementation of behavior modification procedures useful for staff members in long-term care facilities and applications. In Chapter 12, "Pharmacological Interventions Associated With Wandering," medications that affect and are affected by wandering behaviors are described. Chapter 13, "The Alzheimer's Association's Safe Return® Program for Persons Who Wander," provides a succinct overview of a national identification and support program promoting speedy recovery of persons who become lost after being separated from their caregivers. In Chapter 14, "A Home Safety Program for Community-Based Wanderers: Outcomes From the Veterans Home Safety Project," we report findings from the project to develop and evaluate minimum, basic safety actions that should be employed for all persons with dementia living at home. Chapter 15, "Technologies to Manage Wandering," describes new and emerging technologies to assist with assessment of wandering, early detection of elopement, and tracking of persons who are lost. Chapter 16, "Environmental Design," includes a thorough review of current research and best practices with regard to environmental issues impacting wandering in persons with dementia in long-term care. In

Chapter 17, "Evidenced-Based Practice Protocols for Wandering," the challenges associated with identifying evidence-based approaches is discussed, and several best practices are delineated.

The last part, *Future Directions,* includes Chapter 18, "A Research Agenda to Build the Science Associated With Wandering," which identifies methodological issues associated with research in wandering, gaps in research, and an agenda for future research.

Audrey L. Nelson, PhD, RN, FAAN
Donna L. Algase, PhD, RN, FAAN, FGSA

Contributors

James P. Bagian, MD, PE
Chief Patient Safety Officer
Veterans Health Administration
Director, National Center for Patient Safety
Department of Veterans Affairs
Ann Arbor, Michigan

Elizabeth Bass, PhD
Health Economist
VISN8 Patient Safety Research Center
James A. Haley Veterans Affair Medical Center
Tampa, Florida

Elizabeth R. A. Beattie, PhD, RN, FGSA
Regulatory Compliance Associate
University of Michigan
Office of Human Research Compliance Review
Office of the Vice-President for Research
Ann Arbor, Michigan

Cynthia A. Beel-Bates, PhD, RN
Associate Professor
Kirkhof College of Nursing
Grand Valley State University
Grand Rapids, Michigan

Lisa M. Brown, PhD
Assistant Professor
Department of Aging & Mental Health
Louis de la Parte Florida Mental Health Institute
University of South Florida
Tampa, Florida

Margaret P. Calkins, PhD
President
IDEAS, Inc.
Board Chair
IDEAS Institute
Kirtland, Ohio

Steven Charles Castle, MD
Clinical Professor of Medicine
University of California, Los Angeles
School of Medicine
Clinical Director of Geriatrics
Veterans Affair Greater Los Angeles Healthcare
Division of Geriatrics and Gerontology
Geriatric Research Education and Clinical Center
Los Angeles, California

Bettye Rose Connell, PhD
Health Research Scientist
Rehabilitation Research & Development Center
Atlanta Veterans Affair Medical Center
Assistant Professor
Emory School of Medicine
Decatur, Georgia

Joseph M. DeRosier, PE, CSP
Program Manager
National Center for Patient Safety
Department of Veterans Affairs
Ann Arbor, Michigan

James L. Fozard, PhD
Courtesy Full Professor
University of South Florida
School of Aging Studies
Tampa, Florida

Deborah Gavin-Dreschnack, PhD
Health Science Specialist
VISN8 Patient Safety Research Center
James A. Haley Veterans Affair Medical Center
Tampa, Florida

William E. Haley, PhD
Professor and Director
University of South Florida
School of Aging Studies
Tampa, Florida

Rose M. Harvey, DNSc, RN
Adjunct Associate Professor
Bouvé College of Health Sciences
School of Nursing
Northeastern University
Boston, Massachusetts

Kathy J. Horvath, PhD, RN
Associate Director for Education and Evaluation
Veterans Affair New England
Geriatric Research Education Clinical Center
Edith Nourse Rogers Memorial Veterans Hospital
Bedford, Massachusetts

Inez Joseph, PhD, ARNP, NHA
Associate Chief, Nursing Service
James A Haley Veterans Affair Medical Center
Tampa, Florida

William D. Kearns, PhD
Assistant Professor
Department of Aging and Mental Health
Louis de la Parte Florida Mental Health Institute
University of South Florida
Tampa, Florida

Cheryl A. Luis, PhD, ABPP-CN
Associate Clinic Director
Roskamp Institute and Nova Southeastern University
Roskamp Institute Memory Clinic
Tampa, Florida

Nancy Lynn, MSPH
Coordinator of Research Activities
Louis de la Parte Florida Mental Health Institute
University of South Florida
Tampa, Florida

Victor A. Molinari, PhD, ABPP
Professor
Department of Aging and Mental Health
Louis de la Parte Florida Mental Health Institute
University of South Florida
Tampa, Florida

D. Helen Moore, PhD
Health Science Specialist
VISN8 Patient Safety Center of Inquiry
James A. Haley Veterans Affair Medical Center
Tampa, Florida

Monica Moreno
Associate Director, Safety Services
National Alzheimer's Association
Chicago, Illinois

Andrea J. Pe Benito
College of Nursing
University of Florida
Gainsville, Florida

Elizabeth A. Perkins, RNMH, BA
Doctoral Candidate
School of Aging Studies
University of South Florida
Tampa, Florida

Meredeth A. Rowe, PhD, RN
Associate Professor
University of Florida
College of Nursing
Gainesville, Florida

Michelle K. Rutledge, PharmD
Associate Investigator
Health Services Research &
Development Service
VISN8 Patient Safety Research Center
James A. Haley Veterans Affair
Medical Center
Tampa, Florida

Lawrence Schonfeld, PhD
Professor and Chair
Department of Aging and Mental Health
Louis de la Parte Florida Mental Health Institute
University of South Florida
Tampa, Florida

Gwi-Ryung Son Hong, PhD, RN
Assistant Professor
Hanyang University
College of Medicine
Department of Nursing
Seoul, South Korea

Jun-Ah Song, PhD, RN
Assistant Professor
Korea University
College of Nursing
Seoul, South Korea

Laura M. Struble, PhD, RN, GNP
Gerontological Nurse Practitioner and Nurse Educator
Behavioral Health Services
Chelsea Community Hospital
Chelsea, Michigan

Lesley Taylor
Program Analyst
National Center for Patient Safety
Department of Veterans Affairs
Ann Arbor, Michigan

Scott A. Trudeau, MA, OTR/L
Lecturer
Tufts University
Department of Occupational Therapy
Medford, Massachusetts

James Turner
Program Analyst
National Center for Patient Safety
Department of Veterans Affairs
Ann Arbor, Michigan

Carla VandeWeerd, PhD
Assistant Professor
Department of Community and Family Health
College of Public Health
University of South Florida
Tampa, Florida

Ladislav Volicer, MD, PhD, FAAN, FGSA
Courtesy Full Professor
School of Aging Studies MHC 1342
University of South Florida
Tampa, Florida

Lan Yao, PhD, RN
Assistant Research Scientist
University of Michigan School of Nursing
Ann Arbor, Michigan

Acknowledgments

We would like to acknowledge the International Research Consortium on Wandering, for dedication and commitment to this and the many other clinical, research, and educational activities they have approached with enthusiasm and scientific rigor. Members of the Consortium as of August 2006 are named in the following list. For more information on this group and their accomplishments, see http://www.visn8.med.va.gov/patientsafetycenter/wandering/.

Donna L. Algase, PhD, RN, FAAN, FGSA
Shawn Applegarth, MSME
Andrea S. Baptiste, MA
Elizabeth Bass, PhD
Elizabeth R. A. Beattie, PhD, RN
Lisa M. Brown, PhD
Patricia Caldwell, APRN, BC
David Chiriboga, PhD
Bettye Rose Connell, PhD
Susan G. Cooley, PhD
Darlene Davis, MHA, RD, NHA
Joseph M. DeRosier, PE, CSP
Deborah Gavin-Dreschnack, PhD
William E. Haley, PhD
Crista M. Hojlo, PhD, RN, NHA
Kathy J. Horvath, PhD, RN
Inez Joseph, PhD, ARNP, NHA
Bellinda King-Kallimanis, MS
William D. Kearns, PhD
John D. Lloyd, PhD, MErgS, DPS, CPE
Victor A. Molinari, PhD, ABPP
D. Helen Moore, PhD
Audrey L. Nelson, PhD, RN, FAAN
Gail Powell-Cope, PhD, ARNP, FAAN

Meredeth A. Rowe, PhD, RN
Lawrence Schonfeld, PhD
Gwi-Ryung Son Hong, PhD, RN
Carla VandeWeerd, PhD
Ladislav Volicer, MD, PhD, FAAN, FGSA

We would also like to acknowledge the VISN8 Patient Safety Center of Inquiry at the James A. Haley Veterans Administration (Tampa, FL) and the National Center for Patient Safety in the Veterans Health Administration for continued support and resources for improving the safety of veterans who wander.

Several experts in the field agreed to externally review chapters. We appreciate their dedication and scholarly contributions as well. Reviewers include:

Shawn Applegarth, MSME
Tatjana Bulat, MD
Darlene Davis, MHA, RD, NHA
Deborah Gavin-Dreschnack, PhD
Kathy J. Horvath, PhD, RN
William D. Kearns, PhD
D. Helen Moore, PhD
Helen Taylor, RN
Victor A. Molinari, PhD, ABPP
Meredeth A. Rowe, PhD, RN
Lawrence Schonfeld, PhD
Ladislav Volicer, MD, PhD, FAAN, FGSA

The following individuals responded to a national call for best practices or innovations related to wandering assessment or management of wandering. We reviewed many possible submissions and selected a few for inclusion in this book. We wish to recognize the following contributors:

- Kelly Fethelkheir, RN, Bay Pines VA Healthcare System, Bay Pines, Florida
- Fern Pietruszka, PA-C, MPH, Greater Los Angeles VA Nursing Home Care Unit, North Hills, California
- Vivian E. Bugaoan, LCSW, Northport VA Medical Center, Northport, New York

- Judith O'Neal, RN, VA Sierra Nevada Health Care System, Reno, Nevada

Lastly, we wish to recognize Valerie Kelleher for her substantial contributions in communicating with authors, formatting the manuscripts, and checking references and for her editing skills.List of Figures

List of Figures

List of Tables

Evidence-Based Protocols for Managing Wandering Behaviors

PART I

Construct of Wandering

CHAPTER ONE

Wandering Definitions and Terms

Donna L. Algase, D. Helen Moore, Deborah Gavin-Dreschnack, and Carla VandeWeerd

Wandering is a serious concern for family and professional care providers as well as for scientists, clinicians, and policy makers, because the behavior is associated with some of the gravest adverse outcomes in dementia care (e.g., accidents, falls, getting lost, and even death). A growing number of studies reflect this concern focusing on the various aspects of this pervasive and intriguing behavior that include: (1) the nature of wandering—its descriptors, measurement, and natural history; (2) the outcomes of wandering such as getting lost and elopement; (3) wandering-related behaviors such as intrusion, shadowing, or exit seeking; and (4) techniques for wandering management and intervention. It is remarkable, given the increase in contemporary scholarship, that wandering and its related behaviors remains poorly defined. The conundrum of an inaccurate and ambiguous wandering vocabulary has plagued wandering science since its origins several decades ago and persists to this day, to the detriment of scientific discourse and advancement.

Precise definitions work toward improving science, practice, and policy and serve to enhance communication across fields. However, care

---

Aspects of this chapter are based on a journal article, "Mapping the Maze of Terms and Definitions in Dementia-Related Wandering," written by the authors of this chapter and accepted for publication in the *International Journal of Aging and Mental Health*. Blackwell Publishing Co. has granted permission to reprint Figure 1.1 herein and the Compendium of Wandering-Related Terms and Definitions, which appears as Appendix A.

providers, scientists, clinicians, and policy makers who journey even briefly into the literature on wandering quickly learn that a consensus definition for the term is lacking. In many studies, researchers invent their own definitions and fail to place their work within the context of the growing body of wandering studies. Proliferation of definitions to the exclusion of established and valid ones only complicates interpretation and integration of findings across studies, necessities for advancing science and practice and evolving rational policies.

Misuse of wandering-related terms may stem from the aforementioned tendency of authors to draw on their own disciplinary or professional viewpoints when defining the behavior of interest, to the complex multifaceted nature of the behavior itself and to the tendency to confuse the act of wandering—a unique type of locomotion through space engaged in by some cognitively impaired persons—with the potential outcomes of such behavior. Regardless of how the current muddled state of the wandering lexicon is explained, it is essential that any text devoted to the wandering behavior begins with a clear definition of the term.

This chapter includes:

- Stakeholder specific definitions of wandering,
- A compendium of wandering-related terms and definitions and a conceptual map of wandering, and
- Measurement approaches used to estimate the amount and type of wandering.

Hopefully, this approach will foster understanding of wandering by providing readers with definitional, conceptual, measurement and descriptive perspectives on "wandering defined."

DEFINITIONS OF WANDERING

A Scientific Definition of Wandering

The scientific definition of wandering presented here describes the nature of the behavior as it is shaped by four domains: space, time, locomotion, and the drive or impetus for wandering (Algase, Moore, VandeWeerd, & Gavin-Dreschnack, in press). This definitional approach builds on a previous review of wandering measures (Algase, 1999) that describes wandering behavior in terms of its volume (frequency, rate, and duration), geographic pattern, navigational deficits, boundary transgressions, and temporal distribution. The specific methodology used to establish this definition has been previously described (Algase, Moore, VandeWeerd, & Gavin-Dreschnack, in press). This first iteration of a wandering definition may be of potential interest and greatest utility to scientists, because it allows others to independently verify the validity of research results through observation, measurement, or testing:

> wandering is a syndrome of dementia-related locomotion behavior having a frequent, repetitive, temporally-disordered, and/or spatially-disoriented nature that is manifested in lapping, random, and/or pacing patterns, some of which are associated with eloping, eloping attempts, or getting lost unless accompanied. (p. 13)

A Clinical Definition of Wandering

A clinical definition of wandering is one of potential interest and usefulness to clinicians, family, professional care providers, and others who are in direct contact with persons who wander, because the elemental features of the behavior are described and the need for caregiver vigilance implied. The North American Nursing Diagnosis Association (NANDA), an organization that develops, refines, and classifies phenomena of concern to nurses, promulgates the following wandering definition:

> meandering, aimless or repetitive locomotion that exposes a person to harm and is incongruent with boundaries, limits or obstacles. (NANDA, 2001, p. 206)

NANDA further lists some specific wandering behaviors and conditions under which wandering occurs: (1) frequent or continuous movement from place to place, often revisiting the same destination; (2) persistent locomotion in search of "missing" or unattainable people or places; (3) haphazard locomotion; (4) locomotion into unauthorized or private spaces; (5) locomotion resulting in unintended leaving of a premises; (6) long periods of locomotion without an apparent destination; (7) fretful locomotion or pacing; inability to locate significant landmarks in a familiar setting; (8) locomotion that cannot be easily dissuaded or redirected; (9) following behind or shadowing a caregiver's locomotion; (10) trespassing; (11) hyperactivity; scanning, seeking, or searching behaviors; (12) periods of locomotion interspersed with periods of nonlocomotion (e.g., sitting, standing, sleeping); and (13) getting lost (NANDA, 2001).

It is interesting to note that most clinicians who work in the field of dementia care can clearly differentiate wandering locomotion that may or may not be pointless from nonwandering locomotion that has a more obvious endpoint or outcome, such as going to the bathroom to use it or walking to the dining room at the appropriate hour. Likewise preliminary data (Gavin-Dreschnack, VandeWeerd, Moore, & Beattie, 2006) reveals that clinicians correctly recognize wandering as a type of spontaneous, unassisted movement through space, usually walking—but also the wanderer's self-propelled locomotion using a cane, walker, or wheelchair—that from a clinical standpoint occurs at an undesirable or unsuitable time, rate, or location. However when clinicians recount wandering scenarios from memory, they tend to fuse depictions of the behavior with other behavioral symptoms common to dementia, behaviors such as agitation or restlessness; hovering or other stationary standing behavior, such as swaying, rocking, or shifting from foot to foot; searching or scanning behavior, or asking to go "home" or somewhere else; and pacing, as in the back and forth walking of a person who is under pressure, anxious, or irritated. While we have included pacing as a subset of wandering in Figure 1.1, the term is variously described even within literature on wandering, having at times been coupled with aimless wandering as a group of behaviors (Cohen-Mansfield, 1991) or elucidated as a pattern of its own (Martino-Saltzman, Blasch, Morris, & McNeal, 1991). Data have shown that the pattern of relationships among pacing and other dimensions of wandering (persistent walking, spatial disorientation, eloping behaviors, and repetitive walking) differs from that of other wandering, that is, random and lapping (Algase, Beattie, Bogue, & Yao, 2001).

A Policy-Oriented Definition of Wandering

A wandering definition that may aid policy makers and risk managers focuses chiefly on patient safety risks and adverse outcomes. Media reports of accidents, injuries, and deaths of wandering patients, and lawsuits that level charges of unsafe wandering in institutional settings, underscore the need for well-conceptualized policy-oriented definitions.

The Department of Veterans Affairs defines a wandering patient as follows:

> A wandering patient is a high-risk patient who has shown a propensity to stray beyond the view or control of employees, thereby requiring a high degree of monitoring and protection to ensure the patient's safety. (From Management of Wandering and Missing Patient Events, VHA directive 2002–013, p. 1; see Appendix B)

TWO TOOLS FOR EXAMINING WANDERING

The "Compendium" and "Conceptual Map" presented in this section are original to the authors, and the methods used to create them have been elsewhere described (Algase, Moore, Gavin-Dreschnack, & VandeWeerd, accepted). The compendium is an exhaustive listing of wandering-related terms and definitions culled from a review of 183 journal articles on wandering. The conceptual map illustrates the relationship of these terms and definitions. These tools are provided as a general resource and as a guide to terms and concepts found throughout this book.

A Compendium of Wandering-Related Terms and Definitions.

The 121 unique entries in the compendium are credited to the authors who first used or defined the term, as far as could be determined. Although compendium entries were drawn from published work, inclusion of a term or definition does not ensure that it has been validated through research. However the listing is informative for those seeking to gain a broad view of wandering and useful for comparative purposes, such as integrating findings across studies (see Compendium in Appendix A).

A Conceptual Map of Wandering

As the compendium reveals, many wandering-related terms and definitions are similar, while others are quite different from one another. How does one decipher "wandering defined" from this seemingly disjointed linguistic array? In an attempt to answer this question, the authors created a conceptual map of wandering using compendium terms falling into the four domains that shape wandering behavior: space, time, locomotion, and the drive or impetus for wandering. By condensing the list and placing these terms (or groups of terms) into a conceptual map, relationships among them are revealed, supplying a means to assess the extent to which a term represents the concept of wandering, and providing a link between the term and the scientific definition offered earlier in this chapter. The conceptual map appears as Figure 1.1.

The outermost rings of the map represent the domains of locomotion and drive. By locomotion we mean moving oneself through space and time, mostly by walking, but also by propelling a wheelchair or driving a motor vehicle. By drive we mean the internal impetus or reason for moving. All terms in the compendium refer to or imply some feature or aspect of locomotion and thus fall within the locomotion domain. The domain of drive includes terms that imply either its presence (e.g., escapist) or absence (e.g., random). Since all behavior is motivated (or occurs for cause), we positioned terms above the line bisecting the oval for this domain if the term suggested that a wanderer

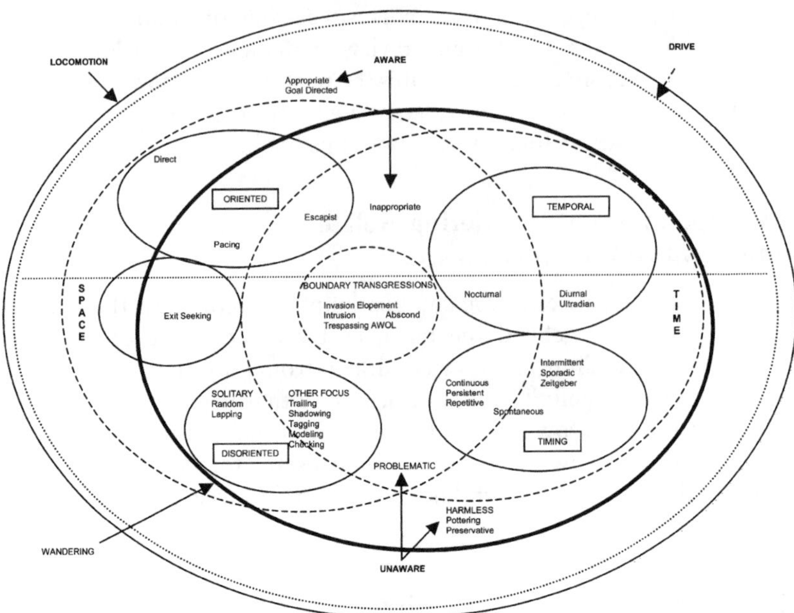

FIGURE 1.1 A conceptual map of wandering.
Source: Algase, Moore, VandeWeerd, & Gavin-Dreschnack, in press.

has awareness of their motivation or drive and below the line if not. However, little information has been gathered from wanderers about their motivations for locomotion, so classification of a term as to awareness of drive is based on authors' clinical judgment and research experience with wanderers (Algase, Moore, Gavin-Dreschnack, & VandeWeerd, accepted).

In the center of the map, two large ovals signify space and time and intersect to create an area where both are represented. Within them are smaller ovals representing subsets of space-and time-related terms. Terms from the compendium are situated within the ovals based on their codes for drive, space, and time.

An oval corresponding to wandering is shown with a thick line encompassing time and space and an area for terms reflecting neither property. To accommodate terms defining nonwandering locomotion (e.g., direct pattern), the oval of the relevant domain extends beyond that representing wandering. An analysis of this conceptual map reveals that terms fitting into the overlap of space and time refer to wandering behaviors that are problematic (i.e., when a wanderer is not aware of drive) or inappropriate to circumstances (i.e., when they are aware).

MEASURES FOR WANDERING

Another path to "wandering defined" obtains to descriptions of how the behavior is measured. This section reviews observational, rating scales and technological methods to assess, quantify, and measure wandering and wandering-related behaviors.

Observational Approaches

An early approach to wandering measurement characterized the geographic patterns of wandering of nursing home residents into four travel patterns using videotape methods (Martino-Saltzman, Blasch, Morris, & McNeal, 1991). Travel patterns are:

- lapping—locomotion that has a circuitous path (closed loop) with at least three legs that (a) return the wanderer to his or her point of origin, and (b) may include brief (several seconds) stops or hesitations as the wanderer changes directional heading along the path;
- pacing—back and forth locomotion between two end points, at which directional heading is reversed;
- random—locomotion along a haphazard path with multiple legs and directional changes and hesitations of up to 30 seconds at any point along the path; and
- direct—locomotion from a point to a destination along a straightforward or uncomplicated path and without significant hesitation.

The Martino-Saltzman methodology has been applied by Algase and colleagues in several descriptive studies of wandering (e.g., Algase, Beattie, Bogue, et al., 2001; Algase, Beattie, & Therrien, 2001; Algase, Kupferschmid, Beel-Bates, & Beattie, 1997). Wandering behavior was observed directly or videotaped according to a time-sampling strategy suited to researcher or observer goals. Individual episodes of locomotion were coded for start and stop time and, at the conclusion of a locomotion episode, for travel pattern. Various technologies ranging from simple paper, pencil, and stopwatch records to computer-based coding programs may be used for coding observations.

From coded observations, a variety of metrics can be generated for individual travel patterns and for wandering overall, which includes all patterns except direct. Both frequency and duration of wandering episodes can be derived from observational data, and both are important to consider, as each parameter may yield a somewhat different picture of

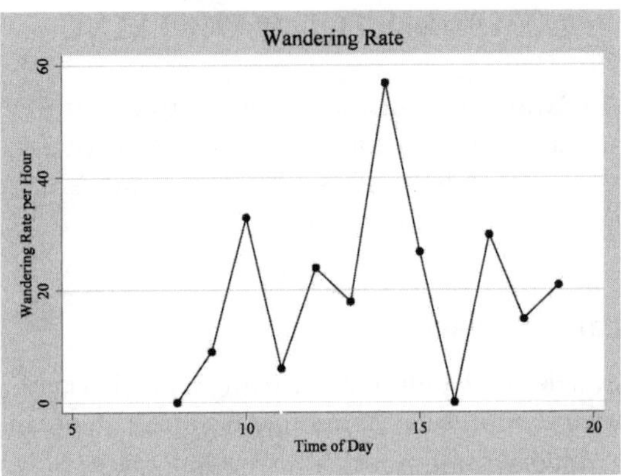

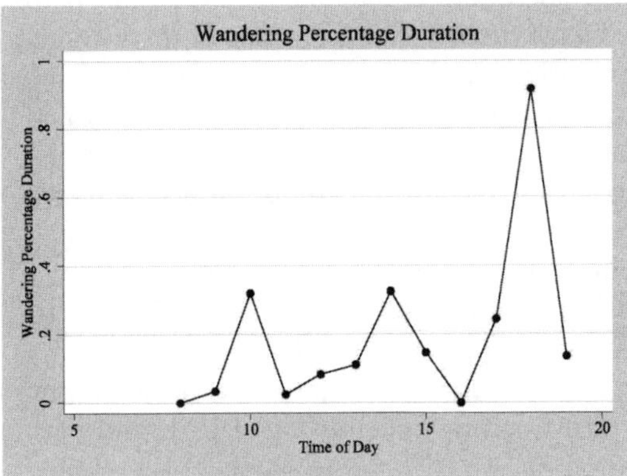

FIGURE 1.2 Wandering rate graph and wandering percentage duration.

wandering. For example, see Figure 1.2. Both frequency (as a sum, mean, or rate of wandering episodes, by pattern or collectively, per unit of time) and duration (as a sum, mean, or percentage of time spent wandering, by pattern or collectively) can be calculated for an observation period or across multiple observation periods, displayed graphically in relation to time of day, and used in statistical procedures.

Rating Scale Approaches

The Algase Wandering Scale was designed originally as a rating scale for formal and informal caregivers to estimate wandering behavior along several dimensions. The original scale was intended to capture the dimensions of amount, temporal distribution, spatial disorientation, eloping behaviors, and wandering patterns. In several studies to evaluate and refine the Algase Wandering Scale, valid and reliable versions were developed for use with residents of long-term care settings and for those living in the community (Algase, Beattie, Bogue, et al., 2001; Song et al., 2003; Algase, Beattie, et al., 2004; Algase, Son, et al., 2004). Both the long-term care and community versions are included in Appendix B.

The Revised Algase Wandering Scale for long-term care (RAWS-LTC) is a 19-item scale composed of three subscales: persistent walking, spatial disorientation, and eloping behaviors. Items are scored from 1 (not a wanderer) to 4 (a problematic wanderer). In validating the scale, a 1-week retrospective timeframe was used as the basis for ratings. Other shorter timeframes may also be applied, depending on the assessor's objectives; however, psychometric properties of the RAWS-LTC for shorter timeframes are unknown and test–retest reliability has not been established. Due to varying lengths of subscales, the overall and subscale scores are calculated as items' means among the items contained within them to enable comparison of scores among subscales. The three subscales consistently demonstrated validity and reliability in studies of earlier versions of the scale across samples composed of residents in nursing homes and assisted living facilities located in the United States, Canada, and Australia.

The RAWS-LTC overall and its persistent walking subscale can differentiate among nonwanderers, occasional wanderers, and nonproblematic and problematic wanderers together as one group. The spatial disorientation subscale can differentiate nonwanderers from occasional wanderers, and nonproblematic and problematic wanderers as one group. The eloping behavior scale can differentiate problematic wanderers from all other groups.

In tests of the original Algase Wandering Scale, the three subscales now comprising the RAWS-LTC were significantly correlated to the hourly rate and the percent and duration of wandering episodes (in proportion to all walking) for overall wandering (random, lapping, and pacing together) and for random pattern wandering alone. Only the persistent walking and eloping behavior subscales were correlated with any of these parameters for lapping and pacing pattern wandering (Algase, Beattie, Bogue, et al., 2001). Means and standard deviations for the RAWS-LTC and its subscales for all groups (nonwanderers, occasional wanderers, nonproblematic wanderers, and problematic wanderers) and overall are shown in Table 1.1, as are the Cronbach's alphas for the overall scale and all subscales.

TABLE 1.1 Mean Item Scores (Standard Deviations) and Cronbach's Alpha of the RAWS-LTC, RAWS-CV

	Overall RAWS	RAWS Subscales				
Group	Overall	Persistent walking	Spatial disorientation	Eloping behaviors	Routinized walking	Negative outcomes
RAWS-LTC						
Nonwanderer (n = 55)	1.61 (.23)	1.91 (.44)	1.50 (.50)	1.18 (.20	N/A	N/A
Occasional wanderer (n = 34)	2.51 (.27)	2.47 (.45)	2.08 (.59)	1.57 (.40)	N/A	N/A
Nonproblematic wanderer (n = 50)	2.54 (.33)	3.08 (.41)	1.77 (.52)	2.42 (.57)	N/A	N/A
Problematic wanderer (n = 8)	2.72 (.36)	3.28 (.39)	2.69 (.54)	2.19 (.67)	N/A	N/A
All groups combined	1.55 (0.54)	2.51 (0.68)	1.99 (0.68)	2.11 (0.51)	N/A	N/A
Cronbach's alpha (N = 147)	.93	.94	.88	.87		

RAWS-CV						
Nonwanderer $n = 112$	1.62 (0.39)	1.68 (0.58)	1.81 (1.06)	1.45 (0.45)	1.80 (0.81)	1.55 (0.64)
Occasional wanderer $n = 68$	2.17 (0.51)	2.38 (0.65)	2.50 (0.96)	2.09 (0.63)	2.44 (0.80)	1.98 (0.73)
Nonproblematic wanderer $n = 34$	2.48 (0.61)	2.93 (0.69)	2.58 (1.13)	2.62 (0.73)	2.76 (0.92)	1.89 (0.67)
Problematic wanderer $n = 36$	2.88 (0.52)	3.29 (0.67)	2.99 (0.98)	3.36 (0.62)	2.97 (0.98)	2.21 (0.90)
All groups combined $N = 250$	2.06 (0.66)	2.28 (0.87)	2.26 (1.11)	2.06 (0.88)	2.28 (0.87)	1.80 (0.75)
Cronbach's Alpha	.95	.94	.88	.87	.89	.76

Expanded from the RAWS-LTC and adapted to community-residing persons with dementia, the revised AWS Community Version (RAWS-CV) is a longer scale with 37 items and 5 subscales: the three contained in the RAWS-LTC, plus routinized walking (indicative of pacing and lapping pattern wandering) and negative outcomes. Items are scored on a Likert scale from 1 (never or unable) to 5 (always) using a 1-week retrospective timeframe for ratings. The RAWS-CV and all its subscales can differentiate among nonwanderers and occasional, nonproblematic, and problematic wanderers. Item means and standard deviations for the overall RAWS-CV and its subscales for each of four subgroups and overall also are shown in Table 1.1, as are Cronbach's alphas for the overall scale and all subscales.

The observational approach used by Algase and colleagues and both versions of the RAWS are consistent with the scientific definition of wandering presented earlier in this chapter. The observational approach can yield information about the frequency, repetition, and temporal distribution of overall wandering and of each wandering pattern. As higher rates and larger proportions of random pattern wandering (as compared to all locomotion) are moderately correlated with spatial disorientation—while lapping and pacing patterns are not (Algase, Beattie, Bogue, et al., 2001)—information about random wandering can also aid in illuminating our understanding of the spatial disorientation aspect of wandering behavior. Both versions of the RAWS have subscales that quantify frequency (persistent walking) and spatial disorientation, as well as eloping behaviors associated with wandering. The RAWS-CV also has a routinized walking subscale that can provide further information concerning the repetitive nature of wandering. Specific items within the persistent walking subscale can also inform us about temporal aspects of wandering. These two approaches to measure wandering can be used to develop valid and reliable understanding of this perplexing behavior and to characterize the impact of interventions for it.

In published studies, investigators have most commonly quantified wandering behavior using observational approaches and rating scales. However few of these methods have undergone rigorous development and validity testing; even among those with strong psychometric properties, authors have recognized a need for further refinements.

Technological Approaches

Researchers have also used a variety of activity monitors and exit-control devices in wandering investigations. Each of these approaches has yielded important insights into the nature of wandering and its consequences. However, neither of these approaches measure wandering directly or exclusively. All activity monitoring devices currently on the market do capture wandering behavior, but likewise detect walking or other motion that is not wandering. At best, these devices can generate an estimate of the amount of locomotion, which may be informative when used in conjunction with other measures. Incorporation of further technological advances into these devices, such as global positioning system (GPS) or radio-frequency identification device (RFID) capability, are needed to render them capable of differentiating wandering from nonwandering locomotion. The use of RFID methods to characterize little understood wandering corollaries (door testing, shadowing, and exit-seeking behaviors) that may serve as antecedents to elopement are currently being pioneered by a team of engineers and clinicians (Kearns & Moore, 2006). This research team advocates RFID methods, because new applications of this standard technology offer the advantage of objective measurement of wandering and related behaviors on an independent, continuous, 24-hour basis as they occur in relationship with the movements of other household residents. This and other studies of activity monitoring devices that have been used to measure wandering are listed at the end of this chapter. Multiple techniques also have been employed to count exiting behaviors, and many more are available commercially and used clinically to establish egress control. Since we consider exiting, eloping, and similar events as outcomes or consequences of wandering, we do not include these techniques and devices as measures of wandering per se. See Chapter 15 for more detail on technologies for managing wandering behaviors.

CONCLUSION

Wandering in dementia is a multifaceted pattern of human activity, a fascinating and elaborate behavior that has historically been difficult to define. Definitional perspectives in this chapter will hopefully provide family and professional care providers, scientists, clinicians, and policy makers with the tools and resources necessary to achieve their individual wandering-related objectives.

REFERENCES FOR STUDIES USING ACTIVITY MONITORING DEVICES TO MEASURE WANDERING

Algase, D. L., Beattie, E. R. A., Lietsch, S. A., & Beel-Bates, C. A. (2003). Biomechanical activity devices to index wandering behavior. *American Journal of Alzheimer's Disease and Other Dementias, 18*(2), 85–92.

Cohen-Mansfield, J., Werner P., Culpepper, W. J., Wolfson, M., & Bickel, E. (1997). Assessment of ambulatory behavior in nursing home residents who pace or wander: A comparison of four commercially available devices. *Dementia & Geriatric Cognitive Disorders, 8*(6), 359–365.

Madsen, J. (1991). The study of wandering in persons with senile dementia. *American Journal of Alzheimer's Disease and Other Dementias, 17,* 21–24.

Scisney-Matlock, M., Algase, D. L., Rogers, A., Yeo, S., Oakley, D., & Young, E. (2000). Measuring behavior: Electronic devices in nursing studies. *Applied Nursing Research, 13*(2), 97–102.

REFERENCES

Algase, D. L. (1999).Wandering in dementia. *Annual Review of Nursing Research, 17,* 185–217.

Algase, D. L., Beattie, E. R. A., Bogue, E., & Yao, L. (2001). The Algase Wandering Scale: Initial psychometrics of a new caregiver reporting tool. *American Journal of Alzheimer's Disease and Other Dementias, 16*(3), 141–152.

Algase, D. L., Beattie, E. R., Song, J. A., Milke, D., Duffield, C., & Cowan, B. (2004). Validation of the Algase Wandering Scale (Version 2) in a cross cultural sample. *International Journal of Aging Mental Health, 8*(2), 133–142.

Algase, D. L., Beattie, E. R. A., & Therrien, B. (2001). Impact of cognitive impairment on wandering behavior. *Western Journal of Nursing Research, 23*(3), 283–295.

Algase, D. L., Kupferschmid, B., Beel-Bates, C. A., & Beattie, E. R. A. (1997). Estimates of stability of daily wandering behavior among cognitively impaired long-term care residents. *Nursing Research, 46*(3), 172–178.

Algase, D. L., Moore, D. H., VandeWeerd, C., & Gavin-Dreschnack, D. (accepted). Mapping the maze of terms and definitions in dementia-related wandering. *International Journal of Aging and Mental Health.*

Algase, D. L., Son, G. R., Beattie, E., Song, J. A., Leitsch, S., & Yao, L. (2004). The interrelatedness of wandering and wayfinding in a community sample of persons with dementia. *Dementia & Geriatric Cognitive Disorders, 17*(3), 231–239.

Cohen-Mansfield, J. (1991). *Instruction manual for the Cohen-Mansfield Agitation Inventory (CMAI).* Rockville, MD: Research Institute of the Hebrew Home of Greater Washington.

Department of Veterans Affairs, Veterans Health Administration (2002). Management of wandering and missing patient events. VHA DIRECTIVE 2002-013, March 4, 2002.

Gavin-Dreschnack, D., VandeWeerd, C., Moore, D. H., & Beattie, E. R. A. (2006, August 21). *Preliminary analysis of focus group data characterizing wheelchair wandering.* Presentation at the International Consortium for Research on Wandering.

Kearns, W., & Moore, D. H. (2006, June 5). *RFID: A novel observational and measurement method in dementia-related wandering.* Poster presentation at the Agency for Healthcare Research and Quality (AHRQ) 2006 Annual Conference on Patient Safety and Health, Washington, D.C.

Martino-Saltzman, D., Blasch, B. B., Morris, R. D., & McNeal, L. W. (1991). Travel behavior of nursing home residents perceived as wanderers and nonwanderers. *Gerontologist, 31,* 666–672.

North American Nursing Diagnosis Association (NANDA). (2001). *Nursing diagnosis: Definitions and classification, 2001–2002* (pp. 206–207). Philadelphia, PA: Author.

Song, J. A., Algase, D. L., Beattie, E. R., Milke, D. L, Duffield, C., & Cowan, B. (2003). Comparison of U.S., Canadian, and Australian participants' performance on the Algase Wandering Scale-Version 2 (AWS-V2). *Research & Theory for Nursing Practice,* 17(3), 241–256.

CHAPTER TWO

Theoretical Models of Wandering

Donna L. Algase, Lan Yao, Cynthia A. Beel-Bates, and Jun-Ah Song

A clear conception and measurable definition of wandering are critical to studies that describe wandering, including the types and variations in presentation and expression of the syndrome. Further, as was discussed in Chapter 1, definitions can provide the structure that enables valid and accurate detection, assessment, and measurement of wandering among individuals with dementia. However, even detailed and elaborate descriptions that are based upon valid measurement approaches are insufficient to explain and predict who will wander, the conditions under which their wandering occurs, and the consequences of unaddressed wandering. Such explanations depend on validated theories that reveal the operative mechanisms, theories that are essential to designing effective interventions targeted to those wanderers and their families most likely to benefit from them.

The goals of Chapter 2 are to differentiate wandering from related concepts and to present a range of current and emerging theories of wandering with an eye toward those that may serve as a basis for evolving effective care strategies. The chapter is organized in four sections. First, wandering is examined in relation to two other categories of related behavior: a) somewhat similar or overlapping ones, such as agitation and restlessness; and b) outcomes of wandering, such as eloping and becoming lost. Second, mechanisms with the potential to explain wandering, at least partially, are presented, along with the scientific evidence supporting the link to wandering. In the third section, mechanisms are integrated into a comprehensive conceptual model of dementia-related behavior: the Need-driven, Dementia-compromised Behavior (NDB) model, specified to wandering. The final section presents a group of other models and theories of wandering, some derived from the NDB model.

WANDERING AND RELATED CONCEPTS

Ideally, defining a behavior like wandering draws a boundary around an observable phenomenon in such a way that it can be used to determine if a behavior fits within the definition, that is, to identify instances of wandering. Conversely, a definition can serve to eliminate behaviors that do not fit, that is, to leave out instances of behavior representing something else. However, labeling—and even empirically validating a definition—does not preclude other investigators, who may perceive the behavior through a different lens, from labeling and defining it, or aspects of it, differently. Such is the case with the phenomenon labeled as wandering in this book. In other words, even with improved clarity and a growing consensus on a scientific definition of wandering, other investigators may include wandering, or some wandering, or locomotion that looks like wandering, within their definitions for similar or related concepts.

The existence of overlapping labels and definitions for wandering and similar phenomena is understandable and expected at this relatively early stage of scientific inquiry into dementia-related behaviors. In fact, this situation exists in many mature sciences when we focus on the outer edges of work in those fields. For example, what was once considered senility or, using the more contemporary term, dementia is now recognized to be a group of diseases that look similar—some still indistinguishable clinically despite years of study—but have differing pathophysiological bases, etiologies, or underlying mechanisms. Experts now assert that Alzheimer's disease (AD), the predominant type of dementia, may actually encompass a group of pathophysiological mechanisms, that is, diseases, leading into a final common pathway that produces the defining pathological features of AD: beta amyloid plaques and neurofibrillary tangles (e.g., Casadesus, et al., 2006; Grammas, Samany, & Thirumangalakudi, 2006; Harman, 2006; McMurtray, Clark, Christine, & Mendez, 2006). While many dementia-related behaviors have been reported and labeled, the community of investigators who study them is yet to adopt a single typology or categorization scheme for organizing these behaviors, though examples have been put forward. Simply put, the most useful typologies for intervention purposes are based on commonality of mechanism or process that gives rise to a related group of behaviors; current understandings of such mechanisms or processes and their interactions are insufficient to yield valid groupings of dementia-related behaviors.

The existence of overlapping or competing conceptual labels for seemingly similar phenomena can also be understood on other grounds. What can be distinguished with terms and definitions may not be as easy to tease apart in physical reality, because multiple phenomena can occur simultaneously. For example, although there are clear diagnostic criteria for dementia and delirium, clinicians familiar with these common conditions of older people are well aware of the difficulty in distinguishing them in patients with whom they are unfamiliar and, further, in determining when they are present simultaneously, as may occur when a person with dementia develops an acute condition. Similarly, there is nothing to say that a person who wanders may not also become restless for a reason unrelated to wandering and, further, that the reason for their restlessness may also have an effect on the way their wandering looks.

Our ability to make distinctions between wandering and other phenomena expressed, at least in part, through locomotor behavior depends not only on defining criteria for each phenomenon, but also on an understanding of the underlying mechanisms driving them and on the potential of these mechanisms to affect one another and, thereby, alter the presentation of wandering and the other co-occurring or related conditions. In the following section, we discuss two types of behaviors that are often poorly differentiated from wandering: (a) those that have manifestations similar to it, and (b) those that are outcomes of it.

MANIFESTATIONS SIMILAR TO WANDERING: AGITATION AND RESTLESSNESS

Agitation

In psychiatric terms, agitation is defined as psychomotor activity, usually nonproductive and repetitious, associated with a feeling of inner tension *(Diagnostic and Statistical Manual of Mental Disorders, 4th ed., text revision)*. Examples include pacing, hand wringing, and an inability to sit still. Cohen-Mansfield originally defined agitation as "inappropriate verbal, vocal, or motor activity . . . judged from the standpoint of an observer rather than that of an elderly person" (Cohen-Mansfield & Billig, 1986). Although not specifying defining criteria, she organized agitation along two dimensions: motor/verbal and aggressive/nonaggressive. Subsequent factor analyses variously revealed three or four subtypes: physically (motor) nonaggressive, physically aggressive, verbally agitated (aggressive and nonaggressive), and sometimes hiding and hoarding (Rabinowitz et al., 2005), which has not been labeled with regard to organizing dimensions. Based on further empirical work, this conception was elaborated to acknowledge (a) a relationship between all agitation subtypes and cognitive functioning, (b) a connection between agitation and other psychological factors, (c) representative of discomfort or discontent for at least some agitated behaviors, and (d) evolving from environmental conditions and need states (Cohen-Mansfield, 1986; 2003).

Cohen-Mansfield and associates (1989) include wandering within the presumably broader concept of *agitation,* particularly as it manifests in dementia. In their widely used instrument, the Cohen-Mansfield Agitation Inventory (CMAI), both wandering and pacing are items contained within the physically nonaggressive subtype of agitation, as is the item: general restlessness. Inclusion of these items is supported in factor analyses of the instrument (Cohen-Mansfield, Marx, & Rosenthal, 1989). However, definitions of restlessness, wandering, and pacing within the instrument are not elaborated. In fact, these authors state that some types of wandering may not be an expression of agitation (Cohen-Mansfield & Billig, 1986), but they do not differentiate them from the types that are.

Restlessness

Restlessness has been defined as a feeling of increased arousal accompanied by an increase in motor activity (Kolanowski, 1991). It can be viewed as the behavioral expression or response to changing, challenging, or threatening conditions (Norris, 1986) and may be accompanied by negative feeling states (e.g., excitement, anxiety, apprehension, impatience, boredom, impending doom or dread) or discomforting physical sensations (e.g., pain, dyspnea). Based on the work of Hebb (1955), Malmo (1959), and Kroeber-Riel (1979), Kolanowski posited that the arousal of restlessness can be seen in terms of activation theory, which casts level of activation as a function of cortical stimulation of the reticular activating system. Further, upward or downward deviations in stimulation from some optimal level induce a drive or aversion (Berlyne, 1960, 1971) that overrides competing stimuli to control behavior. Inputs that can affect arousal include their intensity, size, color, sensory modality, novelty, complexity, degree or suddenness of change, incongruity, and uncertainty (Kolanowski, 1991).

Like wandering, restlessness lacks a standardized definition and is sometimes used interchangeably with the term agitation. While Norris (1978) characterized restlessness as a discontinuous behavior, other authors have differentiated agitation and restlessness only as a matter of degree with agitation being episodic motor or verbal behavior that clearly requires intervention to prevent harm to self or others, while restlessness is a continuous behavioral state that does not pose a danger (Brooke, Questad, Patterson, & Bashak, 1992). Kolanowski (1991) likened restlessness to agitation, noting inclusion of restlessness within the CMAI, and to wandering, based on the common quality of repetitiveness.

Comparison of Wandering, Agitation, and Restlessness

In sum, agitation, restlessness, and wandering share some commonalities. These commonalities are that all three phenomena (a) involve locomotion, which is an essential characteristic for wandering, but not essential for either of the other two phenomena; (b) have a repetitive quality; and (c) represent some disturbed, destabilized, or unsatisfied internal state, condition, or need. Further, comparison of any two phenomena among the three also reveals other areas of overlap (see Table 2.1).

When comparing the descriptions and standardized definition of wandering provided in Chapter 1 and possible mechanisms supporting it (discussed later in this chapter), with those of agitation and restlessness, differences are also apparent, specifically the range and class of behavior included and some defining characteristics. For example, each phenomenon has at least one unique characteristic: a disordered temporal or spatial quality with wandering, some degree of aggression with agitation, and the progressive escalation of involved psychomotor behaviors with restlessness (see Table 2.1).

TABLE 2.1 Features of Wandering, Agitation, and Restlessness

Phenomenon	Wandering	Agitation	Restlessness
Behavioral Class	Locomotor	Motor/verbal	Nonspecific psychomotor
Posited underlying state(s)	Disordered cognition Sensory/perceptual deficit Need-driven	Inner tension Discomfort Discontent	Anticipatory Heightened arousal Suboptimal stimulation
Defining characteristics	Frequent Repetitious Temporally-disordered Spatially-disordered	Nonproductive Repetitious Aggressive or nonaggressive Inappropriate to circumstances	Nonproductive Repetitious Unorganized, diffuse Progressive, small muscle → gross motor → total body

What Explains the Intersection?

As motor behaviors, wandering, agitation, and restlessness intersect at the level of locomotor behavior. In neurology and neuropsychiatry, the purpose of all normal motor behavior is to satisfy needs, which are emotionally based and mediated through the limbic and motor systems (Bachevalier, 1990; Salmon & Lange, 2001). Further, volitional (i.e., cognitively governed) behavior is also expressed through the motor system. Classically, in explaining the basis of locomotion, links between limbic and motor systems are where motivation is translated into action (Mogenson, 1987, 1991; Mogenson, Jones, & Yim, 1980). Skinner and Garcia-Rill (1993) demonstrated that emotion, cognition, and locomotion are anatomically, physiologically, and functionally linked, and they termed these connections the motivational system.

The motivational system supports a view of locomotion consistent with all three phenomena. However, it may not explain all behaviors included within each one. Thus, each phenomenon may have additional etiologies attributable to a broader or more complex set of physiological processes. Further, the limbic system and other brain regions affecting higher order cognitive processes involved in locomotion, such as navigation, are involved in certain dementias (Passini, Rainville, Marchand, & Joanette, 1991; Reid, et al., 1996), thereby affecting the motivational system in, as yet, unclear ways. Thus, the motivational system may explain where wandering, agitation, and restlessness come together, but not where they diverge.

Agitation and restlessness are physical states or conditions based on various, probably differing, physical feelings that are expressed through a wide range of motor behaviors and may include other classes of behavior, such as verbal, or types of behaviors, such as aggressive, which may be both motor and verbal. In contrast, wandering, as defined in this book, is a syndrome limited to one class of behaviors: motor. Within the class of motor behaviors, wandering is further circumscribed as to type: locomotor, that is, those behaviors used to move oneself through space, most commonly walking, but also by means of a conveyance, such as a wheelchair, automobile, or even various forms of public transportation. Also important, wandering is a special subset of locomotor behaviors. This subset is identified by frequent, repetitious, temporal, and spatial characteristics that make locomotion *stand out from what is normally expected* of people having a *similar age and profile of physical and cognitive capabilities*. Thus, not all walking by demented people is wandering, even at the most advanced stages of the disease (Algase, Kupferschmid, Beel-Bates, & Beattie, 1997).

We have also studied the intersection or overlap of these three phenomena empirically in two investigations. In the first study, two subscales of the CMAI (physically aggressive behaviors and physically nonaggressive behaviors) predicted only small to moderate portions of the variance in certain types and parameters of wandering, most notably pacing wandering (Algase, unpublished data). Furthermore, these two subscales also predicted similar portions of the variance in nonwandering locomotion. However, the verbal agitation subscale did not significantly predict any parameter for any type of wandering or nonwandering locomotion. These findings indicate that the locomotor behavior associated with agitation cuts across wandering and nonwandering locomotion similarly, as the motivational system could explain. As to the interaction of wandering and agitation, agitation may serve to increase the frequency or duration of wandering beyond the level a given wanderer may generally exhibit, or it may affect only certain patterns of wandering.

In the second study, observed rates of physically nonaggressive behavior (PNAB) on the CMAI were factor analyzed, resulting in two factors, indicating that the physically nonaggressive subtype of agitation is not a unified condition or state, but may be composed of components or subtypes formed along additional dimensions beyond the physical and nonaggressive ones that bind the PNAB subtype. Factor 1, comprised of pacing or aimless wandering, trying to go to a different place, and handling things inappropriately, could be interpreted as mainly wandering. When correlated to observed rates of wandering, such as lapping, pacing, and random patterns together and individually, Factor 1 correlated moderately with wandering overall and with each pattern individually to a lesser and decreasing degree, supporting this view. Factor 2, comprised of general restlessness, repetitive mannerisms, and inappropriate dressing and disrobing, can be interpreted mainly as restlessness (Algase, Antonakos, Yao, Beattie, & Son, in review). Factor 2 also correlated with overall wandering, but at a substantially lower value and individually only with random wandering.

Together these studies demonstrate that, while agitation may contribute to the type and manner of wandering, it does not adequately characterize wandering overall. Alternatively, there is a more comprehensive explanation. Given that aggression as a unique characteristic of agitation, but absent in the PNAB subtype, the PNAB subtype may not be agitation at all, but a combination of wandering and restlessness, specifically prior to maximum escalation of restlessness. Further, the finding that Factor 2, mainly restlessness, correlated with only random wandering, lends further support to this interpretation, because random wandering has an unorganized or nonproductive (often termed aimless) character, as does restlessness.

BEHAVIORAL OUTCOMES OF WANDERING: ELOPING AND BECOMING LOST

Eloping and becoming lost are the events most commonly and inaccurately equated to wandering, especially by individuals unacquainted with scientific and clinical literature on the topic. Eloping is more commonly understood as the intentional or unintentional leaving of a premises (usually an institutional one) to which the person is assigned or confined without giving others explicit advance notice. Absconding or running away are synonyms. When others are given explicit notice, the more accurate terms for an unapproved leaving are absent without official leave (AWOL) or leaving against medical advice (AMA). Eloping is not unique to persons with dementia, but is limited to people who are subjected to some form of oversight.

If a person with dementia departs from their own residence, they are considered to have left unattended, rather than eloped, as one's own home is not generally a place of confinement. Unattended leaving is not problematic when the person with dementia has the capacity to return unaided as well. Unfortunately, there is always some risk that a subtle decrement in cognitive ability has gone unnoticed or that a chance variation in the environment, such as a detour, will be encountered, both potentially interfering with returning unaided.

Becoming lost is an event during which a person loses their bearings and is unable to execute a pathway to their intended destination, to return to their point of origin, or to connect with a useable source of help. It is an unsettling, even frightening, occurrence with which most mobile people, including those without cognitive impairment, have had experience. Becoming lost can occur within buildings as well as outdoors. When it happens outdoors to a person with dementia, the consequences can be dire. Becoming lost is described in considerable detail in Chapter 10.

As defined in Chapter 1, wandering consists of locomotor behavior and, therefore, is concerned with moving through space. Thus, it may result in eloping or with being or becoming lost when moving about involves reaching a destination or returning to a starting point. However, people with dementia may elope or become lost independent of wandering behavior; conversely, wandering can occur without precipitating either event. We regard eloping and becoming lost as critical and potential, although not inevitable, outcomes of wandering. Table 2.2 compares some features of wandering, eloping, and becoming lost.

PUTATIVE WANDERING MECHANISMS

Over the past three decades, scientists from a number of health-related fields have attempted to explain mechanisms underlying wandering

TABLE 2.2 Features of Wandering, Eloping (and Unattended Leaving), and Becoming Lost

Phenomenon	Wandering	Eloping and unattended leaving	Becoming lost
Conscious choice?	Unknown	Maybe	No
Cognitive state?	Disordered	Varied and nonspecific	Varied and nonspecific
Dangerous?	Possibly	Frequently but not always	Yes
Involves leaving?	Not necessarily	Yes	Not necessarily

behavior. As wandering accompanies cognitive impairment, primarily the dementias, most mechanisms explored are neurologically based. In this section, we summarize major hypotheses that have been investigated. These include the neurologically mediated ones (visual/perceptual deficits, attentional problems, spatial disorientation, movement disorders, rhythm disturbances), as well as other psychosocial factors (personality and behavioral patterns; social and physical environment).

Visual-Perceptual Deficits

Fundamental to many cognitive processes, problems with visual-perceptual processes have been posited as a basis for wandering (Beel-Bates, 2001). Alzheimer's disease has many effects on the visual system because it infiltrates the neuroanatomical substrates of vision, as well as those supporting our ability to construct an internal or cognitive map of our surroundings, that is, the hippocampus (HPC). Specifically affected are eye movement, color vision, depth perception, contrast sensitivity, cortical visuoperception, and visual attention among others (Faust & Belota, 1997).

Impaired figure-ground discrimination, depth perception, and detection of motion decline in AD (Duffy, 1999; Kiyosawa et al., 1989; Mendez, Tomsak, & Remler, 1990; Sadun, Borchert, DeVita, Hinton, & Bassi, 1987; Tetewsky and Duffy, 1999). These deficits contribute to problems with optic flow, the changing patterns one sees during movement (Tetewsky & Duffy, 1999). Elevated thresholds for optic flow are correlated with navigational deficits during ambulation and driving (O'Brien et al., 2001; Tetewsky & Duffy, 1999), which may contribute to wandering.

Attention and Perseveration

Also a basic cognitive process, impaired attention (or concentration) may contribute to wandering behavior. Both attention deficits and perseveration (an inability to disengage attention) have been examined. Recently Chiu and colleagues (2004) demonstrated that distractibility and attentional fatigue predicted getting lost behavior in early AD, an indicator of the spatial disorientation dimension of wandering.

Wandering also may be a form of motor perseveration. Perseveration occurs in AD and with focal damage to the frontal and parietal lobes. Ryan and colleagues (1995) have demonstrated that wanderers with mild AD had a greater degree of perseveration than nonwanderers at similar levels of dementia severity. The perseveration of wanderers was particularly likely to be an ongoing, continuous, or repeated response to a single stimulus, which is associated with damage to the right hemisphere and attention deficits. More studies of attention and wandering are needed across a wider range of dementia to evaluate the impact of attention and perseveration on various patterns and degrees (rate and duration) of wandering.

Spatial Disorientation

Spatial skills depend on visual-perceptual and attentional processes, so it is logical that problems with these basic processes may affect orientation (knowing where one is) and navigation or wayfinding (finding one's way around). Hippocampal regions supporting place learning and recognition are affected by AD (Hyman, Van Hoesen, Damasio, & Barnes, 1984; O'Keefe & Nadel, 1978; Squire, 1992). In one study, neuropsychological tests of memory, visuoconstructive ability, attention, and language impairment in 28 AD subjects showed that only memory and visuoconstructive ability predicted spatial disorientation, operationalized as wandering (Henderson, Mack, & Williams, 1989). Another connection between spatial skills and wandering was suggested when wanderers showed poorer function of the parietal lobes (DeLeon, Potegal, & Gurland, 1984), regions near the HPC involved in spatial and construction tasks, than did nonwandering counterparts with dementia. A positron emission tomography study in vascular dementia showed that wanderers had a relative deficit in regional metabolic rate for glucose in the right parietal lobe (which has a special role in spatial memory), as compared to the left parietal lobe and other brain regions (Meguro et al., 1996). A weakness of these studies is the lack of tests evaluating spatial skills in relation to performance of normal people on tasks in large-scale space. That is, do two-dimensional tests reflect three-dimensional abilities? Further, while these studies establish a relationship between being a wanderer and spatial skill deficits, particular aspects of wandering were not examined in relation to them. Further, in a more recent study using SPECT, wanderers with Alzheimer's disease had poorer perfusion of the *left* temporparietal area, suggesting that neuroanatomical areas less involved with spatial skills are operative (Rolland et al., 2005). As little is known about variation in wandering types and intensity by medical basis for dementia, it may be that types, degrees, and mechanisms of wandering can vary on this basis as well.

A study evaluating wayfinding effectiveness and dimensions of wandering revealed that wayfinding deficits were most highly correlated with the spatial disorientation dimension of wandering on the Algase Wandering Scale and much less so or not at all with persistent walking, eloping behavior, and mealtime impulsivity (Algase et al., 2004). Poor performance on simple wayfinding goals and global wayfinding strategies were the deficits most associated with wandering. Though problems with spatial orientation and problem solving are involved in wandering, they leave some types of, and considerable variance in, wandering unexplained.

Rhythm Disturbance

In aging, and more so in AD, the suprachiasmatic nucleus (SCN) shrinks. This structure, which has been called the biological clock, mediates rhythms associated with the light–dark (or circadian) cycle, such as sleep and activity. The effect of SCN shrinkage is a flattening or even obliteration of diurnal variation. Flattening of the circadian rhythm reflects more hours during which activity occurs and, often, advancement of acrophase, which shifts the highest rates of activity to later in the day.

Subjects with AD have a lower amplitude circadian rhythm for motor activity (i.e., more hours with activity and greater nighttime activity) and a delayed acrophase in body temperature compared to healthy controls (Satlin, Volicer, Stopa, & Harper, 1995). However, among AD subjects, a subgroup had even greater differences in the acrophases for activity and temperature cycles and a greater proportion of nighttime activity, indicating greater impairment in the SCN (Satlin et al., 1991). Wanderers display increased nighttime locomotor activity. In more recent work by Algase, Antonakos, Beattie, Yao, and Beel-Bates (2006, unpublished data), the distribution of wandering episodes, graphed as hourly rates and durations, indicate several possible patterns in the distribution of daytime wandering, not all of which show a delay in acrophase. Further studies are needed to examine circadian disturbances in other dementias and to equate disturbances with patterns and dimensions of wandering.

Movement Disorder

We have all observed wanderers in a state of seemingly perpetual motion and whose wandering will not be deterred. While not as fully elaborated as the hypothesis of spatial disorientation, movement disorders have been suggested as a possible basis for such wandering.

In addition to its role in spatial orientation, the HPC also plays a role in locomotor output. Damage to the HPC affects the mobility gradient, which shifts animals to higher levels of motor activity and shorter stop periods (Whishaw, 1994). Because testing requires implanting of electrodes, human studies have been limited to only case reports and do not include demented wanderers. However, to the extent that damage to the HPC in humans produces a mobility gradient, it may be among mechanisms specifically affecting the amount of wandering in dementia.

Likening wandering to the restlessness of schizophrenia, Weller (1987) postulated that the reduction of acetylcholine in AD may result in a relative excess of dopamine. Positron emission tomography has provided evidence to support this hypothesis (Meguro et al., 1996).

Personality and Behavioral Patterns

Personality and prior behavior patterns were actually the first explanatory hypothesis offered for wandering, advanced in 1982 by Monsour and Robb. These investigators demonstrated, through a retrospective approach using family members as informants, that wanderers were more likely to have had an outgoing personality and to have reacted to stressful conditions using motor activity, such as walking. A preserved social façade has also been reported among wanderers (Dawson & Reid, 1987).

In more recent years, theorists on personality have shown that personality may appear to change in dementia, but demented individuals maintain their position on personality factors relative to one another (Chatterjee, Strauss, Smyth, & Whitehouse, 1992; Kolanowski & Whall, 1996; Siegler et al., 1991; Strauss & Pasupathi, 1994). Using this observation, Thomas (1997) has shown that wanderers, or at least those individuals with dementia having higher levels of motor output, are more extroverted and open than nonwanderers.

In a recent dissertation, Song (2003) obtained an opposite outcome. Using a larger sample and a continuous (versus categorical) measure of wandering, and controlling for level of cognitive impairment and mobility status, extraversion was inversely related to wandering overall, and more to the three dimensions of wandering, spatial disorientation, eloping behavior, and attention shifting. In addition to methodological differences accounting for the discrepant results of these two studies, Song pointed out that, according to Costa and McRae (1992), introversion (low extraversion) should be considered the absence—not the opposite—of extraversion; thus low extraversion indicates being reserved (not unfriendly), independent (not a follower), and preferring to be alone.

Thus, wandering may be an attempt to use established internal and external strategies for preserving self-identity. This interpretation is consistent with one of the earliest studies of wandering where wanderers had significantly greater nonsocial or alone behavior (Snyder, Rupprect, Pyrek, Breckhus, & Moss, 1978) and with findings of Linton and colleagues (1997), who also failed to confirm Thomas's results.

Social Environment

Environmental factors of any type have been examined in only a few studies of wandering. What is known is that wanderers have poorer language skills than nonwanderers and lower levels of social interaction (Dawson & Reid, 1987; Snyder et al., 1978). Lacking language skills and social interaction, wandering may be a means to engage others by drawing attention to themselves or by locating and lingering near others. This hypothesis is further supported by observational studies. Accordingly, most episodes of wandering end within two feet of other people (Algase, 1992; Algase & Cheng, 1992). Further, those that end in social interaction have a longer lag time to the next episode, whereas those that end near other people, but not in engagement with the wanderer, have shorter lag times, suggesting that social interaction addresses a felt need to ambulate and reduces further wandering in the short run.

Considered as a type of foraging or searching, wandering is a possible means of coming upon what one needs, either directly by finding it or indirectly by increasing visibility and thereby calling attention to oneself and one's apparent need for assistance (Algase, Moore, VandeWeerd, & Gavin-Dreschnack, in press). This function of wandering has been demonstrated empirically (Choi, 1999).

Physical Environment

Through our observations of hundreds of wanderers over numerous studies, we have noted that certain environmental factors may affect the expression of wandering. Noise, light, and commotion seem to attract wandering behavior, and we are currently investigating these factors. Our observations about noise and light have already been confirmed in one study by Cohen-Mansfield and associates (1991). However, in another study conducted by Cohen-Mansfield and colleagues (1998), more restful and homelike areas (termed enhanced environments) not only attracted wanderers, but quelled their wandering to an extent. Recently, the environmental quality of ambiance, which reflects human preferences for engaging and soothing environments, was demonstrated to increase sitting and decrease walking among people with dementia (Yao & Algase,

2006), with the engaging dimension accounting for the most variance in activity level.

THE NEED-DRIVEN, DEMENTIA-COMPROMISED BEHAVIOR MODEL OF WANDERING

While a growing body of empirical evidence illustrates that a number of mechanisms explain some wandering, each mechanism has been investigated individually, and interactions among potential mechanisms are thus far not well understood. Further, because of limitations in the way that wandering or wanderers were identified in most studies of these mechanisms, the specific types or dimensions of wandering that are affected by each mechanism have not been explicated fully. This state of knowledge called for development of a more comprehensive theory of wandering that took a broader range of mechanisms and their interactions into account.

In the mid-1990s, three groups of investigators, collectively known as the Need-driven, Dementia-compromised Behavior Collaborative Research Group (NDB-CRG), collaborated to evolve a predictive model of these behaviors and launched efforts to investigate them in an interactive way. These groups were: Algase and colleagues (Antonakos, Beattie, Beel-Bates, DeCicco, Kolanowski, Son, Song, & Yao), at the University of Michigan, whose focus was wandering; Whall and colleagues (Antonakos, Colling, DeCicco, Kim, Kolanowski, & Son), also at the University of Michigan, whose focus was aggressive behavior; and Beck and colleagues (Lambert, O'Sullivan, & Richards) at the University of Arkansas for Medical Sciences, whose focus was problematic vocalizations.

Using a synthesis approach to integrate findings of studies that isolated contributing factors or supported underlying mechanisms for these behaviors, the NDB-CRG developed the Need-driven Dementia-compromised Behavior (NDB) Model (Algase et al., 1996). This work represented a fundamental shift in then current thinking about such behaviors (Donaldson, 2000) because emphasis on their problematic nature for formal and informal caregivers was replaced with a view taken from the perspective and context of the person with dementia. Further, the NDB model acknowledged the widely held tenet that behavior is motivated or purposeful at some level. Even if motivation is unknown to, or inaccessible, or inexpressible by a person with dementia, their behavior should be taken to represent the most integrated and functional response to ambient conditions and need states that one is capable of expressing.

NDB Model Components

At the most abstract level, the NDB model posits two groups of interacting factors that result in need-driven behaviors: background and proximal (see Figure 2.1). Background factors, consisting of cognitive status, general health, personal characteristics (personality and behavioral response to stress), and sociodemographic factors, are seen as stable (in the short run) and forming an internal context that alters, limits, or otherwise affects the way in which people with dementia are able to perceive, experience, and/or interact with their environment. Consequently, background factors affect the impact of proximal factors on dementia-compromised behaviors. For example, a health condition (a background factor) that limits mobility would compromise one's ability to move away from a noxious environmental condition (proximal factor) and might result in a behavior other than walking, such as aggression. Background factors are thought to identify individuals at risk for or likely to demonstrate wandering or other need-driven behaviors under the right conditions.

Proximal factors, consisting of personal need states, both physiological and psychological, and environmental conditions, both physical and social, are seen as dynamic or in a state of flux. Proximal factors are understood to represent the conditions under which dementia-compromised behaviors occur among individuals at risk for them. For example, wandering might be a search for food in response to hunger, or screaming a response to pain.

Both groups of factors are hypothesized to have direct effects on or produce need-driven dementia-compromised behaviors (NDBs). Further,

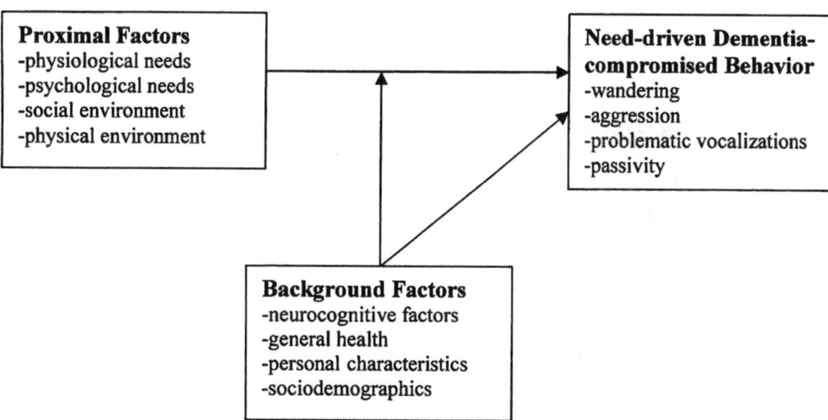

FIGURE 2.1 The Need-driven Dementia-compromised Behavior (NDB) Model.

background factors are thought to moderate or mediate the effects of proximal factors, that is, they form a context within which proximal factors are perceived or experienced. For example, visual-perceptual deficits would alter the amount and quality of visual input from the environment, thereby reducing cues that aid in interpreting and navigating the environment. Major propositions of the NDB model are presented in Table 2.3.

At a less abstract level, each background and proximal factor encompasses a group of related characteristics or conditions. This is the level at which mechanisms underlying various NDBs may begin to diverge. In other words, not all characteristics or conditions may be operative for every NDB or, if operative, may have differing or opposing effects from one behavior to another. Table 2.4 lists and defines the characteristics and conditions representing each background and proximal factor when the model is specified to wandering (NBD-W). Presently, the list is nearly identical for all NDBs, with the greatest variation occurring in the proximal factors for social and physical environment, based upon descriptive studies of individual behaviors, and known differences in the expression of these behaviors. For example, wandering could be expected to occur in a setting with a complex physical design, whereas problematic vocalizations or aggression may be unaffected by such complexity. Further, speed of caregiving, a social environment variable in the NDB, is not included in the NDB-W, since wandering is not usually precipitated by caregiving activities as aggression and problematic vocalizations are known to be.

Also operating at this level of abstraction are covariations and interactions among factor components, both known and unknown. Considered as independent components, irrespective of any NDB, some covariations and interactions among components are likely general within the NDB model, potentially operative across all NDBs. For example, within some

TABLE 2.3 Major Propositions of the NDB Model

1. Background factors constitute relatively stable, slowly changing characteristics of the person with dementia.
2. Proximal factors are more fluid or dynamic features of the person and of the immediate environment.
3. Proximal factors occur and are perceived by the person with dementia in the context of existing background factors.
4. Both background and proximal factors play an independent role in the occurrence of NDBs.
5. Both background and proximal factors interact or combine in some sequence to produce NDBs.

TABLE 2.4 Background and Proximal Factors, Components, and Definitions of the NDB-W Model

Factors and Components	Definitions
BACKGROUND FACTORS	
Neurocognitive factors	
• Memory	The mental capacity of retaining and reviving facts, events, and impressions, or of recalling or recognizing previous experiences.
• Attention	The mental capacity of maintaining selective or sustained concentration.
• Language Skills	The communicating ability that involves the use of sounds, grammar, and vocabulary, according to a system of rules.
• Visual-spatial skills	The ability pertaining to the perception of the spatial relationships between objects in one's field of vision.
• Mobility	The quality of moving freely in a place or moving to and from a certain position or place.
General Health	Overall condition of a person's body (e.g., comorbidity, ADL & IADL, and motor ability)
Personal characteristics	
• Personality	Distinctive qualities of a person, especially those distinguishing personal characteristics that make one socially appealing.
• Stress response	A certain way of reacting to internal or external pressure.
Sociodemographics	
• Age	The length of time, measured by years from birth, during which a person has existed.
• Gender	The sex of a person, male or female.
• Occupation	A person's usual or principal work or business, especially as a means of earning a living, prior to illness.
PROXIMAL FACTORS	
Physiological need states	
• Hunger	A strong desire or need for food.
• Thirst	A sensation of dryness in the mouth and throat related to a need or desire to drink.

(Continued)

TABLE 2.4 Background and Proximal Factors, Components, and Definitions of the NDB-W Model (Continued)

• Pain	A distressing sensation in a particular part of the body.
• Elimination	Bodily discharges including urine and feces.
Psychological need states	
• Positive	Good feeling or emotion, especially as manifested by facial expression or body language.
• Negative	Bad feeling or emotion, especially as manifested by facial expression or body language.
Social and Physical Environment	
• Social Interaction	A dynamic, mutual, or reciprocal action and reaction a person displays with the companionship of others.
• Staff mix and ratio	The number and type of personnel charged with the nursing care for a person.
• Ambiance	The mood, character, quality, tone, or atmosphere of an environment (e.g., own rooms, hallways, dining rooms, activity rooms) where a person belongs.
• Crowding	The number of and distance from other people within a defined area.
• Complexity	The association and assemblage of physical features of an environment (e.g., a physical design of a facility).
• Ambient conditions	The combination of light level, sound level, temperature, and humidity within a location.

range, memory covaries with attention, regardless of any NDB. However, it is also likely that the extent of covariation and interaction among factor components may result in the expression of differing NDBs. For example, mobility status may be high or low for individuals with a strong motor-type response to stress, that is, it does not covary with a motor-type stress response. However, mobility status may interact with a motor-type stress response, that is when mobility status is low, locomotor responses to stress are inexpressible. In this case, persons who would normally respond to stress by walking are less able or unable to do so and may resort to other types of responses (verbal, aggressive, or passive).

Model Testing

Although the NDB model has gained significant popularity clinically and scientifically, published tests of the model (and the NDB-W) as a whole are lacking, although such testing is underway. However, some confidence can be placed in the major relationships posited in the model, as they are based on earlier studies of individual factors and mechanisms. What remains largely unknown is the covarying and interactive effects of multiple factors and components considered simultaneously on the occurrence of NBDs individually and collectively and on the specific manner in which NDBs are affected by them, for example, by pattern, dimension, and severity (rate, duration) of wandering.

While not a test of the entire NDB model, one study has examined background factors as predictors of NDBs among residents with dementia in long-term care settings (Algase, Beck, Whall, & NDB-CRG, 2003). Residents were classified by positive history on three NDBs: wandering, aggression, and vocalizations. Participants with a positive history of NDBs (singly and combined) were compared to those without NDBs. Background factors were used to predict membership in each grouping. Distinct risk profiles emerged for each NDB group, as shown in Table 2.5. These results show that NDBs may co-occur in any combination and are differentially affected by background factors.

DERIVED AND OTHER WANDERING MODELS

The NDB and NDB-W models are serving to advance scientific understanding of wandering and other dementia-related behaviors and to develop the evidence-base for guiding clinical practice. However, as all models do, they have limited application. Several other models have also been proposed, some derived from the NDB/NDB-W models and others based on different conceptions altogether. These models are presented briefly in the following section.

Wandering as a Rhythm: A Descriptive Model

Prior to 1988, few studies of wandering or wanderers had been conducted. Neither measures for wandering nor criteria for identifying wanderers had been validated. Taking a heuristic approach to the problem, Algase and Tsai (1991) developed an early model of wandering, as both an approach to measurement and to intervention.

TABLE 2.5 Background Characteristics by NDB (Single and Combined) Compared to No NDBs

All	Only	With Vocalizers	With Aggressors	With Vocalizers and Aggressors
Wanderers				
Younger age Lower MMSE Lower aggressive stress response Higher verbal stress response	Younger age Lower aggressive stress response	Lower MMSE Better mobility Higher verbal stress response	Better mobility Higher neuroticism	Younger Lower MMSE Better mobility Higher verbal stress response Lower openness
Vocalizers				
More likely female Lower MMSE Poorer mobility Higher verbal stress response	More likely female Lower MMSE Poorer mobility Higher verbal and motor stress response Lower neuroticism	N/A	More likely female Poorer mobility Lower extraversion	N/A
Aggressors				
Lower MMSE, Poorer mobility Lower extraversion Higher verbal stress response	Poorer mobility Lower extraversion Higher verbal stress response, conscientiousness		N/A	N/A

Model Components

Accordingly, wandering was portrayed as a nonlinear ultradian rhythm, that is, one whose cycle is shorter than 24 hours. Each wandering cycle was composed of a locomoting and nonlocomoting phase (see Figure 2.2). In addition to characterizing the length and phases of the cycle, application of rhythm theory to wandering allows investigation into the nature of the rhythm. Nonlinear rhythms are of two types: limit cycle, like a flexible spring, in which physiological phenomena repeat at regular intervals, like respiration or heart beat; or relaxed oscillation, like a siphon, in which physiological phenomena build to a critical point and then release, like elimination. Wandering was posited as the latter type.

For measurement purposes, a rhythmic view of wandering provided a powerful means to delimit wandering episodes when combined with Martino-Saltzman and colleagues' (1991) inefficient travel patterns (random, lapping, pacing), and thereby to count and time cycles and phases. Other metrics, such as the ratio of locomoting or nonlocomoting phase duration to overall cycle duration, were also made possible through this approach.

Rhythm theory also posits that nonlinear rhythms in particular are paced either internally by endogenous physiological pacers or externally by one or more exogenous ones, termed zeitgebers (or triggers). For wandering, pacers may be either endogenous, that is, with a physiological excess or deficit, or exogenous, for example, triggered by noise. Pacers or zeitgebers were viewed as targets for intervention.

Model Tests

Several descriptive studies of wandering were conducted within a rhythm view and general cycle and phase parameters estimated for random, lapping, and pacing pattern wandering, as well as for direct walking (nonwandering). Table 2.6 shows some summary data for 25 wanderers from two long-term care settings who were each observed for 24 hours (Algase et al., 1997). Selected stimuli, such as the presence and proximity of people, were also examined within this view, as discussed previously in this chapter.

The Nature of Visuospatial Skills in Wandering in Persons With AD: A Structural Model

Drawing on the fields of neuroscience, environmental psychology, ophthalmology, and nursing, Beel-Bates (2001) synthesized a microlevel

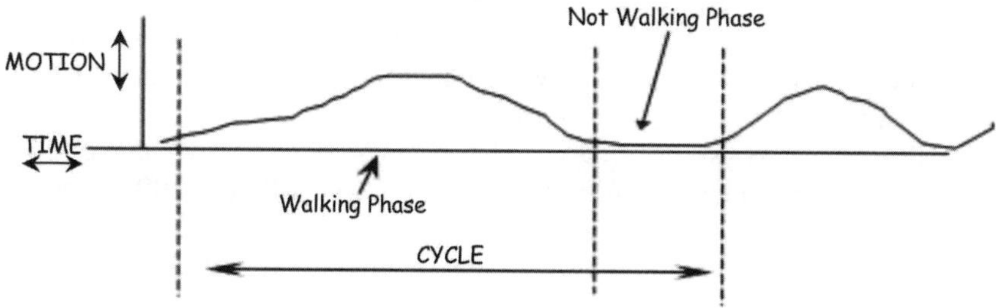

FIGURE 2.2 Wandering as a rhythm.

TABLE 2.6 Wandering Cycle Parameters Over a 24-Hour Period (N = 25)

	Average hourly cycle rate (mean)	Average hourly locomoting-phase duration (mean minutes)	Average % of cycle for locomoting phase (mean)
Random pattern	0.63	2.29	40.1%
Lapping pattern	0.11	2.00	19.3%
Pacing pattern	0.08	0.62	20.8%
Overall wandering	0.82	2.18	36.1%
Direct pattern (nonwandering)	0.92	1.32	28.9%

structural model to represent the cascade of visual skills and steps of cognitive map formation that support effective wayfinding and, when disrupted, lead to faulty wayfinding and wandering (see Figure 2.3).

Model Components

In brief, the NDB model elaborates on mechanisms operative for the background factor of visual-spatial skills. Accordingly, fundamental visual processes (visual attention, peripheral vision, and contrast sensitivity) are essential to support image segmentation, a two-step process by which the "whereness" and "whatness" properties of a picture plane (2-D or 3-D) are analyzed. Image segmentation and object recognition are depicted as parallel and interacting processes of the brain's locator and contour systems respectively, consistent with the dual pathways of the visual system. The locator and contour systems convey information from the dual visual systems to the HPC, where spatial memories are formed and stored as a cognitive map, an abstract representation of the scene or place that draws upon other stored information about the place. Based on the map, an individual elects a direction and a pathway to navigate in a familiar setting or to form a new map in an unfamiliar setting. Navigation is an essential activity for map formation.

Brain regions essential to visual processes that support image segmentation are affected in AD, as is the HPC. Beel-Bates (2001) posits a resulting inability to form or use cognitive maps. In Figure 2.3, the steps in the cascade that may be affected are illustrated with dashed lines. Breakdown at any point weakens the ability to form and use cognitive maps, which are the basis for normal wayfinding. Beel-Bates's model is an elegant integration of information across several fields to present a

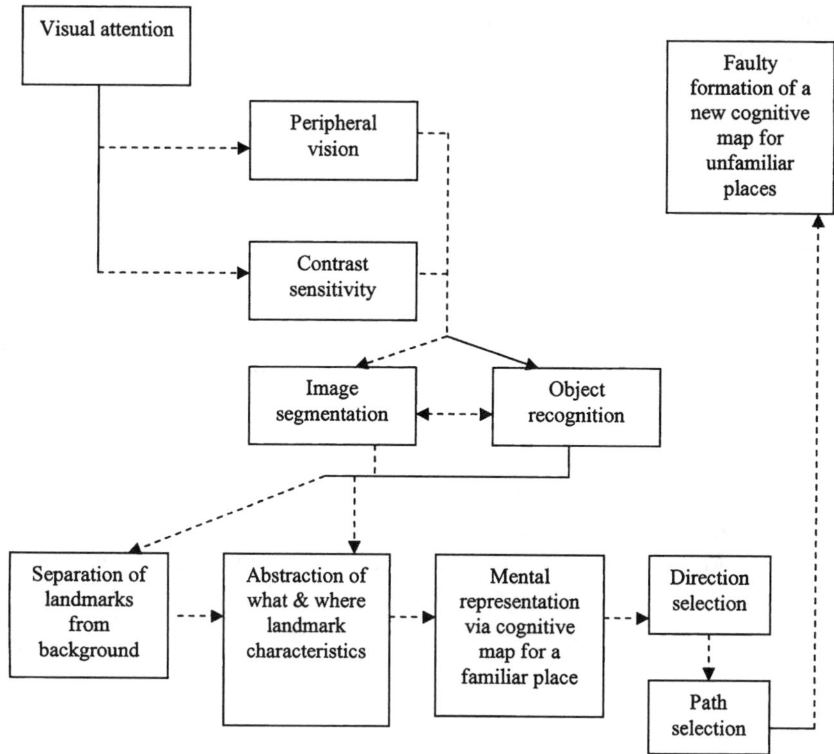

FIGURE 2.3 Nature of visuospatial skills in wandering in persons with AD.

detailed and comprehensive view of the relationship between vision, cognitive mapping, and wayfinding that can go awry to result in some wandering, specifically the spatially disordered locomotion.

Implications of the model within the context of the NDB-W model, and more specifically in relation to its modifiable proximal factors (and thus intervention), has yet to be elaborated. However, concepts such as crowding and complexity of the physical environment are likely candidates for further study in conjunction with the Beel-Bates's model.

Locomoting Responses to Environment in Elders With Dementia: A Noncognitive Model of Wandering

Also derived from the NDB-W, Yao (2004) proposed a significant shift in considering neurocognitive contributions to wandering from an emphasis on cognition to emotion. Using a theory synthesis approach, Yao modeled a mechanism mediating person–environment interaction in dementia that is embedded in the interaction of background and proximal factors of the NDB model. Accordingly, Yao based her Locomoting Responses to Environment in Elders with Dementia (LRE-EWD) model, shown in Figure 2.4, on the five propositions of the NDB model (Table 2.3) along with the following assumptions drawn from psychology and neuroscience:

1. Behavior is the outcome of cognitive and emotional processing of environmental information.
2. Bodily responses have primary relationship with emotions rather than cognition (LeDoux, 1996).
3. Motor response is one type of emotional response (Adolphs, 1999) and a fundamental issue associated with all basic emotions (Davidson, 1993; Ekman, 1992; Panskepp, 1998).
4. Emotional responses are mostly adaptive.
5. Although the primary reaction to the environment, emotion yields rigid and automatic responses, whereas cognition yields flexible and optimal ones.

Model Components

The model depicts affect (emotion) and cognition as separate, though interrelated systems. In an environmental encounter, stimuli are processed first (faster) via the affective system and do not depend on the cognitive system before yielding a global, generalized effect. Such effects relate to preferences and to approach–avoidance of behavioral tendencies (Ulrich, 1983). Configurations of environmental stimuli that characterize preferences (or

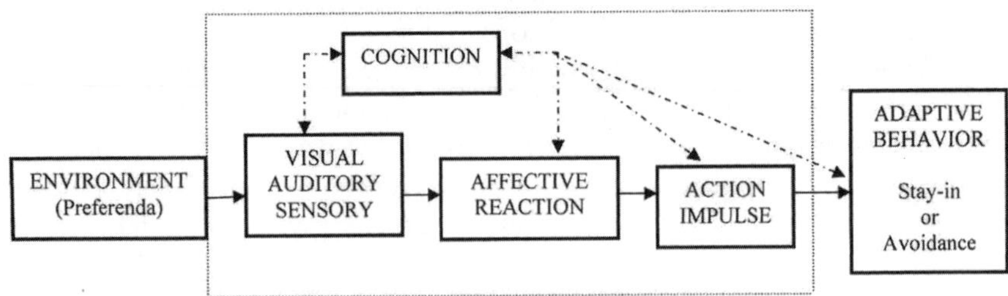

FIGURE 2.4 Locomoting Responses to Environment in Elders With Dementia (LRE-EWD).
Source: Yao, 2004

preferenda, Zajonc, 2001) are often too vague or global to be specifically identified features, but are highly effective in eliciting affect.

After triggering the affective system, preferenda then triggers the cognitive system where stimuli and the setting are evaluated for significance to well-being via recognition, identification, and much more extensive information processing (Ulrich, 1983). Cognitive evaluation of actual or anticipated outcomes of the encounter are influenced by experience (learned associations, expectations, memories) and refine the initial affective response from which other emotions may be generated (Ulrich). Cognitive processing may lead to carrying out, suppressing, or denying the initial reaction of the affective system, which primes the individual for locomotion.

In the case of dementia, impairment of the cognitive system degrades the quality of stored information available for cognitive evaluation (Hamann, Monarch, & Goldstein, 2000) such that weak, distorted, or no cognitive modification of the initial response occurs. As dementia progresses, the influence of cognition over emotion becomes weaker or absent, leaving emotional responses as the dominant ones. Ambulatory behavior becomes an emotional response to the environment. Unfavorable environments would spur avoidance (walking away) and favorable ones would incite approach (walking toward or staying in).

Model Test

The LRE-EWD model has been tested in research, and results support the model. In the test, the concept of preferenda was operationalized as environmental ambiance.

Implications

Yao's model breaks new ground for approaches to wandering and other NDBs. It also offers an explanation for the sometimes conflicting views of wandering (harmful vs. helpful, seeking vs. leaving, attracting attention vs. avoiding or withdrawing) and for the increase in wandering with advancing cognitive impairment apart from its spatially-disordered nature.

Risky Wandering and Adverse Outcomes: A Longitudinal Predictive Model

At once both a strength and limitation of the NDB-W is its focus on minute-by-minute factors that precipitate wandering. However, such a view does not illuminate our understanding of how wandering develops over the course of dementia. Another limitation of this model is its inattention to outcomes of wandering, that is, to the types and amounts of wandering that result in adverse outcomes for wanderers and an undesirable impact on caregivers. To address these shortcomings, the Risky Wandering and Adverse Outcomes (RWAO) model was developed by Algase and colleagues (2004).

Model Components

This putative model (Figure 2.5) was synthesized from elements of the NDB model (Algase et al., 1996) and the stress process model of caregiving (Perlin, Mullan, Semple, & Skaff, 1990). The RWAO model depicts an interactive relationship over time between wanderers and their caregivers (CGs) affecting outcomes for both. This relationship is best characterized as a caregiving process during which the wanderer develops increasing dependency, and the caregiver assumes growing responsibility. Whether or not adverse outcomes develop for wanderers or CGs follows from a stress response view. The model specifies relationships among concepts leading directly and indirectly to adverse outcomes for both parties.

According to the RWAO model, wandering includes frequency/persistence, spatial disorientation, mealtime impulsivity, and nighttime walking. These behaviors may lead to immediate adverse outcomes for wanderers (those following from specific wandering episodes), such as inadequate food intake, fatigue, falls and fractures, and eloping. Immediate adverse outcomes can lead to cumulative adverse outcomes due to pile-up of unmanaged or poorly managed wandering, for example, poor nutritional status, or to escalation of its immediate adverse outcomes, such as death as a consequence of eloping.

Similarly, characteristics of the CG shape their responses to wandering and caregiving. These characteristics, when insufficiently matched to the demands of the caregiving situation, can lead to adverse outcomes for CGs, such as, reduced physical, mental, financial, and social resources; sleep deprivation; loss of privacy; and social isolation. If unchecked, adverse outcomes for CGs lead to cumulative adverse outcomes for wanderers due to a decline in caregiver performance over time.

Also affecting adverse outcomes for either party are two sets of mediating variables: contributing factors and CG strategies. Derived from the NDB background factors, contributing factors typify the characteristics of the person with dementia and constitute risk factors for wandering behavior. When viewed over time, the stable nature of background factors in the NDB model becomes dynamic for some factors. Thus, contributing factors become either enduring (or predisposing) or dynamic (enabling and neurocognitive) in long-term view represented in the RWAO model. Predisposing factors are characteristics of the person with dementia that

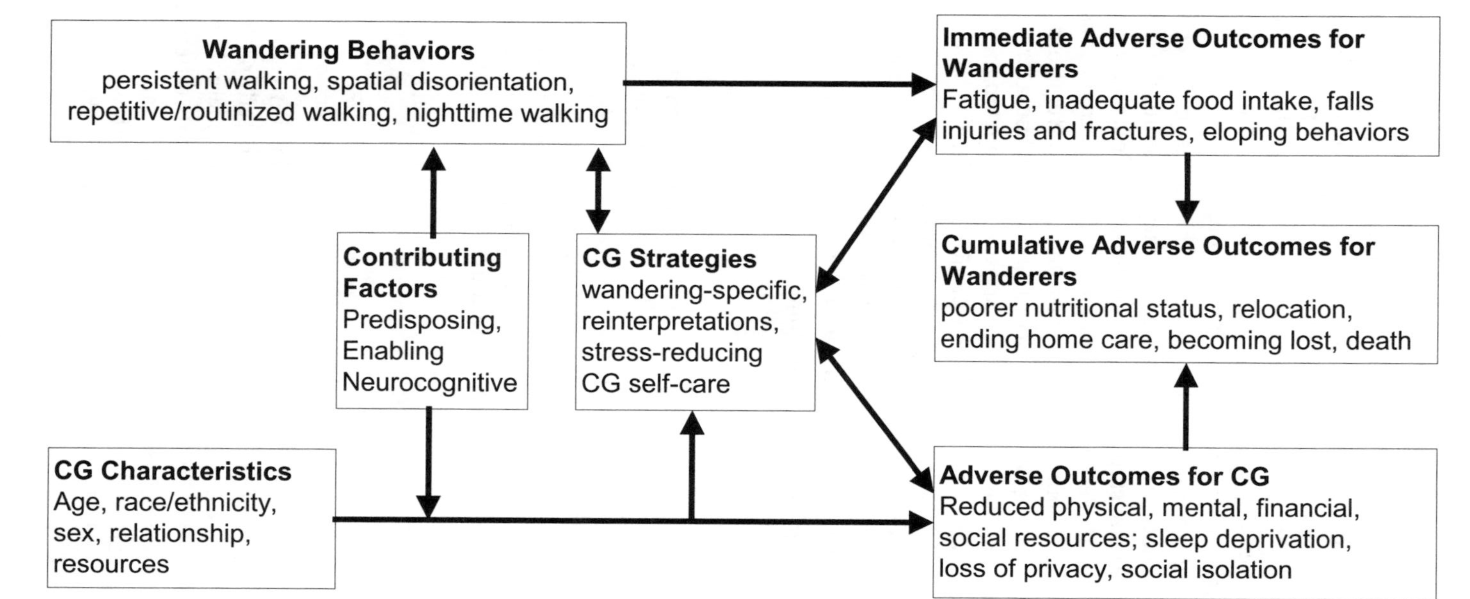

FIGURE 2.5 Putative model of Risky Wandering and Adverse Outcomes (RWAO).

operate to shape long-standing or habitual patterns of behavior, for example, gender, personality, and behavioral response to stress. Enabling factors are those that support (or detract from) locomotor ability (e.g., general health, mobility status) and thus, capability to wander. Neurocognitive factors are domains of thinking and behavior directly involved in a specific dementing process. Dynamic (enabling and neurocognitive) factors are potentially amenable to intervention.

Contributing factors may also influence the effects of CG characteristics on adverse outcomes for caregivers as they may alter the character of the dyadic relationship or the caregiving load (Perlin et al., 1990). CG strategies, which Perlin and colleagues call coping, are actions taken to manage the problem (wandering or its immediate adverse outcomes), to change the meaning of the problem (thereby redefining demands of caregiving), or to manage symptoms of stress resulting from the problem (adverse outcomes for CG). Within our putative model, CG strategies are shaped directly by CG characteristics and these, in turn, affect adverse outcomes for CG. Over time, these strategies affect and are affected by wandering behaviors and immediate outcomes for wanderers, due to the changing nature of wandering behavior in response to intervention, or as a manifestation of progressive dementia.

Model Implications and Tests

The RWAO model provides a basis for studies aimed to describe and explain factors (and their sequencing) that lead to the emergence, management, and outcomes of specific types of wandering. Such information would be of substantial benefit in screening for those at risk and in the design, timing, and targeting of interventions to mitigate development of wandering or its adverse outcomes. To date, no formal tests of the RWAO model have been completed, although projects to do so have been developed.

CONCLUSION

The ultimate goal of developing theories on wandering is to advance the design, testing, and targeting of effective, evidence-based intervention. While the scientific study of wandering is young, considerable progress has been made in an important step toward this goal: differentiating wandering from similar phenomena, both conceptually and operationally. Further progress in explaining the complexity of wandering has been gained through development of the NDB model. The NDB model integrates multiple individual mechanisms operative in wandering into a coherent, testable model that can enable identification of persons at risk for wandering and the conditions under which those at risk will manifest various types and degrees of the behavior. A full test of the NDB model for its adequacy in explaining wandering is underway; at this time, only a partial test of the model has been accomplished. Risk factors for wandering were shown to vary depending upon the co-occurrence of one or more other need-driven behaviors.

The NDB model has also made other important contributions to the study of wandering. While not yet fully validated, it has fostered theoretical thinking about wandering and spawned development of other models. These models, together with the NDB model, in time will provide the refined and valid theories needed to support rigorous intervention studies. Such studies will lead to practice improvements that will benefit wanderers and their families.

REFERENCES

Adolphs, R. (1999). The human amygdale and emotion. *Progress in Clinical Neuroscience, 5*(2), 125–127.

Algase, D. L. (1992). A century of progress: Today's strategies for managing wandering behavior. *Journal of Gerontological Nursing, 18*(11), 28–34.

Algase, D. L., Antonakos, C., Beattie, E., Yao, L. & Beel-Bates, C.A. (2006). Unpublished data from *Wandering: Background and Proximal Factors.* National Institute of Nursing Research, 1R01NR04569.

Algase, D. L., Antonakos, C., Yao, L., Beattie, E.R.A., Son, G. R. (2007). *Are wandering and physically-non-aggressive agitated behaviors equivalent?* Manuscript submitted for publication.

Algase, D. L., Beattie, E., & Son, G. (2004). *Wandering, adverse outcomes, and caregiver strategies.* Grant application, 1RO1NR009244, National Institutes of Nursing Research.

Algase, D., Beck, C., Kolanowski, A., Whall, A., Berent, S., Richards, K., et al. (1996). Need-driven dementia-compromised behavior: An alternative view of disruptive behavior. *American Journal of Alzheimer's Disease, 11*(6), 10–19.

Algase, D., Beck, C., Whall, A., & the NDB Collaborative Research Group. (2003). Exploring NDB background factors as predictors of wandering, aggression and problematic vocalizations. *The Gerontologist (Program Abstracts), 43*(SI 1), 83–84.

Algase, D. L., & Cheng, J. (1992). Antecedent and consequent activity as pacers for wandering cycles. *The Gerontologist (Program Abstracts), 31,* 144.

Algase, D. L., Kupferschmid, B., Beel-Bates, C. A., & Beattie, E.R.A. (1997). Estimates of stability of daily wandering behavior among cognitively impaired long-term care residents. *Nursing Research, 46*(3), 172–178.

Algase, D. L., Moore, D. H., VandeWeerd, C., & Gavin-Dreschnack, D. (in press). Mapping the maze of terms and definitions in dementia-related wandering. *Aging and Mental Health.*

Algase, D. L., Son, G. R., Beattie, E., Song, J. A., Leitsch, S., & Yao, L. (2004). The interrelatedness of wandering & wayfinding in a community sample of persons with dementia. *Dementia & Geriatric Cognitive Disorders, 17*(3), 231–239.

Algase, D. L., & Tsai, J. (1991). Wandering as a rhythm. *The Gerontologist, 31* (Special Issue), 140.

Bachevalier, J. (1990). Ontogenetic development of habit and memory formation in primates. *Annals of the New York Academy of Sciences, 608,* 457–477.

Beel-Bates, C. A. (2001). Visuospatial function in ambulatory aged women with probable Alzheimer's disease: A multiple case study (Doctoral dissertation, University of Michigan, 2001). *Dissertation Abstracts International, 62,* 157.

Berlyne, D. (1960). *Conflict arousal and curiosity.* New York: McGraw-Hill.

Berlyne, D. (1971). *Aesthetics and psychobiology.* Engelwood Cliffs, NJ: Prentice-Hall.

Brooke, M. M., Questad, K. A., Patterson, D. R., & Bashak, K. J. (1992). Agitation and restlessness after closed head injury: A prospective study of 100 consecutive admissions. *Archives of Physical Medicine and Rehabilitation, 73*(4), 320–323.

Casadesus, G., Garrett, R., Webber, K. M., Hartzler, A. W., Atwood, C. S., Perry, G., et al. (2006). The estrogen myth: Potential use of gonadotropin-releasing hormone agonists for the treatment of Alzheimer's disease. *Drugs in R & D, 7*(3), 187–193.

Chatterjee, A., Strauss, M. S., Smyth, K. A., & Whitehouse, P. J. (1992). Personality changes in Alzheimer's disease. *Archives of Neurology, 48,* 486–491.

Chiu, Y. C., Algase, D., Whall, A., Liang, J., Liu, H. C., Lin, K. N., et al. (2004). Getting lost: Directed attention and executive function in early Alzheimer's disease patients. *Dementia and Geriatric Cognitive Disorders, 17,* 174–180.

Choi, J. (1999). Wandering as a goal-seeking behavior: Examining wanderers' negotiation with the physical environment. *Architectural Research* Journal of Architectural Institute of Korea, *1*(1) *11–16.*

Cohen-Mansfield, J. (1986). Agitated behaviors in the elderly II. A conceptual review. *Journal of the American Geriatric Society, 34*(10), 722–727.

Cohen-Mansfield, J. (2003). Agitation in the Elderly: Definitional and theoretical conceptualizations. In D. P. Hay, D. T. Klein, L. K. Hay, G. T. Grossberg, & J. S. Kennedy (Eds.), *Agitation* (pp. 1–22). Washington, DC: American Psychiatric Publishing, Inc.

Cohen-Mansfield, J., & Billig, N. (1986). Agitated behaviors in the elderly I. A conceptual review. *Journal of the American Geriatric Society, 34*(10), 711–721.

Cohen-Mansfield, J., Marx, M., & Rosenthal, A. (1989). A description of agitation in a nursing home. *Journal of Gerontology, 44*(3), M77–84.

Cohen-Mansfield, J., & Werner, P. (1998). The effects of an enhanced environment on nursing home residents who pace. *Gerontologist, 38*(2), 199–208.

Cohen-Mansfield, J., Werner, P., Marx, M., & Freedman, L. (1991). Two studies of pacing in the nursing home. *Journal of Gerontology, 46,* 77–83.

Costa, P. T., & McRae, R. (1992). *Revised NEO personality inventory and NEO five-factor inventory, professional manual.* Odessa, FL: Psychological Assessment Resources.

Davidson, R. J. (1993). The neuropsychology of emotion and affective style. In M. Lewis & J. M. Haviland (Eds.), *Handbook of emotion* (pp. 143–154). New York: Guilford.

Dawson, P., & Reid, D. W. (1987). Behavioral dimensions of patients at risk of wandering. *Gerontologist, 27*(1), 104–107.

DeLeon, M. J., Potegal, M., & Gurland, B. (1984). Wandering and parietal signs in senile dementia of Alzheimer's type. *Neuropsychobiology, 11,* 155–157.

Donaldson, S. K. (2000). Breakthroughs in scientific research: The discipline of nursing, 1960–1999. *Annual Review of Nursing Research, 18,* 247–311.

Duffy, C. J. (1999). Visual loss and Alzheimer's disease: Out of sight, out of mind. *Neurology, 52,* 10–11.

Ekman, P. (1992). An argument for basic emotions. *Cognition and Emotion, 6*(3/4), 169–200.

Faust, M. E., & Belota, D. A. (1997). Inhibition of return and visuospatial attention in healthy older adults and individuals with dementia of the Alzheimer's type. *Neuropsychology, 11,* 13–29.

Grammas, P., Samany, P. G., & Thirumangalakudi, L. (2006). Thrombin and inflammatory proteins are elevated in Alzheimer's disease microvessels: Implications for disease pathogenesis. *Journal of Alzheimer's Disease, 9*(1), 51–58.

Hamman, S. B., Monarch, E. S., & Goldstein, F. C. (2000). Memory enhancement for emotional stimuli is impaired in Alzheimer's disease. *Neuropsychology, 14*(1), 82.

Harman, D. (2006). Alzheimer's disease pathogenesis: Role of aging. *Annals of the New York Academy of Sciences, 1067,* 454–460.

Hebb, D.O. (1955). Drives and the CNS (conceptual nervous system). *Psychological Review, 62,* 243–254.

Henderson, V., Mack, B., & Williams, B. W. (1989). Spatial disorientation in Alzheimer's disease. *Archives of Neurology, 46,* 391–394.

Hyman, B. T., Van Hoesen, G. W., Damasio, A. R., & Barnes, C. L. (1984). Alzheimer's disease: Cell-specific pathology isolates the hippocampal formation. *Science, 225*(4667), 1168–1170.

Kiyosawa, M., Bosley, T. M., Chawluk, J., Jamieson, D., Schatz, N. J., Savino, P. J., et al. (1989). Alzheimer's disease with prominent visual symptoms. *Ophthalmology, 96*(7), 1077–1086.

Kolanowski, A. M. (1991). Restlessness in the elderly: A concept analysis. In P. L. Chinn (Ed.), *Anthology on Caring* (pp. 345–353). New York: National League for Nursing.

Kolanowski, A. M., & Whall, A. (1996). Life-span perspective on personality in dementia. *Image: The Journal of Nursing Scholarship, 28*(4), 315–320.

Kroeber-Riel, W. (1979). Activation research: Psychological approaches in consumer research. *Journal of Consumer Research, 5,* 340–350.

LeDoux, J. E. (1996). *The emotional brain: The mysterious underpinnings of emotional life.* New York: Simon & Schuster.

Linton, A. D., Matteson, M. A., & Byers, V. (1997). The relationship between premorbid lifestyle and wandering behaviors in institutionalized people with dementia. *Clinical and Experimental Research, 9*(6), 415–418.

Malmo, R. B. (1959). Activation: A neurological dimension. *Psychological Review, 66*(6), 367–386.

Martino-Saltzman, D., Blasch, B. B., Morris, R. D., & McNeal, L. W. (1991). Travel behavior of nursing home residents perceived as wanderers and nonwanderers *Gerontologist, 31*(5), 666–672.

McMurtray, A., Clark, D. G., Christine, D., & Mendez, M. F. (2006). Early-onset dementia: Frequency and causes compared to late-onset dementia. *Dementia & Geriatric Cognitive Disorders, 21*(2), 9–64.

Meguro, K., Yamaguchi, S., Yamazaki, H., Itoh, M., Yamaguchi, T., Matsui, H., et al. (1996). Cortical glucose metabolism in psychiatric wandering patients with vascular dementia. *Psychiatry Research, 67*(1), 71–80.

Mendez, M. F., Tomsak, R. L., & Remler, B. (1990). Disorders of the visual system in AD. *journal of Clinical Neuro-ophthalmology, 1,* 62–69.

Mogenson, G. J., Jones, D. L., & Yim, C. Y. (1980). From motivation to action: Functional interface between the limbic system and the motor system. *Progress in Neurobiology, 14,* 69.

Monsour, N., & Robb S. S. (1982). Wandering behavior in old age: A psychosocial study. *Social Work, 27*(5), 411–416.

Norris, C. (1978). Restlessness. In C. Carlson & B. Blackwell (Eds.), *Behavioral concepts and nursing intervention* (pp. 141–153). New York: J.B. Lippincott Co.

Norris, C. (1986). Restlessness: A disturbance in rhythmicity. *Geriatric Nursing, 7*(6), 302–306.

O'Brien, H. L., Tetewsky, S. J., Avery, L. M., Cushman, L. A., Makous, W., & Duffy, C. J. (2001). Visual mechanisms of spatial disorientation in Alzheimer's disease. *Cerebral Cortex, 11,* 1083–1092.

O'Keefe, J., & Nadel, L. (1978). *The hippocampus as a cognitive map.* Oxford: Clarendon Press.

Panskepp, J. (1998). *Affective neuroscience: The foundations of human and animal emotions.* New York: Oxford University Press.

Passini, R., Rainville, C., Marchand, N., & Joanette, Y. (1995). Way-finding in dementia of the Alzheimer's type: Planning abilities. *Journal of Clinical and Experimental Neuropsychology, 17,* 820–832.

Perlin, L. I., Mullan, J., Semple, S., Skaff, M., (1990). Caregiving and the stress process: An overview of concepts and their measures. *Gerontologist, 30*(5), 583–591.

Rabinowitz, J., Davidson, M., DeDeyn, P. P., Katz, I., Brodaty, H., & Cohen-Mansfield, J. (2005). Factor analysis of the Cohen-Mansfield Agitation Inventory in three large samples of nursing home patients with dementia and behavioral disturbance. *American Journal of Geriatric Psychiatry, 13,* 991–998.

Reid, W., Brow, B., Creasey, H., Grayson, D., McCusker, E., Bennett, H., et al. (1996). Age at onset and pattern on neuropsychological impairment in mild early-stage Alzheimer's disease. A study of community-based population. *Archives of Neurology, 53*(10), 1056–1061.

Rolland, Y., Payoux, P., Lauwers-Cances, V., Voison, T., Esquerre, J., & Velles, B. (2005). A SPECT study of wandering behavior in Alzheimer's disease. *International Journal of Geriatric Psychiatry, 20,* 816–820.

Ryan, J. P., McGowan, J., McCaffrey, N., Ryan, G. T., Zandi, T., & Brannigan, G. G. (1995). Graphomotor perseveration and wandering in Alzheimer's disease. *Journal of Geriatric Psychiatry & Neurology, 8,* 209–212.

Sadun, A. A., Borchert, M., DeVita, E., Hinton, D. R., & Bassi, C. J. (1987). Assessment of visual impairment in patients with Alzheimer's disease. *American Journal of Ophthalmology, 104*(2), 113–120.

Salmon, D. P., & Lange, K. L. (2001). Cognitive screening and neuropsychological assessment in early Alzheimer's disease. *Clinical Geriatric Medicine, 17*(2), 229–254.

Satlin, A., Teicher, M. H., Lieberman, H. R., Badessarini, R. J., Volicer, L., & Rheaume, Y. (1991). Circadian locomotor activity rhythms in Alzheimer's disease. *Neuropsychopharmacology, 5*(2), 115–126.

Satlin, A., Volicer, L., Stopa, E. G., & Harper, D. (1995). Circadian locomotor activity and core-body temperature rhythms in Alzheimer's disease. *Neurology of Aging, 16*(5), 765–771.

Siegler, J. C., Welsh, K. A., Dawson, D. V., Fillenbausm, G. G., Earl, N. L., Kaplan, E. B., et al. (1991). Ratings of personality change in patients being evaluated for memory disorders. *Alzheimer's Disease and Associated Disorders, 5*(4), 240–250.

Skinner, R. D., & Garcia-Rill, E. (1993). Mesolimbic interactions with mesopontine modulation of locomotion. In P. W. Kalivas & C. D. Barnes (Eds.), *Limbic motor circuits and neuropsychiatry.* Ann Arbor, MI: CRC Press, 152–167.

Snyder, L. H., Rupprect, P., Pyrek, J., Breckhus, S., & Moss, T. (1978). Wandering. *The Gerontologist, 18,* 272–280.

Song, J. (2003). Relationship of premorbid personality and behavioral response to stress to wandering behavior of residents with dementia in long-term care facilities (Doctoral dissertation, University of Michigan, 2003).

Squire, L. R. (1992). Declarative and nondeclarative memory: Multiple brain systems supporting learning and memory. *Journal of Cognitive Neuroscience: Special Issue: Memory Systems, 4,* 232–243.

Strauss, M. E., & Pasupathi, M. (1994). Primary caregivers' descriptions of Alzheimer's patients' personality traits: Temporal stability and sensitivity to change. *Alzheimer's Disease and Associated Disorders, 8*(3), 166–176.

Tetewsky, S. J., & Duffy, C. J. (1999). Visual loss and getting lost in Alzheimer's disease. *Neurology, 52,* 958–965.

Thomas, D. W. (1997). Understanding the wandering patient: A continuity of personality perspective. *Journal of Gerontological Nursing, 23*(1), 16–24.

Ulrich, R. S. (1983). Aesthetic and affective response in natural environment. In I. Altman & J. F. Wohlwill (Eds.), *Human behavior and environment: Advances in theory and research* (Vol. 6, pp. 85–125). New York: Plenum Press.

Weller, M. P. (1987). A biochemical hypothesis of wandering. *Medicine, Science & the Law, 27*(1), 40–41.

Whishaw, I. Q. (1994). "Short stops" in rats with fimbria-fornix lesions: Evidence for change in the mobility gradient. *Hippocampus, 4,* 577–582.

Yao, L. (2004). Locomoting responses to environment in elders with dementia: A model construction and preliminary testing (doctoral dissertation, University of Michigan, 2004).

Yao, L., & Algase, D. (2006). Environmental ambiance as a new window on wandering. *Western Journal of Nursing Research, 28*(1), 89–104.

Zajonc, R. B. (2001). Mere exposure: A gateway to the subliminal. *Current Directions in Psychological Science, 10*(6), 224–228.

CHAPTER THREE

Epidemiology of Wandering

Ladislav Volicer

Wandering behavior is recognized as an important problem by family members, health care workers, and policy makers and was the subject of many research studies. Despite the terminology problem described in Chapter 1, these studies provide important information that forms a basis for future studies. The purpose of this chapter is to review epidemiological studies of wandering and describe factors related to wandering and consequences of wandering behavior.

INCIDENCE AND PREVALENCE OF WANDERING

Wandering is most common in individuals who suffer from dementia, although it may occur also in other conditions. The significance of the wandering problem in dementia is best documented by caregivers themselves, who report wandering is a problem in more then 70 percent of cases (Rabins, Mace, & Lucas, 1982). Research studies provide inconsistent information about prevalence of wandering, because most of the studies are cross-sectional and do not take into consideration that the incidence of wandering depends on the duration and severity of dementia (Klein et al., 1999). Another problem with the research methodology is inconsistency in the definition of wandering behavior, with wandering sometimes improperly combined with agitation (Devanand et al., 1997).

A cross-sectional study involving data obtained nationally from 134 VA nursing homes included 15,092 male residents having moderate to severe cognitive impairment, using data from the Minimum Data Set (MDS).

This study explored the extent of and factors associated with wandering behaviors upon nursing home admission in a male VA population. The prevalence of wandering over a 4-year period was found to be 6.5 percent. Frequency of wandering was associated with socially inappropriate behavior, resistance to care, use of antipsychotic medication, independence in locomotion/ambulation, and dependence in activities of daily living associated with basic hygiene. A multivariate logistic regression model using these variables was found accurate in predicting wandering behavior (Schonfeld et al., in press).

Longitudinal studies indicate that wandering behavior starts on the average 10 months after diagnosis of dementia in 40 percent of individuals (Jost & Grossberg, 1996), but eventually occurs in 80 percent of all patients with dementia (Hope et al., 2001). Cross-sectional studies find prevalence of wandering between 15 and 28 percent (Kiely, Morris, & Algase, 2000; Klein et al., 1999; Rolland et al., 2006), with wandering characteristics similar in nursing homes and assisted living facilities (Beattie, Song, & LaGore, 2005).

PROGRESSION OF WANDERING BEHAVIORS

The character of wandering changes with the progression of dementia. Initially, wandering consists of walking for an appropriate reason but then repeated several times. This may be caused by an impairment of short-term memory causing the individual to forget that the task was already accomplished. Next, attempts to leave home occur at inappropriate times and may be thwarted by a caregiver. A study targeting caregivers of individuals with dementia found that 69 percent of caregivers who were interviewed reported that their family member wandered out of the house at some point (Calkins & Namazi, 1991). Disorientation regarding time of the day or lack of realization that the person would be lost if they left the home are factors that might be associated with such wandering.

As dementia progresses, individuals become less able to do household or garden chores, but they may still walk around trying to accomplish them. In the English literature, this behavior was called "pottering" (Hope et al., 2001). Individuals may also indulge their walking habit excessively and eventually walk aimlessly in their environment. They also may trail or shadow their caregiver. Wandering at night is also quite common, occurring in more than half of those who wander. Most individuals exhibit several types of wandering for an average of 3.2 wandering-related behaviors as measured by the "Pressure Behavioural Examination" (Hope et al., 2001). With further progression of dementia, many individuals develop gait difficulties that limit their wandering behavior.

Longitudinal perspectives reveal the expression of wandering as a dynamic rather than a static phenomenon, fluctuating over time and change in cognitive and functional status. A separate analysis of the Devanand cohort (Devanand et al., 1997) showed that wandering increased from a baseline rate of 39 percent to a peak of 57 percent at 3 years and then declined to 46 percent at study conclusion at 5 years, this against a backdrop of steady decline in cohort scores of cognition (Holtzer et al., 2003).

FACTORS RELATED TO WANDERING BEHAVIORS

Demographic Factors

The typical wanderer has been profiled as relatively young within the older population, more cognitively impaired, might have experienced sleep problems, had a more active premorbid lifestyle, used more psychotropic medications, and more likely to be a man (Lai & Arthur, 2003). Studies show that wandering is more common among men (Kiely et al., 2000; Rowe, Feinglass, & Wiss, 2004), and one study reported increased wandering with increased age (Cooper, Mungas, & Weiler, 1990). Premorbid activity level is not related to the incidence of wandering (Linton, Matteson, & Byers, 1997), but wandering may be related to premorbid personality. Personality questionnaires administered to informant surrogates of wanderers and nonwanderers determined that wanderers were perceived to be higher on the factors of extroversion and agreeableness (Thomas, 1997). In a study of nursing home residents, pacing (intense wandering that is difficult to redirect) was related to past life-threatening experiences (Cohen-Mansfield, Werner, Marx, & Freedman, 1991). Black and Latino community dwelling individuals with dementia have higher prevalence of wandering than whites (Sink, Covinsky, Newcomer, & Yaffe, 2004). Some limited research suggests that wandering characteristics do not differ between different countries (Song et al., 2003).

Wanderers who reside in a nursing home differ from other residents by fewer medical diagnoses, better appetites, and shorter durations of stay (Cohen-Mansfield et al., 1991). However, policy changes in the long-term care sector and in health care financing since 1991 may influence the profile for nursing home wanderers toward an older, sicker, largely female, and predominantly wheelchair bound population, although confirmations of these trends remains anecdotal. Wandering is positively related to cognitive impairment and to past life-threatening experiences. Short- and long-term memory deficits and antipsychotic medications increased the likelihood of wandering; the presence of pneumonia, constipation, functional impairment, and female gender decreased likelihood (Kiely et al., 2000). Men in nursing homes were found more likely to wander than women, 59 percent versus 41 percent (Ott, Lapane, & Gambassi, 2000).

In community-dwelling settings, persons who wander exhibit a greater frequency of wandering associated with more severe levels of impairment in cognition, day-to-day functioning, and behavior (Logsdon et al., 1998). Functional impairment and disruptive behavior were the strongest independent predictors of wandering occurring within the past week in this sample. Community-dwelling wanderers in France have more severe cognitive impairment, less autonomy, and increased likelihood of being undernourished (Rolland et al., 2006).

Type of Dementia

Some studies indicate that wandering is more common in individuals diagnosed with Alzheimer's disease than in individuals with other types of dementia (Klein et al., 1999; Thomas, 1997). However, one study found a higher incidence of wandering in fronto-temporal dementia than in Alzheimer's disease or vascular dementia (Bathgate, Snowden, Varma, Blackshaw, & Neary, 2001). Another study using autopsy verified diagnoses reported that patients with Lewy body dementia were more likely to wander than patients with Alzheimer's disease, especially earlier in the disease course (Knuffman, Mohsin, Feder, & Grossberg, 2001).

Type of Cognitive Impairment

Aside from spontaneous, independent locomotion through space, cognitive impairment is the only descriptor universally applicable to all wanderers (Algase & Struble, 1992). Of the many reported correlates of wandering, the association between cognitive impairment and wandering has received the broadest empirical confirmation (Kiely et al., 2000; Logsdon et al., 1998), although it must be kept in mind that not all cognitively impaired people wander.

Detailed psychological testing showed that wandering is associated with greater graphomotor perseveration, while spatial orientation and attention or concentration were similar in both wanderers and nonwanderers (Ryan et al., 1995). There is also some indication that involvement of a specific brain area is related to wandering behavior in individuals with Alzheimer's disease. Using single photon emission computed tomography (SPECT) imaging, it was found that despite similar clinical dementia severity, wanderers with Alzheimer's disease had more severely reduced regional blood flow in the parietal-temporal lobe than subjects without wandering behavior (Rolland et al., 2005). The parieto-temporal area is correlated with visuospatial function. However, in a study of patients with similar severity of vascular dementia, wanderers had higher cerebral metabolic rate for glucose in bilateral frontal lobes, left parietal lobe, left temporo-parieto-occipital region, left occipital lobe, and cerebellum than nonwanderers (Meguro et al., 1996). More recent investigation indicates that spatial disorientation is related to some aspects of wandering but not to repetitive walking and mealtime impulsivity (Algase et al., 1996).

Psychopathology and Medication

A French study found that wandering was associated with delirium, aggressiveness, irritability, depression, anxiety, euphoria, apathy, and disinhibition in individuals with Alzheimer's disease living in the community (Rolland et al., 2006). Wandering was also more common in individuals with dementia who had delusions (Lachs, Becker, Siegal, Miller, & Tinetti, 1992). However, presence of these symptoms may just indicate greater severity of dementia, which is independently associated with increased wandering. Wandering is associated with neuroleptic use (Klein et al., 1999), but it is not clear if side effects of drugs (e.g., akathisia) are actually the etiology or if the wandering is related to the psychiatric problems for which the drugs are used.

Circadian Changes

Nocturnal wandering was found related to sleep disturbance (Klein et al., 1999), perhaps caused by a disruption of circadian rhythms. Circadian rhythms have been found to be disturbed in both normal aging and in progressive degenerative dementias. In Alzheimer's disease, a study using constant routine protocol found that the endogenous circadian phase is delayed compared to healthy elderly subjects. There was also dissociation of the activity and core body temperature rhythms (Harper et al., 2005). Patients with fronto-temporal dementia had less nocturnal activity and phase delay in their core body temperature than patients with Alzheimer's disease, but their activity rhythm was highly fragmented and uncoupled from the rhythm of core body temperature (Harper et al., 2001).

Patients with postmortem diagnosis of dementia with Lewy bodies manifest similar delay of circadian phase but greater disturbance of locomotor activity circadian rhythms than patients with Alzheimer's disease (Harper et al., 2004). This may be related to increased wandering in patients with Lewy bodies dementia mentioned previously (Knuffman et al., 2001).Wandering behavior may be also part of the sundowning syndrome that is associated with more circadian phase delay, less correlation of circadian temperature rhythm with the 24-hour cycle, and with lower amplitude of the circadian temperature (Volicer, Harper, Manning, Goldstein, & Satlin, 2001).

Factors Related to Elopement

Elopement may be caused by lack of effective precautions to prevent elopement despite history of elopement intentions or attempts, lack of awareness by the staff of resident location, and ineffective use of alarm devices intended to alert staff to elopement attempts (Aud, 2006). Elopement also happens when the caregiver is distracted or asleep, the individual with dementia is home alone, or when they are being transported by professional services (Rowe & Glover, 2001). Chapter 10 describes factors associated with elopement in community-based settings, while Chapter 9 describes elopement in institutional settings (acute care and long-term care).

CONSEQUENCES OF WANDERING

Wandering is not always an undesirable behavior. Wandering provides physical exercise that is beneficial for maintaining independent mobility, appetite, and a normal sleep pattern. A study found that nursing home residents who pace have fewer medical diagnoses and better appetite than residents who do not pace (Cohen-Mansfield et al., 1991). It concluded that pacing is a reflection of good health within the nursing home population and that caregivers may want to encourage rather than inhibit this behavior. However, many studies indicate that pacing also exposes individuals to adverse consequences. Chapter 6 provides more detail about the impact of wandering behaviors on functional status, including walking.

Getting Lost

Wandering off the unit or out of a facility is the fourth most common adverse event in long-term care settings, occurring at a rate of 3/100 beds per year (Gurwitz, Sanchez-Cross, Eckler, & Matulis, 1994). A longitudinal 5-year study of 104 community living individuals with dementia showed that almost half of them had to be brought back at least once, five of them were at prolonged and persistent risk of getting lost, and only one third never demonstrated any apparent risk of getting lost (McShane et al., 1998). Probability of getting lost was increased if the size of the area available for walking was small. Probability of getting lost was not related to the amount of time the subject spent walking, but it was decreased by better topographic memory (McShane et al., 1998). A national study showed that only 4 percent of memory-impaired individuals who wander away from home are able to return unassisted, and even individuals who take independent walks on a regular basis may become lost and unable to return home (Rowe & Glover, 2001). On the basis of this data, it is concluded that all persons with dementia are at risk for getting lost, regardless of age, past behavior, and sex, although men are at higher risk of getting lost and dying (Rowe et al., 2004). Chapter 10 provides more detail about precipitating events, wandering behavior, and search strategies for persons who become lost in the community.

Change of Residency

Attempts to leave the house increases risk of institutionalization almost five times in community living individuals with dementia, especially in individuals who attempt to leave despite locked doors (McShane et al., 1998). Frequent wandering is an independent factor contributing to earlier discharge of individuals from assisted living to nursing home settings (Kopetz et al., 2000). Administrators of assisted living facilities describe two types of wandering: wandering within the building and wandering out of the building. Wandering within the building was seen as a minor problem, but wandering outside was a serious concern that necessitated transfer to a nursing home. The administrators reported that alarming the door does not work well in assisted living because there is fewer staff available to respond to an alarm. Automatic locking of a door when the wandering resident approaches was not seen as a solution either, because the door was getting locked often even when the resident did not try to get out and other residents were unable to come in or out before the staff came and reset the door (Aud, 2004).

Malnutrition

Individuals who pace can walk almost constantly, covering distances as long as 25 miles a day (Hope et al., 2001). Such behavior affects their nutritional state, because they are unable to sit down for meals, and because pacing increases significantly their caloric requirements. A study found that individuals who were pacing required an additional 1600 Kcal a day to maintain their nutritional status (Rheaume, Riley, & Volicer, 1987). Undernourishment of individuals who wander was also described in a French study (Rolland et al., 2006). Individuals who pace are also in danger of foot injury if they are not provided with well-fitted comfortable shoes. Chapter 6 provides more detail about the impact of wandering behaviors on functional status, including feeding.

Caregiver Stress

Wandering is stressful for caregivers of individuals with dementia. Caregiving distress was increased significantly with greater frequency of wandering in a population-based sample of 193 individuals with Alzheimer's disease living in the community (Logsdon et al., 1998). Among caregivers of demented individuals who attended day services, caregivers of the mobile patients reported greater burden than caregivers of nonmobile patients, with wandering identified as the most important stress factor (Miyamoto, Ito, Otsuka, & Kurita, 2002). Chapter 2 includes a discussion of caregiver stress in the Model of Risky Wandering.

Falls and Mortality Rate

Wanderers are at increased risk of falling (Kiely, Kiel, Burrows, & Lipsitz, 1998), and falls are the most frequently reported adverse events for residents with dementia in institutional settings (Gurwitz et al., 1994). Those who do fall are more likely to sustain fractures, especially hip fractures (Snyder, Rupprecht, Pyrek, Breckhus, & Moss, 1978). Hip fractures increase mortality rate with more than 50 percent death rate after hospitalization for hip fracture (Morrison & Siu, 2000). Wandering increased almost two-fold the mortality rate of individuals with dementia living either in a community or a nursing home, even after statistical analysis controlled for age and severity of dementia (Suh, Kil Yeon, Shah, & Lee, 2005). Mortality rate is substantially increased in individuals with dementia who get lost. In one study, the percentage of individuals who eloped from a long-term care facility and were found dead was 16–22 percent, which is higher than the percentage of individuals with dementia who reside in these facilities, estimated at 5 percent (Rowe et al., 2004). Another study found that 80 percent of elopements involved chronic wanderers, 45 percent occurred in the first 48 hours after admission, and elopement resulted in death in 70 percent of the cases (Rodriguez, 1993). A mortality rate of 45 percent was reported in another study (Hill, 1991), which suggested that risk depends on the time elapsed before the resident is found. Research conducted in the mid-Atlantic states found that all residents discovered within 24 hours of disappearance survived, while only 54 percent of those requiring greater than 24 hours to be found survived (Koester & Stooksbury, 1995).

Increased Health Care Costs

Alzheimer's disease is an expensive disease to treat, and the same is true for other progressive degenerative dementias. The cost of treatment in the

United States has been estimated to be as high as $29.1 billion annually. The annual direct cost for a patient with Alzheimer's disease in the community was estimated to be over $6,000 and indirect cost over $52,000 (Small, McDonnell, Brooks, & Papadopoulos, 2002). Long-term care costs in a nursing home ranges from $110 to $210 per day or $40,000 to $75,000 per year. Since wandering is very often a precipitant either for institutionalization or transfer from a less expensive assisted living facility to a nursing home, wandering greatly increases the costs of health care for individuals with dementia. Ten percent of lawsuits against long-term care settings involve elopement at an average expense of $100,000 per case (Foxwell, 1994). When the charge is wrongful death, awards range from $180,000 to $1.5 million (Rodriguez, 1993).

CONCLUSION

Research on the epidemiology of wandering documents the widespread incidence and significant consequences this behavior poses for family members, health care workers, and policy makers. Several factors are related to wandering, the most important of them is a cognitive impairment that impairs judgment of special orientation. Consequences of wandering include risk to the individual, increased caregiver burden, and societal costs. Wandering poses a significant safety challenge for care providers.

REFERENCES

Algase, D. L., Beck, C., Kolanowski, A., Whall, A., Berent, S., Richards, K., et al. (1996). Need-driven dementia-compromised behavior: An alternative view of disruptive behavior. *American Journal of Alzheimer's Disease, 11*(6), 10–19.

Algase, D. L., & Struble, L. (1992). Wandering: What, why and how? In K. Buckwalter (Ed.), *Geriatric mental health nursing: Current and future challenges* (pp. 61–74). Thorofare, NJ: Slack.

Aud, M. A. (2004). Residents with dementia in assisted living facilities. The role of behavior in discharge decisions. *Journal of Gerontological Nursing, 30*(6), 16–26.

Aud, M. A. (2006). Dangerous wandering: Elopements of older adults with dementia from long-term care facilities. *American Journal of Alzheimer's Disease and Other Dementia, 19*(6), 361–368.

Bathgate, D., Snowden, J. S., Varma, A., Blackshaw, A., & Neary, D. (2001). Behaviour in frontotemporal dementia, Alzheimer's disease and vascular dementia. *Acta Neurol. Scand., 103*(6), 367–378.

Beattie, E.R.A., Song, J.-A., & LaGore, S. (2005). A comparison of wandering behavior in nursing homes and assisted living facilities. *Research and Theory for Nursing Practice, 19*(2), 181–196.

Calkins, M. P., & Namazi, K. H. (1991). Caregiver's perceptions of the effectiveness of home modifications for community living adults with dementia. *American Journal of Alzheimer's Care and Research, 6*, 25–29.

Cohen-Mansfield, J., Werner, P., Marx, M. S., & Freedman, L. (1991). Two studies of pacing in the nursing home. *Journal of Gerontology, 46*(3), M77–M83.

Cooper, J. K., Mungas, D., & Weiler, P. G. (1990). Relation of cognitive status and abnormal behaviors in Alzheimer's disease. *Journal of the American Geriatrics Society, 38*(8), 867–870.

Devanand, D. P., Jacobs, D. M., Tang, M. X., Del Castillo-Castaneda, C., Sano, M., Marder, K., et al. (1997). The course of psychopathologic features in mild to moderate Alzheimer disease. *Archives of General Psychiatry, 54*(3), 257–263.

Foxwell, L. G. (1994). Elopement—Exposure and control. *Journal of Long-Term Care Administration, 21*(4), 8–12.

Gurwitz, J. H., Sanchez-Cross, M. T., Eckler, M. A., & Matulis, J. (1994). The epidemiology of adverse and unexpected events in the long-term care setting. *Journal of the American Geriatrics Society, 42*(1), 33–38.

Harper, D. G., Stopa, E. G., McKee, A. C., Satlin, A., Fish, D., & Volicer, L. (2004). Dementia severity and Lewy bodies affect circadian rhythms in Alzheimer disease. *Neurobiology of Aging, 25*(6), 771–781.

Harper, D. G., Stopa, E. G., McKee, A. C., Satlin, A., Harlan, P. C., Goldstein, R., et al. (2001). Differential circadian rhythm disturbances in men with Alzheimer disease and frontotemporal degeneration. *Archives of General Psychiatry, 58*(4), 353–360.

Harper, D. G., Volicer, L., Stopa, E. G., McKee, A. C., Nitta, M., & Satlin, A. (2005). Disturbance of endogenous circadian rhythm in aging and Alzheimer's disease. *American Journal of Geriatric Psychiatry, 13*(5), 359–368.

Hill, K. (1991). *Predicting the behavior of lost persons.* Fairfax, VA: NASAR.

Holtzer, R.,Tang, M. X., Devanand, D. P., Albert, S. M.,Wegesin, D. J., Marder, K., et al. (2003). Psychopathological features in Alzheimer's disease: Course and relationship with cognitive status. *Journal of the American Geriatrics Society, 51*(7), 953–960.

Hope, T., Keene, J., McShane, R. H., Fairburn, C. G., Gedling, K., & Jacoby, R. (2001). Wandering in dementia: A longitudinal study. *International Psychogeriatrics, 13*(2), 137–147.

Jost, B. C., & Grossberg, G. T. (1996). The evolution of psychiatric symptoms in Alzheimer's disease: A natural history study. *Journal of the American Geriatrics Society, 44*(9), 1078–1081.

Kiely, D. K., Kiel, D. P., Burrows, A. B., & Lipsitz, L. A. (1998). Identifying nursing home residents at risk for falling. *Journal of the American Geriatrics Society, 46*(5), 551–555.

Kiely, D. K., Morris, J. N., & Algase, D. L. (2000). Resident characteristics associated with wandering in nursing homes. *International Journal of Geriatric Psychiatry, 15*(11), 1013–1020.

Klein, D. A., Steinberg, M., Galik, E., Steele, C., Sheppard, J.-M., Warren, A., et al. (1999). Wandering behaviour in community-residing persons with dementia. *International Journal of Geriatric Psychiatry, 14*(4), 272–279.

Knuffman, J., Mohsin, F., Feder, J., & Grossberg, G. T. (2001). Differentiating between Lewy body dementia and Alzheimer's disease: A retrospective brain bank study. *Journal of American Medical Directors Association, 2*(4), 146–148.

Koester, R. J., & Stooksbury, D. E. (1995). Behavioral profile of possible Alzheimer's patients in Virginia search and rescue incidents. *Wilderness and Environmental Medicine, 6*(1), 34–43.

Kopetz, S., Steele, C. D., Brandt, J., Baker, A., Kronberg, M., Galik, E., et al. (2000). Characteristics and outcomes of dementia residents in an assisted living facility. *International Journal of Geriatric Psychiatry, 15*(7), 586–593.

Lachs, M. S., Becker, M., Siegal, A. P., Miller, R. L., & Tinetti, M. E. (1992). Delusions and behavioral disturbances in cognitively impaired elderly persons. *Journal of the American Geriatrics Society, 40*(8), 768–773.

Lai, C. K., & Arthur, D. G. (2003). Wandering behaviour in people with dementia. *Journal of Advanced Nursing, 44*(2), 173–182.

Linton, A. D., Matteson, M. A., & Byers, V. (1997). The relationship between premorbid life-style and wandering behaviors in institutionalized people with dementia. *Aging, 9*(6), 415–418.

Logsdon, R. G., Teri, L., McCurry, S. M., Gibbons, L. E., Kukull, W. A., & Larson, E. B. (1998). Wandering: A significant problem among community-residing individuals with Alzheimer's disease. *Journal of Gerontology, Series B: Psychological Sciences and Social Sciences, 53*(5), P294–P299.

McShane, R., Gedling, K., Keene, J., Fairborn, C., Jacoby, R., & Hope, T. (1998). Getting lost in dementia: A longitudinal study of a behavioral symptom. *International Psychogeriatrics, 10*(3), 253–260.

Meguro, K., Yamaguchi, S., Yamazaki, H., Itoh, M., Yamaguchi, T., Matsui, H., et al. (1996). Cortical glucose metabolism in psychiatric wandering patients with vascular dementia. *Psychiatry Research: Neuroimaging, 67*(1), 71–80.

Miyamoto, Y., Ito, H., Otsuka, T., & Kurita, H. (2002). Caregiver burden in mobile and non-mobile demented patients: a comparative study. *International Journal of Geriatric Psychiatry, 17*(8), 765–773.

Morrison, R. S., & Siu, A. L. (2000). Survival in end-stage dementia following acute illness. *Journal of the American Medical Association, 284*(1), 47–52.

Ott, B. R., Lapane, K. L., & Gambassi, G. (2000). Gender differences in the treatment of behavior problems in Alzheimer's disease. SAGE Study Group. Systemic Assessment of Geriatric drug use via Epidemiology. *Neurology, 54*(2), 427–432.

Rabins, P. V., Mace, N. L., & Lucas, M. (1982). The impact of dementia on the family. *Journal of the American Medical Association, 248*(3), 333–335.

Rheaume, Y., Riley, M. E., & Volicer, L. (1987). Meeting nutritional needs of Alzheimer patients who pace constantly. *Journal of Nutrition in the Elderly, 7*(1), 43–52.

Rodriguez, J. (1993). Resident falls and elopements: Cost and controls. *Nursing Homes, 42,* 16–17.

Rolland, Y., Gillette-Guyonett, S., Nourhashemi, F., Andrieu, S., Cantet, C., Payoux, P., et al. (2006). Wandering and Alzheimer's type disease. Descriptive study. *Revue Medecine Interne, 24*(Suppl. 3), 333s–338s.

Rolland, Y., Payoux, P., Lauwers-Cances, V., Voisin, T., Esquerre, J. P., & Vellas, B. (2005). A SPECT study of wandering behavior in Alzheimer's disease. *International Journal of Geriatric Psychiatry, 20*(9), 816–820.

Rowe, M. A., Feinglass, N. G., & Wiss, M. E. (2004). Persons with dementia who become lost in the community: A case study, current research, and recommendations. *Mayo Clinic Proceedings, 79*(11), 1417–1422.

Rowe, M. A., & Glover, J. C. (2001). Antecedents, descriptions and consequences of wandering in cognitively impaired adults and the Safe Return (SR) program. *American Journal of Alzheimer's Disease and Other Dementia, 16*(6), 344–352.

Ryan, J. P., McGowan, J., McCaffrey, N., Ryan, G. T., Zandi, T., & Brannigan, G. G. (1995). Graphomotor perseveration and wandering in Alzheimer's disease. *Journal of Geriatric Psychiatry and Neurology, 8*(4), 209–212.

Schonfeld, L., King-Kallimanis, B., Brown, L. M., Davis, D. M., Kearns, W. D., Molinari, V. A., et al. (in press). *Wandering behaviors in VA nursing home care units. Journal of the American Geriatrics Society.*

Sink, K. M., Covinsky, K. E., Newcomer, R., & Yaffe, K. (2004). Ethnic differences in the prevalence and pattern of dementia-related behaviors. *Journal of the American Geriatrics Society, 52*(8), 1277–1283.

Small, G. W., McDonnell, D. D., Brooks, R. L., & Papadopoulos, G. (2002). The impact of symptom severity on the cost of Alzheimer's disease. *Journal of the American Geriatrics Society, 50*(2), 321–327.

Snyder, L. H., Rupprecht, P., Pyrek, J., Breckhus, S., & Moss, T. (1978). Wandering. *The Gerontologist, 18*(3), 272–280.

Song, J.-A., Algase, D. L., Beattie, E.R.A., Milke, D. L., Duffield, C., & Cowan, B. (2003). Comparison of U.S., Canadian, and Australian participants' performance on the Algase Wandering Scale-Version 2 (AWS-V2). *Research and Theory for Nursing Practice, 17*(3), 241–256.

Suh, G. H., Kil Yeon, B., Shah, A., & Lee, J. Y. (2005). Mortality in Alzheimer's disease: A comparative prospective Korean study in the community and nursing homes. *International Journal of Geriatric Psychiatry, 20*(1), 26–34.

Thomas, D. W. (1997). Understanding the wandering patient. A continuity of personality perspective. *Journal of Gerontological Nursing, 23*(1), 16–24.

Volicer, L., Harper, D. G., Manning, B. C., Goldstein, R., & Satlin, A. (2001). Sundowning and circadian rhythms in Alzheimer's disease. *American Journal of Psychiatry, 158*(5), 704–711.

CHAPTER FOUR

Neuropsychological Correlates of Wanderers

Cheryl A. Luis and Lisa M. Brown

INTRODUCTION

Neuropsychological evaluation is often used to characterize the nature and extent of neurobehavioral changes associated with a dementia syndrome. Its usefulness extends to predicting future changes, such as the potential for cognitive decline or improvement and likelihood of concomitant behavioral or personality changes. For example, older adults who perform lower than expectation on tests assessing free recall of verbal memory are at risk for subsequent development of Alzheimer's disease (AD) (Petersen et al., 1997). Deficits on measures assessing performance of attention, visual constructive ability, and verbal fluency in individuals diagnosed with AD have been shown to predict subsequent psychosis (Paulsen et al., 2000). Logically, it seems reasonable that performance on neuropsychological measures would be useful in identifying individuals who are at increased risk of wandering, a particularly troubling behavior that is often exhibited by those with dementia. Knowledge of neuropsychological correlates of wandering behaviors could potentially aid clinicians and caregivers in predicting those who are most likely to wander and thus assist in the timely development of appropriate interventions.

Although relatively few studies have addressed the usefulness of neuropsychological evaluation in the prediction of wandering, the results so far do indicate a relationship between cognitive changes and wandering. To put wandering and cognition into context, this chapter provides an overview of the research based on neuropsychological concepts frequently used to describe and evaluate the brain behavior relationship.

Although the majority of studies employed cognitive screening measures that are commonly used to detect the presence of cognitive impairment in older adults, more recent research has turned to neuropsychological assessment to better elucidate how the brain controls and produces wandering behaviors.

This chapter also reviews what is currently known about the wandering cognition relationship and highlights how methodological approaches, settings, assessments, samples, and definitions of wandering influence reported research findings. The material presented is organized according to functional categorizations common to neuropsychological evaluation (e.g., measures of global decline, visuospatial functioning, attention, executive functioning, language, and memory). Within each of these sections is a description of existing studies. An overview of the existing literature is useful for both researchers and clinicians alike, because it forms a foundation of evaluation issues to consider when studying or treating persons at risk for wandering, and argues for the need for more well-executed studies.

COGNITIVE DEFICITS

A number of studies have examined the potential relationship between wandering behaviors and cognition (Burns, Jacoby, & Levy, 1990; Chiu et al., 2004; Cooper, Mungas, & Weiler, 1990; Edgerly & Donovick, 1998; Henderson, Mack, & Williams, 1989; Hope et al., 2001; McShane et al., 1998; Passini, Rainville, Marchand, & Joanette, 1995; Ryan et al., 1995). Wandering has been reported to be associated with global (i.e., overall) decline in cognitive function, visual-spatial deficits, dysexecutive signs, memory impairment, and language dysfunction. Each of these domains are reviewed below in greater detail along with supporting literature.

Global Decline

Cross-sectional studies examining wandering behaviors in dementia have reported a positive correlation between general cognitive decline and wandering. For example, Burns et al. (1990) examined the frequency of behavioral and psychiatric symptoms in 178 patients who were diagnosed with possible or probable AD. Nearly 20 percent exhibited wandering behavior as defined by caregiver report of increased walking. Furthermore, increasing prevalence rates were associated with higher Clinical Dementia Rating Scale (CDR) scores (Hughes, Berg, Danziger, Cohen, & Martin, 1982). Similarly, Cooper et al. (1990) reported that abnormal behaviors, including wandering, were associated with lower Mini-Mental Status Examination (MMSE) scores (Folstein, Folstein, & McHugh, 1975). These researchers also report a relationship between wandering and advancing age. Overall, the correlations and effect sizes in regard to the association between global decline and wandering in these studies were modest.

Earlier studies also found weak associations among wandering and dementia severity (Cohen-Mansfield, 1986; Teri, Borson, Kiyak, & Yamagishi, 1989). Reliance on retrospective report to determine both frequency of wandering and level of cognitive ability is a major limitation of another study (Cooper et al., 1990). In addition, these studies used one brief screening measure, such as the MMSE or CDR, as their measure of cognitive function (Burns et al., 1990; Cooper et al., 1990).

Holtzer et al. (2003) examined the occurrence of wandering behaviors (and other behavioral and psychiatric disturbances) longitudinally during the course of AD. Researchers observed 236 patients diagnosed with probable AD biannually for up to 5 years. The primary measure of cognition was an extended version of the MMSE. Wandering behaviors increased as a function of time, suggesting that behaviors were associated with increasing disease severity.

Edgerly and Donovick (1998) conducted one of the few studies that examined the relationship between wandering and cognition. A variety of neuropsychological measures were used, including a standard measure of global intellectual ability (Information subtest of the Wechsler Adult Intelligence Scale—Revised; WAIS-R); verbal and visual memory tests (i.e., the 9-item California Verbal Learning Test, Revised; CVLT-R); the recall measure on the Benton Visual Retention Test (BVRT); visual spatial ability (BVRT copy); language skills (i.e., Controlled Oral Word Association Test, The Token Test); and the MMSE. In this study, wandering was defined as exit attempts from unit, observed activity level, and staff ratings on a checklist of navigational ability. In comparison to infrequent wanderers (rated low), frequent wanderers (rated high) performed more poorly on WAIS-R Information, BVRT, and CVLT (5-trial total score). Despite modest to high correlations among the neuropsychological measures, the MMSE was the best predictor of staff ratings of wandering, suggesting that global deterioration may be the best predictor. High rated wanderers had an average MMSE cut score of 11, while low wanderers had an average MMSE cut score of 17. The small sample size (N = 29) and disproportionate number of females limits generalizability of these findings.

To date, the most conclusive study regarding the relationship between global cognitive function (MMSE) and dementia-related wandering comes from a longitudinal study describing the natural history of wandering. Using a prospective design, Hope and colleagues (2001) followed 86 patients who were diagnosed with a clinical diagnosis of AD or vascular dementia and examined their autopsy findings at their time of death. Wandering behavior was carefully operationalized. The Present Behavioral Examination (PBE), a validated instrument of behavioral change that assesses 12 items (increased walking, trailing, puttering, attempts to leave home, aimless walking, etc.), was administered along with a clinical interview every 4 months by two trained clinicians (kappa = .89). Regular interviews with caregivers using the PBE following institutionalization were also conducted (at 4-month intervals) up until time of death. In general, wandering behaviors were associated with global cognitive decline and occurred in the moderate to late stage of the disease (defined by MMSE mean cut scores of 13 and 4, respectively). However, the data revealed a pattern of progression beginning with "....excessive but appropriate walking, attempts to leave home, and puttering (in which there seems some purpose) through to clear hyperactivity that becomes increasingly aimless and inappropriate" (Hope et al., 2001, p. 142). Retrospective reports may therefore omit early wandering behavior such as excessive but appropriate walking, as this may not be perceived as troubling by caregivers. Caregiver distress should be considered as an important component of the definition of wandering.

Visuospatial Impairment

Other investigators have contended that wandering behaviors reflect focal neurological damage involving the brain regions that are implicated in spatial functions. Henderson, Mack, and Williams (1989) postulated that wandering behaviors represent a behavioral correlate of spatial disorientation and thus reflect greater pathological changes in the right hemisphere. These authors used caregiver report on four items (wandering, getting lost indoors, getting lost on familiar streets, and being unable to recognize familiar surroundings) on a 5-point Likert scale (never occurs = 1 to occurs daily or more often = 5) to define wandering and to calculate a spatial disorientation index. The 28 ambulatory, community-dwelling individuals diagnosed with AD who were included in the study were administered a brief neuropsychological battery including measures of memory (5-item delayed recall), attention (digit span), language (object naming), visuospatial ability (clock and house drawing), and the MMSE. Nearly 40 percent of the sample exhibited at least three of the four wandering behaviors. Using stepwise multiple regression, the 5-item delayed recall and drawing tasks emerged as significant predictors of higher spatial disorientation index score. The authors hypothesized that right inferior parietal damage combined with memory impairment "may be a primary determinant of spatial disorientation in individuals with AD" (p. 394). Similar findings were reported earlier by de Leon, Potegal, and Gurland (1984).

Attentional and Executive Impairment

Spatial disorientation was not, however, found to distinguish wanderers from nonwanderers in a study using AD subjects with mild impairment (Ryan et al., 1995). In this study of 15 subjects, graphomotor perseverations on the Bender Visual Motor Gestalt Test and Clock Drawing Test differentiated wanderers from nonwanderers. These authors concluded that spatial disorientation per se may not underlie behavior but rather an inability to shift visual attention. Attentional impairments are often associated with declines in executive abilities. Reduced executive functioning may therefore play a role in wandering as well. Chiu and colleagues (2004) reported that getting lost in both familiar and unfamiliar surroundings was associated with declining directed attention abilities in early stage AD.

In another sample of patients with mild to moderate AD, Passini et al. (1995) used trained observers to document performance and decision-making processes in reaching a specified destination. Based on qualitative analyses, the AD patients, in comparison to the normal elderly controls, exhibited poor structured planning. These patients' performances were characterized by difficulty forming and retaining a plan of action, problems with inhibiting competing stimuli (as defined by impulsively getting off track), and inability to stop a search sequence following arrival at destination. The latter was conceptualized as a form of perseveration. Taken together, these findings suggest that wandering (as defined by getting lost), when present early in the course of AD, reflects executive dysfunction, suggestive of disruption in striatal-frontal circuits.

Memory and Language

Deficits in memory and language functions have also been shown to predict wandering. A longitudinal, prospective study was conducted by McShane and colleagues (1998) examining the predictive ability of neuropsychological measures for getting lost. Study participants (104 community-dwelling AD and vascular dementia subjects with a mean MMSE of 14.9, SD = 7.1) were followed every 4 months for a minimum of 5 years. At each follow-up visit, a standardized assessment of walking behaviors for the previous 4 weeks was conducted by trained raters. Although tests of delayed object recall, visual constructive ability, and immediate and delayed topographic memory (i.e., ability to recall a short route modeled by examiner) differentiated those subjects who went on to develop getting lost behaviors, immediate topographic memory was the only measure that emerged as a significant predictor of subsequent wandering behavior. The robustness of prediction was rather modest, however (positive predictive value = 44%). Topographic memory tasks tap spatial memory; as such, they are therefore also related to visuospatial abilities. Early research revealed that wanderers, in contrast to nonwanderers, demonstrated greater cognitive impairment in recent and remote memory, orientation to time and place, and ability to respond appropriately to a given conversation topic (Snyder, Rupprecht, Pyrek, Brekhus, & Moss, 1978).

CONCLUSION

Taken together, the aforementioned studies offer some *tentative* findings regarding the association of cognitive function and wandering behaviors. Wandering behaviors, particularly disruptive ones such as aimless walking or getting lost, are associated with greater levels of overall cognitive impairment and are therefore more likely to occur during the moderate to late stages of dementia syndrome (most studies in AD patients). Individuals with bilateral or greater right hemisphere involvement may be at higher risk for developing wandering behaviors. During the early stage of the disease, wandering behaviors that are perceived as troubling by caregivers may reflect impairment in executive abilities. However, the studies reviewed in this chapter do not demonstrate that specific cognitive deficits or global cognitive decline is the cause of wandering.

Methodological issues, including nebulous definitions of wandering that are often determined by invalidated measures or retrospective account, varying sample characteristics (e.g., AD versus dementia, community dwelling versus nursing home), and brief screening measures of cognitive abilities instead of comprehensive and well-validated neuropsychological measures, obfuscate these findings. Few studies to date have examined the relationship between the development of wandering-like behaviors and neuropsychological impairment in a prospective longitudinal cohort of well characterized patients (e.g., AD only).

Currently, little is known regarding possible confounding variables, such as caregiver burden in perception of wandering as a problematic behavior, or factors such as depression, medication, sensory loss, and pain, all of which are known to affect behavior and cognition in dementia patients (Marin et al., 1997). A well-defined, objective measure of wandering has been developed (Algase, Beattie, Bogue, & Yao, 2001), and its usefulness in a variety of settings and patient populations is under investigation (Beattie, Song, & LaGore, 2005; Son, Song, & Lim, 2006). Such a measure serves as an important step in clarifying our understanding of the relationship between wandering and cognition.

REFERENCES

Algase, D. L., Beattie, E. R., Bogue E. L., & Yao, L. (2001). The Algase wandering scale: Initial psychometrics of a new caregiver reporting tool. *American Journal of Alzheimer's disease and other dementias, 16*(3), 141–152.

Beattie, E. R., Song, J., & LaGore, S. (2005). A comparison of wandering in nursing homes and assisted living facilities. *Research and Theory for Nursing Practice, 19*(2), 181–196.

Bowen, J. D., Malter, A. D., Sheppard, L., Kukull, W. A., McCormick, W. C., Teri, L., et al. (1996). Predictors of mortality in patients diagnosed with probable Alzheimer's disease. *Neurology, 47*(2), 433–439.

Burns, A., Jacoby, R., & Levy, R. (1990). Behavioral abnormalities and psychiatric symptoms in Alzheimer's disease: Preliminary findings. *International Psychogeriatrics, 2*(1), 25–36.

Chiu, Y. C., Algase, D., Whall, L., Liang, J., Liu, H. C., Lin, K. N., et al. (2004). Getting lost: Directed attention and executive functions in early Alzheimer's disease patients. *Dementia and Geriatric Cognitive Disorders, 17*(3), 174–180.

Clyburn, L. D., Stones, M. J., Hadjistavropoulos, T., & Toukko, H. (2000). Predicting caregiver burden and depression in Alzheimer's disease. *Journals of Gerontology Series B: Psychological Science and Social Sciences, 55*(1), 2–13.

Cohen, C. A., Gold, D. P., Shulman, K. I., Wortley, J. T., McDonald, G., & Wargon, M. (1993). Factors determining the decision to institutionalize dementing individuals: A prospective study. *Gerontologist, 33*(6), 714–720.

Cohen-Mansfield, J. (1986). Agitated behaviors in the elderly II: Preliminary results in the cognitively deteriorated. *Journal of the American Geriatrics Society, 34*(10), 722–727.

Cooper, J. K., Mungas, D., & Weiler, P. G. (1990). Relation of cognitive status and abnormal behaviors in Alzheimer's disease. *Journal of the American Geriatrics Society, 8*(38), 867–870.

de Leon, M. J., Potegal, M., & Gurland, B. (1984). Wandering and parietal signs in senile dementia of Alzheimer's type. *Neuropsychobiology, 11*(3), 155–157.

Edgerly, E. S., & Donovick, P. J. (1998). Neuropsychological correlates of wandering in persons with Alzheimer's disease. *American Journal of Alzheimer's Disease, 13*(6), 317–329.

Eustace, A., Coen, R., Walsh, C., Cunningham, C. J., Walsh, J. B., Coakley, D., et al. (2002). A longitudinal evaluation of behavioral and psychological symptoms of probable Alzheimer's disease. *International Journal of Geriatric Psychiatry, 17*(10), 968–973.

Folstein, M. R., Folstein, S. E., & McHugh, P. R. (1975). "Mini-mental state." A practical method for grading the cognitive state of patients for the clinician. *Journal of Psychiatric Research, 12*(3), 189–198.

Henderson, V. W., Mack, W., & Williams, B. W. (1989). Spatial disorientation in Alzheimer's disease. *Archives of Neurology, 46*(4), 391–394.

Holtzer, R., Tang, M. X., Devanand, D. P., Albert, S. M., Wegesin, D. J., Marder, K., et al. (2003). Psychopathological features in Alzheimer's disease: Course and relationship with cognitive status. *Journal of the American Geriatrics Society, 7*(51), 953–960.

Hope, R. A., & Fairburn, C. G. (1990). The nature of wandering in dementia: A community-based study. *International Journal of Geriatric Psychiatry, 5*(4), 239–245.

Hope, T., Keene, J., McShane, R. H., Fairburn, C. G., Gedling, K., & Jacoby, R. (2001). Wandering in dementia: A longitudinal study. *International Psychogeriatrics, 13*(2), 137–147.

Hughes, C. P., Berg, L., Danziger, W. L., Cohen, L. A., & Martin, R. L. (1982). A new clinical scale for the staging of dementia. *British Journal of Psychiatry, 140,* 566–572.

Kiely, D. K., Morris, J. N., & Algase, D. L. (2000). Resident characteristics associated with wandering in nursing homes. *International Journal of Geriatric Psychiatry, 15*(11), 1013–1020.

Marin, D. B., Green, C. R., Schmeidler, J., Harvey, P. D., Lawlor, B. A., Ryan, T. M., et al. (1997). Noncognitive disturbances in Alzheimer's disease: Frequency, longitudinal course, and relationship to cognitive symptoms. *Journal of the American Geriatrics Society, 45*(11), 1331–1338.

McShane, R., Gedling, K., Keene, J., Fairburn, C., Jacoby, R., & Hope, T. (1998). Getting lost in dementia: A longitudinal study of behavioral symptoms. *International Psychogeriatrics, 10*(3), 253–260.

O'Donnell, B. F., Drachman, D. A., Barnes, H. J., Petersen, K. E., Swearer, J. M., & Lew, R. A. (1992). Incontinence and troublesome behaviors predict institutionalization in dementia. *Journal of Geriatric Psychiatry and Neurology, 5*(1), 45–52.

Passini, R., Rainville, C., Marchand, N., & Joanette, Y. (1995). Wayfinding in dementia of the Alzheimer's type: Planning abilities. *Journal of Clinical and Experimental Neuropsychology, 17*(6), 820–832.

Paulsen, J. S., Salmon, D. P., Thal, L. J., Romero, R., Weisstein-Jenkins, C., Galasko, D., et al. (2000). Incidence of and risk factors for hallucinations and delusions in patients with probable AD. *Neurology, 54*(10), 1965–1971.

Petersen, R. C., Smith, G. E., Waring, S. C., Ivnik, R. J., Kokmen, E., & Tangelos, E. G. (1997). Aging, memory, and mild cognitive impairment. *International Psychogeriatrics, 9*(Suppl 1), 65–69.

Ryan, J. P., McGowan, J., McCaffrey, N., Ryan, G. T., Zandi, T., & Brannigan, G. G. (1995). Graphomotor perseveration and wandering in Alzheimer's disease. *Journal of Geriatric Psychiatry and Neurology, 8*(4), 209–212.

Sloane, P. D., Mitchell, C. M., Preisser, J. S., Phillips, C., Commander, C., & Burker, E. (1998). Environmental correlates of resident agitation in Alzheimer's disease special care units. *Journal of the American Geriatrics Society, 46*(7), 862–869.

Snyder, L. H., Rupprecht, P., Pyrek, J., Brekhus, S., & Moss, T. (1978).Wandering. *The Gerontologist, 18*(3), 272–280.

Son, G. R., Song, J., & Lim, Y. (2006). Translation and validation of the Revised-Algase Wandering Scale (community version) among Korean elders with dementia. *Aging and Mental Health, 10*(2), 143–150.

Teri, L., Borson, S., Kiyak, H. A., & Yamagishi, M. (1989). Behavioral disturbance, cognitive dysfunction, and functional skill. Prevalence and relationship in Alzheimer's disease. *Journal of the American Geriatrics Society, 37*(2), 109–116.

PART II

Assessment

CHAPTER FIVE

Assessment of Wandering Behaviors

Donna L. Algase

A thorough and accurate assessment provides the strongest data to guide intelligent care of an individual who wanders. Such an assessment is best guided by an organizing protocol and carried out using standardized assessment tools. Such a protocol and assessment tools are described in this chapter. The chapter is organized according to the four purposes of the WING Assessment Protocol (WING-AP):

- to determine the *wandering* status (W) of an individual with dementia,
- to identify *influencing* factors (I),
- to screen for presence or risk of possible *negative* outcomes (N), and
- to determine *goals* for care (G).

THE WING-AP FOR INDIVIDUALS WITH DEMENTIA

Wandering can occur at all levels of cognitive impairment and in any setting where individuals with dementia reside and receive care. The WING-AP is a systematized theory-based approach to detect wandering and to set and prioritize appropriate goals for care. It was designed for application across all care settings and levels of dementia severity.

No professional standards have yet been established concerning the scope and frequency of wandering assessments. Yet, the progressive nature of dementia and changing character of wandering across disease stages (Hope et al., 2001; McShane et al., 1998) warrants that all at-risk persons be assessed. Thus, *individuals with an identified dementia who are capable of locomotion, whether independently or with assistance,* are the target group for assessment. Assessments should be conducted whenever an at-risk individual initially enters a care setting or system and at periodic intervals thereafter, as the status of their condition dictates. In the following sections of this chapter, the WING-AP is elaborated for each purpose.

W: Wandering Status

Because wandering is a risky behavior with the potential for serious consequences, the first order of importance is to determine if an individual with dementia currently wanders, or has done so in the past. This entails careful separate interviews of the family member and the individual with dementia, if able. Individual interviews can provide a fuller picture as responses are not influenced by the presence of the other party.

In conducting an assessment, it is important to note that many caregivers and individuals with dementia may not relate well to the term *wandering*. For some it carries a stigma or negative connotation; for others a very narrow meaning, namely eloping; and for others still no meaning at all in relation to dementia, that is, they have no reason to recognize that some locomotion of the individual with dementia may be aberrant and could become dangerous. Further, wandering is often a reason for relocation to a long-term care setting (Cumming, Cumming, Titus, Schmelzle, & MacDonald, 1982; Klein et al., 1999; Lam, Sewell, Bell, & Katona, 1989; McShane et al., 1998; Moak, 1990; Rockwood, Stolee, & Brahm, 1991; Sanford, 1975; Vieweg, Blair, Tucker, & Lewis, 1995). Thus, when the assessment is associated with such placement, some caregivers may fear that a positive history of wandering will render the affected individual ineligible for admission, and an individual with dementia may sense that a difficult behavior could precipitate loss of one's own home. Therefore, choosing terms other than wandering or using descriptions of wandering rather than terms is helpful for obtaining complete and accurate information.

An initial assessment of wandering status not only serves the purpose of determining current and prior wandering status, but also provides a baseline for comparison to future assessments, enabling identification and trajectory of behavior change over time, which can be used for timing anticipatory guidance to caregivers.

Assessing Wandering Status

Overall, an assessment of *wandering status* should include information about the amount of walking one does; the times, places, and reasons one walks; and whether or not walking has assumed any unusual patterns, problematic characteristics, or deviations from prior walking habits of the individual with dementia. In addition, it is important to determine if the individual drives a car or uses public transportation independently, is in the habit of going out alone, has ever become lost, or acknowledges any degree of spatial disorientation. Assessing current behavior is a good place to start and can be used as a point of reference for simultaneous assessment of prior behavior by comparison. Inclusion of (1) a quantifiable or objective measure of current wandering status, (2) three consecutive days of monitored activity level, and (3) a standardized performance test of spatial ability are recommended. These three elements capture the full spectrum of wandering as defined in this book.

The structure of the WING-AP for assessing wandering status is shown in Table 5.1. Areas to be assessed are listed in the first column, and corresponding interview questions and approaches to objective measurement (as available) are listed in subsequent columns of the same row. Interview questions are phrased for caregivers, but can also be adapted for use with the individual with dementia, as degree of cognitive impairment and ability to communicate may permit. Open-ended and structured questions are offered to illustrate possible ways to elicit information, but other similar ones developed by an interviewer for a particular care setting or purpose may serve equally well.

Several objective approaches to assessing wandering status appear in Table 5.1. The Revised Algase Wandering Scale (RAWS), both long-term care (-LTC) and community versions (-CV), were discussed in Chapter 1 and are contained in Appendix B, along with information on administering, scoring, and interpreting the scale. Scores may be graphed, as shown in Figures 5.1 (for the RAWS-LTC) and 5.2 (for the RAWS-CV) to reveal where scores are consistent with those of nonwanderers, sporadic wanderers, wanderers, or problematic wanderers, based on psychometric evaluations of the scales (Algase, Beattie, Bogue, & Yao, 2001; Algase, Beattie et al., 2004; Algase, Son et al., 2004). Blank graphs for each version of the RAWS are contained in Appendix B.

In Figures 5.1 and 5.2, the arrows indicate the range within which about two-thirds of individuals in each category will score: nonwanderer (black arrow), occasional wanderer (blue), wanderer (green), and problematic wanderer (red). Similarly, the colored bars indicate the average score for individuals in each category. Because scores for each category can overlap, a particular score for an individual will sometimes fall within

TABLE 5.1 Assessment Approaches for Wandering Status Using the WING-AP

Locomotion	Suggested Interview Questions	Objective Measures
Amount of walking	How much does *name of individual with dementia* walk daily? Do you think *name* walks: ___only enough to do what must be done ___a little more than that ___an average amount for age and health status ___more than average ___excessively	Revised Algase wandering scale (RAWS)-LTC and -CV, persistent walking subscale Digital pedometer with activity log Observation log
Time of walking	What time of the day does *name* walk the most? ...the least? When does *name* walk most (repeat for least): ___in the morning ___in the early afternoon ___in the late afternoon ___in the evening ___during the night	Individual questions within RAWS-LTC and -CV persistent walking subscale Digital pedometer with activity log Observation log
Walking qualities	Tell me about anything unusual that you may have noticed about *name's* walking? Have you noticed any of the following about *name's* walking: ___follows you or other caregiver around ___appears to get off-track on his/her way to a place ___walks the same route over and over again	AWS-CV, repetitive walking subscale

	___paces back and forth ___walks only certain routes, never deviates ___has changed his/her walking habits or behaviors	
Driving status	Tell me about when *name* drives a car? Does *name* drive a car? ___alone ___only if accompanied ___no longer drives ___never drove	n/a
Public conveyances	Tell me about when *name* might use a taxi, bus, train, or other public transportation? Does *name* use public transportation? ___alone ___only if accompanied ___no longer uses public transportation ___never uses public transportation	n/a
Reasons for walking or driving or using a public conveyance	For what reasons does *name* go walking outside, drive alone, or use public transportation alone? Does *name* go walking or driving alone: ___for entertainment or exercise ___to run errands ___to keep appointments ___to work or volunteer ___to visit family or friends ___other____________ ___no longer walks or drives alone	

(Continued)

TABLE 5.1 Assessment Approaches for Wandering Status Using the WING-AP (Continued)

Locomotion	Suggested Interview Questions	Objective Measures
Common destinations	What places might *name* walk or drive to? ___grocery, other store, or business ___church ___home of family or friend (who?) ___just around the neighborhood ___a distant place, ____________	n/a
Becoming lost	Tell me about a recent time *name* got lost when out alone.	RAWS-LTC and -CV, eloping subscale
	How many times has *name* gotten lost when out walking or driving? ___hasn't gotten lost ___only once ___only a few times ___repeatedly	
Spatial disorientation	Tell me about any signs you've noticed that *name* is having trouble recognizing where s/he is.	RAWS-LTC and -CV, spatial disorientation subscale
	Have you noticed that *name* has trouble: ___finding his/her way to/from a well known place ___finding his/her way around the neighborhood ___finding his/her way around the house	Demonstration of ability to locate specific destinations in a familiar environment

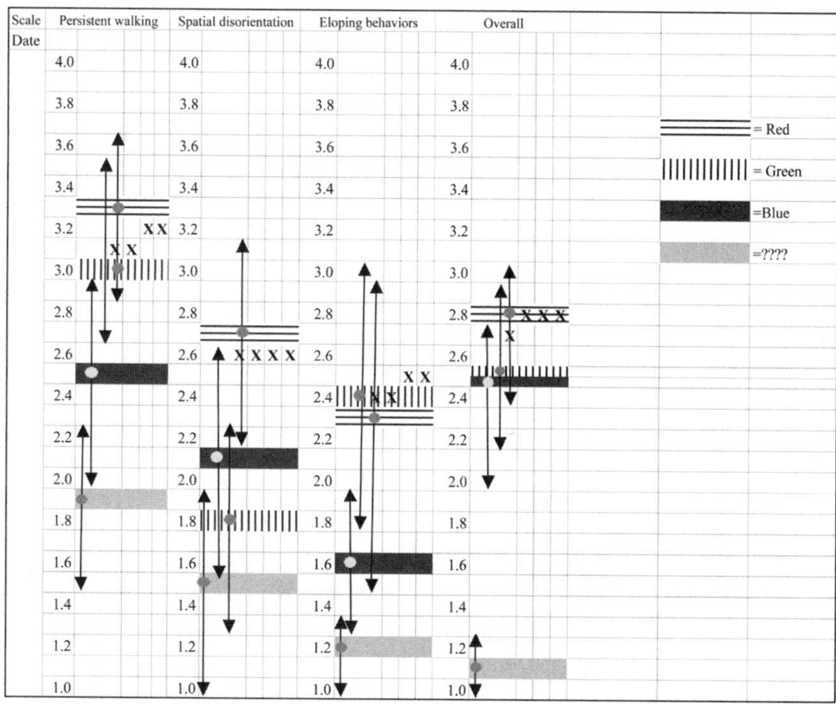

FIGURE 5.1 AWS-LTC scores graphed over four assessments.

the range of more than one category. To interpret such a score, determine which colored bar it is closest to and consider that the most likely, but not definite, category to which they belong. Categories are provided as a guide to interpretation and are not definitive.

While several types of activity monitors have been used to assess the amount of wandering (Algase, Beattie, Lietsch, & Beel-Bates, 2003; Cohen-Mansfield, Werner, Culpepper, Wolfson, & Bickel, 1997; Madson, 1990), none are commonly used outside research settings. Alternatively, if the individual with dementia has no gait disturbance and will wear a pedometer, inexpensive digital pedometers are widely available and can provide similar data. If using a pedometer, care must be taken to assure that it is properly set and is registering steps accurately, as older people may have a shuffling gait or make insufficient impact when walking to register their steps on the instrument. It is best if the person can wear the pedometer around the clock for 72 hours but if the pedometer is bothersome to the person, leaving it off during sleep is permissible. Readings are taken at predetermined intervals and written on a log. The pedometer should be set to zero at the beginning of each day and reset to zero each

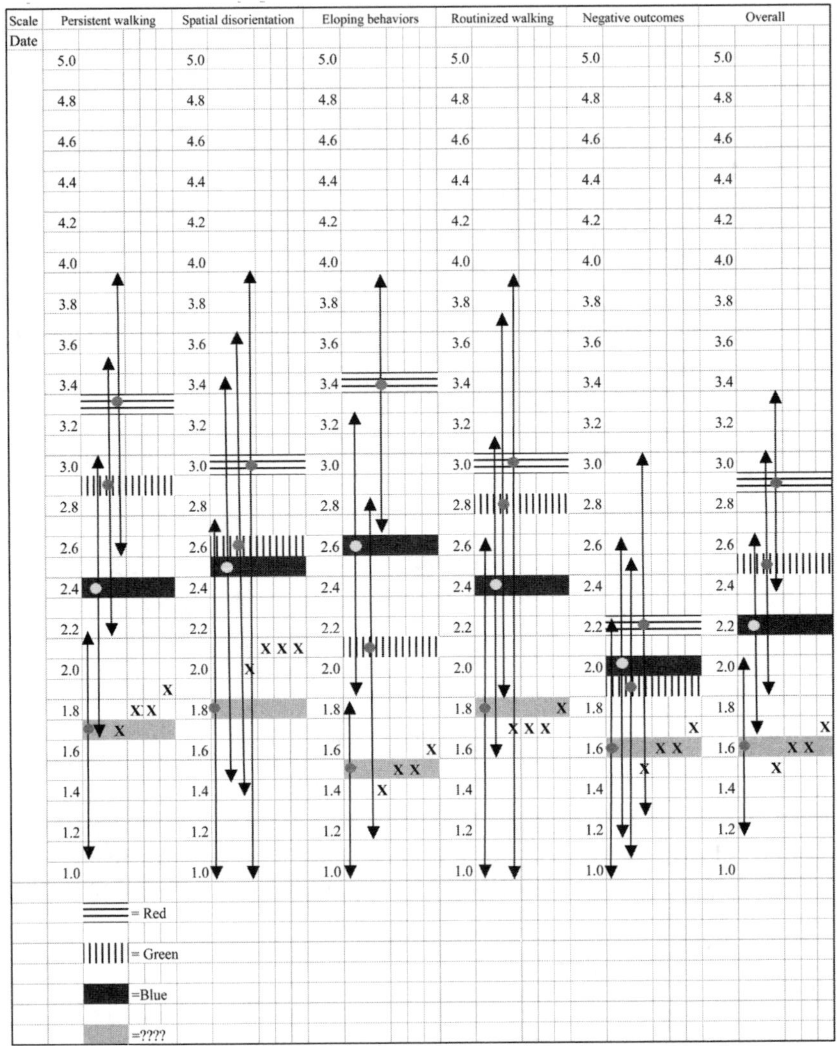

FIGURE 5.2 AWS-CV scores graphed over four assessments.

time it is read to limit loss of data. In residential care settings, readings can be taken as often as hourly, but every three hours may provide an adequate picture. To assist caregivers in the home, the log can be designed for longer intervals. Suggested intervals after the start of each day are at noon (or lunch time), at 6:00 P.M. (or dinner time), at bedtime, and upon arising, if the pedometer is worn overnight. Table 5.2 shows sample logs. For a visual view of the information, readings can be graphed.

TABLE 5.2 Examples of One-Day Pedometer Logs

Pedometer Log—Residential Care Setting				Pedometer Log—Home Setting		
q hr.	Reading	q 3-hr.	Reading	Suggested times	Clock time	Reading
Date:	3/27/06		3/27/06	Date: 3/27/06		
0600	000	0600	000	Upon arising	7 A.M.	000
0700	115	0900	716	At lunch time	11:30 A.M.	652
0800	67	1200	856	At dinner time	5:00 P.M.	820
0900	534	1500	324	Bedtime	10:00 P.M.	414
etc.	...	etc.	...	Upon arising	7:15 A.M.	56
24-hrs. total	...		...			1942

If a pedometer is unfeasible or not available, direct observation can be substituted. However, it is a more tedious and time-consuming approach for the nursing staff or caregiver. If nursing staff are making the observations, it is suggested that one person be assigned to watch the individual for a consistent amount of time (no less than 10 minutes) out of each hour during their shift, with staff being assigned around the clock for three days. Rather than recording the actual number of times the person walked or the actual duration of their walking, a rating system may give an accurate enough picture for clinical purposes. An example is shown as Table 5.3. If a caregiver is making the observations, the information may be more useful and the approach more reliable if a simplified version of the rating system is provided for them to use, collapsing the hourly times into larger blocks of time, such as early morning (awakening until breakfast), morning (breakfast to lunch time), early afternoon (lunch time to dinner time), late afternoon (dinner time until 7:00 P.M.), evening (7:00 P.M. until bedtime), and during the night. See Table 5.4 for a suggested format. Observers should be made aware that frequency represents the number of individual instances of walking, and duration represents the proportion of time spent walking. It is possible to have only one or a few instances of long duration, as well as several instances constituting only a limited duration. It is not necessary for observers to try to differentiate walking and wandering, as other aspects of the assessment will aid in making an overall judgment about wandering status. Three days of observation will enable evaluation of any stable temporal pattern for walking.

Other characteristics of an individual's walking can also be noted during observations. Behaviors such as following others around (shadowing), walking back and forth (pacing), or walking with no apparent destination of for no clear reason are examples. If observed, notes should be made of these characteristics.

Finally, an assessment for spatial disorientation is important to include. Some items on the RAWS address spatial disorientation, but a performance measure can provide insight into the types of wayfinding errors that an individual makes in pursuing specific locations. In the home, a person can be asked to show the way to the kitchen, bathroom, or other location that is not directly observable from the place of the interview (Liu, Gauthier, & Gauthier, 1991). In a residential setting, some time is needed for a newly admitted person to acclimate to the surroundings before a performance test is done; one month is the suggested interval. Staff can also make note of the type of difficulties a new resident is having in learning their surroundings.

I: Influencing Factors

In the WING-AP, *influencing factors* are those that go toward determining if and when wandering behavior will be expressed. Information about these factors is useful (1) for forecasting who will wander, (2) for identifying conditions under which they are likely to do so, and (3) in

TABLE 5.3 Example of a One-Day Observation Log in a Residential Care Setting

Observation Log: Residential care setting		
Time	Frequency	Duration
	A = 0 B = 1x C = several times D = many time	A = 0 B = < ¼ of time C = ¼ < ½ of time D = > ½ of time E = continuous
0600–0700	C	C
0700–0800	B	B
0800–0900	C	D
and so on		

TABLE 5.4 Example of a One-Day Observation Log in a Home Setting

Observation Log: Home setting			
Time		Frequency	Duration
Suggested	Clock time of reading	A = 0 B = 1x C = several times D = many times	A = 0 B = minimal time B = < ¼ of time C = ¼ < ½ of time D = > ½ of time E = continuous
Awake	6:30 am	–	–
Awake to breakfast	8:30 am	B	B
Breakfast to lunch	12:00	D	D
Lunch to dinner	5:00 pm	C	B
Dinner to 7:00 p.m.	7:30 pm		
7:00 pm to bedtime	10:30 pm		
Bedtime to awakening	6:30 am		

identifying possible targets for intervention, if necessary. There are three categories of influencing factors: risk factors, precipitating factors, and reinforcing factors. While choice of these factors is theory-based and the guiding theories are synthesized from available research findings, not all factors have been adequately evaluated as predictors of actual types and degrees of wandering.

Risk factors are those characteristics of individuals with dementia that indicate which individuals have an increased likelihood of being or becoming a wanderer. Ideally, choice of these factors would be based on a validated theory or an empirically determined set of predictors. As earlier chapters in this book have shown, a number of possible predictors have been identified and some carry the weight of empirical evidence. However, studies are few, samples are generally nonrandom and small, and results are sometimes conflicting. At this state of the science on wandering, erring on the side of caution, within the limits of available resources, is the recommended approach. In other words, the safest approach is to collect information about all putative risk factors, if affordable.

According to the model of risky wandering and adverse outcomes (RWAO) discussed in Chapter 2, risk factors can be thought of as enduring or dynamic (Algase, 2004). Enduring risk factors are generally immutable characteristics that predispose a person to wander because they shape long-standing or habitual behavior in general. While not usually subject to change, information about enduring risk factors can give a good picture of behavior considered normal or usual for a given individual. These factors include personality (Song, 2003; Thomas, 1997), dominant behavior pattern under stressful conditions (Monsour & Robb, 1982), and gender. On the other hand, dynamic risk factors are potentially amenable to change or intervention and are of two types: enabling and neurocognitive. Enabling risk factors are those that support (or detract from) locomotor ability, and thus, wandering; these include mobility and health status (Cohen-Mansfield, Werner, & Marx, 1991), functional ability and pain (Kovach, Weisman, Chaudbury, & Calkins, 1997), vision (Beel-Bates, 2001; Duffy, 1999), and medications (Holtzer et al., 2003). Neurocognitive risk factors are domains of thinking and behavior directly involved in a specific dementing process: these are identified by dementia diagnosis, including results of medical tests and examinations that pinpoint areas of brain involvement (specifically the hippocampus and parietal lobes, especially the right lobe) (deLeon, Potegal, & Gurland, 1984; Hyman, Van Hoesen, Damasion, & Barnes, 1984; Meguro et al., 1996; Squire, 1992) and results of neurological and neuropsychological testing for attention (Chiu et al., 2004), perseveration (Ryan et al., 1995), memory and visuo-construction skills (Henderson, Mack, & Williams, 1989), language skills (Algase, 1992a; Dawson & Reid, 1987), and wayfinding effectiveness (Algase, Son et al., 2004).

Precipitating factors are those circumstances or events that are associated with the onset of specific wandering episodes. These may be environmental conditions, either physical or social, or internal conditions, such as physiological needs or psychological states (e.g., feelings and moods) of the individual with dementia, as posited in the NDB model (Algase et al., 1996).

Reinforcing factors are those conditions, usually environmental, associated with cessation of specific wandering episodes or with elongation of elapsed time until the next wandering episode (Algase, 1992b). A reinforcing factor may be the converse of a precipitating factor, such as when food intake satisfies the physiological need of hunger, but reinforcing factors are not always so. For example, during an episode of wandering, an individual with dementia may come upon a pleasing view or friendly person that attracts their attention and interrupts their wandering; subsequent wandering episodes may occur in an effort to re-elicit this pleasant experience.

Assessing Influencing Factors

Risk Factors. Many alternatives exist for assessing enduring and dynamic risk factors, including structured interviews, clinical assessment strategies, and objective measures. Although much assessment of enduring and dynamic risk factors can be accomplished through a structured interview, objective measures provide an easier means for comparing change over time and, if standardized, for pegging results to a reference group. Some suggested approaches are shown in Table 5.5. Some objective measures are only available commercially and are so indicated in the table. Some alternatives are available on the Web; these are also indicated in the table.

Because enduring risk factors are not expected to change significantly over time, the WING-AP directs that information about them be collected only once. However, information about dynamic risk factors requires periodic updating. In general, the factors that change in association with advancing dementia (e.g., functional ability, neurocognitive factors) should be reassessed approximately every six months, as most dementias progress slowly. Dynamic risk factors that are not associated with dementia per se (e.g., pain, general health status) could change suddenly and should be reassessed for their impact on wandering whenever a change in their status is noted or suspected.

Precipitating and Reinforcing Factors. As dementia advances, affected individuals become less and less able to perceive, identify, and communicate their needs and preferences. Knowledge of precipitating and reinforcing factors can give insight into possible reasons for wandering that are likely amenable to intervention when accurately identified. However, precipitating and reinforcing factors are not always apparent to family members, who are often untrained in or unaccustomed to purposeful observation of behavior patterns. Consequently, interview questions should be carefully crafted to elicit relevant information concerning these factors. While an interview may not initially yield information about all relevant precipitating and reinforcing risk factors, it can serve to heighten family members' awareness of possible factors and, in subsequent interviews, more detailed information often is obtained. In residential settings, such as nursing homes or assisted living facilities, information about precipitating factors can be obtained through careful, systematic observation of the individual with dementia by professional and direct care staff. Assessment of precipitating and reinforcing factors should be ongoing as these can change in response to advancing dementia and to changes in the environment or as new information from family may be obtained.

TABLE 5.5 Assessment Approaches for Influencing Factors Using the WING-AP

Influencing Factors	Suggested Interview Questions	Objective Measures
Risk Factors		
Enduring (assess once)		
Personality	How would you describe *name's* lifelong personality? During *name's* adult years, would you say s/he is an extrovert? __Y __N ....is open to new ideas? __Y __N ......is overly anxious? __Y __N ....is attentive to detail? __Y __N ......is agreeable? __Y __N	NEO Five Factor Inventory (Costa & McRae, 1992) Online personality test: http://www.humanmetrics.com/cgi-win/JTypes1.htm
Enabling (assess q 6 six mo. if dementia-related; assess as needed if not dementia-related)		
Mobility[1]	See functional ability	See functional ability
Health status[2]	Please describe *name's* general state of health. Would you say *name's* is generally: ____excellent ____good ____fair ____poor	Review medical record for problems affecting mobility, stamina, nutritional status, pain.
Functional ability[1]	Please describe *name's* ability to take care of his/herself. OR What help would/does *name* need to stay in their own home?	Any common screening instrument for ADL and IADL, such as the Katz (Katz, Ford, Moskowitz & Jaffe, 1963) or Lawton & Brody (1969).

	Does *name* need help to do any of the following: _____manage check book _____manage own medications _____shop _____use the phone _____cook _____do laundry	For specific information on the types of assistance needed, observation of performance is suggested.
	Does *name* need help to do any of the following: _____dressing _____bathing and hygiene _____toileting _____feeding _____walking	
Pain[2]	What painful conditions does *name* have that you are aware of? Does *name* regularly use any prescribed or over the counter drugs for pain? If so, what are they?	Assessing Pain in Dementia (Horgas, 2003) available at: http://www.hardfordgn.org/publications/trythis/assessingpain.pdf#=search=92662pain%20asssessment%dementia%20
Vision[1]	Has *name* had a visual examination since developing dementia? If so, where are results available?	Recommend professional assessment of acuity, peripheral vision, and contrast sensitivity. Observation for apparent difficulty
Medications[2]	Has name ever been prescribed any medications to manage symptoms or behaviors associated with dementia? If so, what are/were they?	Review medical record for neuroleptics, sedatives/hypnotics, anti-depressants, digoxin (Also, see Chapter 12)

(Continued)

TABLE 5.5 Assessment Approaches for Influencing Factors Using the WING-AP (Continued)

Influencing Factors	Suggested Interview Questions	Objective Measures
Neurocognitive (assess q 6 six mo.)		
Type and Stage of Dementia	Has *name* received a medical evaluation for dementia from a geriatrician or neurologist? If so, where are medical records available? What type of dementia does *name* have? When was the diagnosis made?	Mini-mental status exam (Folstein, Folstein & McHugh, 1975) Clinical Dementia Rating Scale (Hughes, Berg, Danziger, Cohen, & Martin, 1982)
Neuropsychological function	Has *name* received a neuropsychcologlcal evaluation for dementia? If so, where are medical records available?	Review records for results of tests addressing memory, attention, executive functioning, and language skills.
Predisposing Factors		
Physical environment	Can you tell me about any conditions in the environment that seem to affect *name's* walking patterns? Have you noticed any changes in *name's* walking patterns when the following conditions are present: ____high temperature and humidity ____darkness ____noise ____crowding ____high activity level ____when conditions are restful/comfortable ____when conditions are engaging	Direct observation is the current approach to gaining information about walking and the physical environment. Observations in various locations and under various conditions give the best picture of effects on walking. The individual can also be asked to validate an observation.

Social environment	Can you tell me about any conditions in social conditions that seem to affect *name's* walking patterns? Have you noticed any changes in *name's* walking patterns when the following conditions are present: ____when a directive is given ____when people are brusk ____when people are condescending ____when people are in a hurry	Direct observation is the current approach to gaining information about walking and social interactions. Observations with various individuals and categories of individuals (e.g., nurses, housekeeping; familiar vs. unfamiliar) and under various various conditions (casual, bathing, eating, structured activity, incidental) give the best picture of effects on walking. The individual can also be asked to validate an observation.
Physiological needs	Have you noticed any changes in *name's* walking behavior that signals a particular want or need? Does name's walking behavior change when: _____it's time to go to the bathroom _____it's time to eat _____s/he's tired _____s/he is in pain	The individual can also be asked to validate an observation. Direct observation is the current approach to gaining information about walking physical needs. Observations in various situations and at various times gives the best picture of effects on walking. The individual can also be asked to validate an observation.
Psychological needs	Have you noticed any changes *in name's* walking behavior that signals a particular emotional or psychological issue?	Direct observation is the current approach to gaining information about walking emotional or psychological needs. Observations in various situations give the best picture of effects on walking.

(Continued)

TABLE 5.5 Assessment Approaches for Influencing Factors Using the WING-AP (Continued)

Influencing Factors	Suggested Interview Questions	Objective Measures
	Does *name's* walking behavior change when s/he is: _____bored _____overwhelmed/over stimulated _____anxious _____angry _____sad _____happy _____contented	The individual can also be asked to validate an observation.
Precipitating and Reinforcing Factors		
Precipitating	Have you noticed any thing that seems to increase, decrease or change *name*'s walking behavior?	Observations about the physical and social environment may provide insight into precipitating factors.
Reinforcing factors	Have you noticed any thing that seems to satisfy *name*'s need to walk?	Observations about the physical and social environment may provide insight into reinforcing factors.

[1] Risk factors associated with dementia

[2] Risk factors not associated with dementia per se

N: Negative Outcomes

Consistent with the RWAO model (Algase, 2004), two categories of negative outcomes for the individual with dementia are included in the WING-AP: immediate and cumulative. *Immediate outcomes* are the negative consequences for the individual with dementia that can occur in the short run, at times even associated with a single wandering episode. Such outcomes include fatigue, inadequate food intake (Rheaume, Riley & Volicer, 1987), falls and injuries (Buchner & Larson, 1987; Keily, Kiel, Burrows, & Lipsitz, 1998), exit attempts, unescorted exits, and getting lost outside the home (Rowe & Glover, 2001; Soverini & Borghesi, 1968). *Cumulative outcomes* are the negative consequences for the individual with dementia that build up over time, some mounting from inattention to immediate outcomes. Cumulative outcomes include nutritional status (Rheaume et al., 1987) and relocation within the community or to a residential care facility (Cancro, 1968).

It bears mentioning that not all outcomes of wandering are negative. Because walking is a form of exercise, wandering—a form of walking—may bring about some of the benefits associated with exercise; however, these benefits may be offset by accompanying declines in social and language skills (Snyder, Rupprecht, Pyrek, Breckhus, & Moss, 1978). Neither should it be assumed that if wandering presents no obvious negative consequences, there is no reason for concern. If wandering (or some wandering) represents an unmet need, it signals for attention to the need. It is also important to recognize that spatial disorientation is an unsettling experience and may induce fear or anxiety in wanderers who are uncertain of their location or the pathway to a desired destination. In the converse, efforts to avoid fear or anxiety associated with spatial disorientation may limit the amount of walking that a person with dementia does. Finally, some consequences of wandering are cumulative, and inattention to wandering in the short run may lead to such consequences.

Assessing for Negative Outcomes

As shown in Table 5.6, structured interviews and some assessment tools can generate information about both immediate and cumulative outcomes. However, especially in residential care settings, careful observation often yields the clearest picture about immediate outcomes such as fatigue, food intake, and exiting behaviors. For wanderers, negative outcomes need ongoing monitoring, especially those that may lead to cumulative outcomes.

TABLE 5.6 Assessment Approaches for Negative Outcomes Using the WING-AP

Outcomes	Suggested Interview Questions	Objective Measures
Immediate Outcomes		
Fatigue	How do you think *name's* walking affects his/her level of fatigue? Do you think *name's* walking affects _____fatigue level _____sleep patterns	SF36, vitality scale Ware & Sherbourne (1992)
Inadequate food intake	Tell me about the way *names's* walking affects his/her eating patterns. Has *name's* walking ever: _____interfered with ability to stay at the table _____interfered with completing a meal _____increased his/her appetite?	Rating each meal for % of food consumed over a one-week period
Falls and injuries	Can you describe any falls or injuries that have resulted from *name's* walking? Has *name's* walking resulted in: _____falls _____injuries	Direct observation Count times individual trips alert system over a one week period.
Exit attempts	Can you describe efforts name has made to leave a location or home despite your effort to keep him/her there? Has *name* tried to leave home alone against your wishes?	Direct observation Count times individual trips alert system over a one week period.

Unescorted exits	Can you tell me about any times that *name* walked away?	Direct observation Review incident report for any elopements
	Can you tell me about any times that *name* got separated from you (or others) when out together?	Specific items on the RAWS
Getting lost outside of home	Can you tell me about any times that *name* got lost?	Specific items on the RAWS-CV
	Has *name* ever gotten lost since developing dementia?	
Cumulative Outcomes		
Nutritional status	Do you think *name's* weight has changed since developing dementia? ...in relation to his/her walking?	Mini Nutritional Assessment (Vellas, Garry & Guigoz, 1999)
	Has *name* lost weight since developing dementia?	Weight trend BMI trend
	Do you think his/her walking is affecting his/her weight?	
Relocation	Are you considering a relocation for *name?* Or What is the reason for *name's* relocation to ___?	n/a
	Is *name's* walking a reason for relocation?	

G: Goals for Care

To determine goals for care, analyzing information obtained through assessment to determine wandering status is the next step. A summary of such status, along with information about influencing factors and negative outcomes, guides selection and prioritization of goals for care.

Determining Wandering Status

The individual's wandering status can be stated as currently present, historically positive (and continuing or not), or currently negative. If wandering is present, the data should be summarized to describe and document wandering in terms of its frequency, repetitiveness, temporal distribution, and spatial character. Converting pedometer readings and observational logs to graphs is helpful for this purpose. If data are conclusive, the level of wandering (occasional, nonproblematic, or problematic) can be assigned and is helpful for establishing goals and priorities. Wandering status can be summarized using a format as shown in Table 5.7.

If wandering is not present, information about enduring and dynamic characteristics may suggest whether or not wandering behavior is likely to develop. A positive history of wandering or eloping behaviors is the strongest indicator, especially in combination with (1) enabling factors that support independent locomotion, (2) absence of those that detract from such locomotion, and (3) an advancing level of cognitive impairment. Individuals matching these characteristics should be considered at the greatest risk for developing wandering behavior in the future and warrant careful monitoring for signs of its onset.

Selecting and Prioritizing Goals for Care

Six goals for the care of persons who wander have been suggested (Algase, 1998). These include:

- assuring safety
- aiding navigation
- minimizing restrictions
- using preserved skills
- supporting abilities
- affording comfort

The first three goals are related most directly to wandering; the remaining goals may apply as well to individuals with dementia who

TABLE 5.7 Summary of Wandering Status

Initial assessment date:	Re-assessment date:	Re-assessment date:
Wandering Status		
_____Present, no prior hx	_____Present, no prior hx	_____Present, no prior hx
_____Positive hx	_____Positive hx	_____Positive hx
____continuing	____continuing	____continuing
____not continuing	____not continuing	____not continuing
____recurring	____recurring	____recurring
_____Negative	_____Negative	_____Negative
Probable Wandering Level		
_____Problematic	_____Problematic	_____Problematic
_____Nonproblematic	_____Nonproblematic	_____Nonproblematic
_____Occasional	_____Occasional	_____Occasional
_____Nonwanderer	_____Nonwanderer	_____Nonwanderer
Wandering Characteristics		
Frequency		
_____high	_____high	_____high
_____medium	_____medium	_____medium
_____low	_____low	_____low
_____seldom	_____seldom	_____seldom
Duration		
_____>50%	_____>50%	_____>50%
_____25% < 50%	_____25% < 50%	_____25% < 50%
_____< 25%	_____< 25%	_____< 25%
_____m inimal	_____minimal	_____minimal
Temporal pattern (check all that apply)		
_____early morning	_____early morning	_____early morning
_____morning	_____morning	_____morning
_____early afternoon	_____early afternoon	_____early afternoon
_____late afternoon	_____late afternoon	_____late afternoon
_____evening	_____evening	_____evening
_____nighttime	_____nighttime	_____nighttime
Spatial disorientation		
_____none	_____none	_____none
_____none in familiar place	_____none in familiar place	_____none in familiar place
_____mild	_____mild	_____mild
_____moderate	_____moderate	_____moderate
_____severe	_____severe	_____severe

(Continued)

TABLE 5.7 Summary of Wandering Status (Continued)

Initial assessment date:	Re-assessment date:	Re-assessment date:
Eloping Behaviors		
_____lurks at doorways _____enters off-limit areas _____follows others out _____tries locks and handles _____positive hx eloping	_____lurks at doorways _____enters off-limit areas _____follows others out _____tries locks and handles _____positive hx eloping	_____lurks at doorways _____enters off-limit areas _____follows others out _____tries locks and handles _____positive hx eloping
Other features		
_____repetitive _____paces _____laps _____random _____shadows _____disrupts meals	_____repetitive _____paces _____laps _____random _____shadows _____disrupts meals	_____repetitive _____paces _____laps _____random _____shadows _____disrupts meals
Risk Level for Future Wandering (check all that apply)		
_____positive wandering hx _____independently mobile _____mod. cog. impair-men _____severe cognitive imp. Risk level: _____high _____medium _____low	_____positive wandering hx _____independently mobile _____mod. cog. impairment _____severe cognitive imp. Risk level: _____high _____medium _____low	_____positive wandering hx _____independently mobile _____mod. cog. impairment _____severe cognitive imp. Risk level: _____high _____medium _____low

do not wander. However, these latter three goals are included in the description here because they may point to a need for interventions that are specific for wanderers.

The goal of *assuring safety* is aimed to prevent negative outcomes of wandering. It calls for interventions that prevent foreseeable problems related to eloping, such as fall risks, weight loss, and poor nutritional status. This is an especially important goal when wanderers display high frequency and duration of wandering, spatial disorientation, eloping behaviors, and visual or mobility problems.

The goal of *aiding navigation* has the outcome of improved functioning. This goal calls for interventions that enhance spatial orientation and wayfinding, reduce distractions and overstimulation to conserve limited cognitive capacity while wayfinding, and increase visibility for destinations or locations used to support functioning and self-sufficiency, such as toilets. Many useful suggestions and supporting evidence for such interventions are included in Chapter 16 on environmental design. This goal is important for wanderers who are spatially disoriented and have poor attention, executive functioning, and vision.

The goal of *minimizing restrictions* addresses quality of life as it is concerned with freedom of movement, lack of unnecessary sedation, and the exercise of choices and preferences insofar as possible. This goal calls for interventions that use the least restrictive, yet effective, alternative in addressing problems arising from wandering and that preserve the dignity, personhood, and individuality of the wanderer. While this goal is relevant to all wanderers, and to nonwanderers as well, it is especially important for those with problematic wandering as they are the ones for whom restrictions are most likely to be imposed.

The goals of *using preserved skills* and *supporting abilities* prevent excess disability and have the outcome of improved or sustained functioning. Preserving skills calls for interventions that build on the individual's strengths. If walking has been a means for releasing stress, then efforts to reduce a high degree of wandering may be counterproductive. Identification and mitigation of the stressor are desirable, but not always possible. Further, interventions that prevent or forestall negative outcomes, such as assuring adequate intake of food and fluids, would also be indicated. The goal of preserving skills is relevant to all wanderers, and nonwanderers as well, but is particularly important for wanderers who, prior to the onset of dementia, purposefully used walking as a means of self-help or health promotion. Supporting abilities calls for interventions that enable the person with dementia to do as much for themselves as possible. If the basis of one's wandering is to explore, and thereby to gain (or sustain) familiarity with and comfort in their surroundings, then limiting wandering, especially through restraint, prevents some possible benefits of wandering and contributes to iatrogenesis.

The goal of *affording comfort* has the outcome of an improved quality of life. Interventions that enhance communication of needs, whether physical or psychological, and take action to meet them fulfill this goal. This goal can benefit all persons with dementia, however, it is especially important for wanderers who are unable to communicate their needs and for whom wandering is a means to attract attention and assistance.

CONCLUSION

In this chapter, the WING-AP was described and operationalized through identification of pertinent assessment tools and approaches. Based on theory and supported with available empirical evidence, the WING-AP affords a comprehensive and systematic approach to assess individuals with dementia as to wandering, its influencing factors, and its negative outcomes. Further, the WING-AP supports selection and prioritization of goals pertinent to the individual's wandering status, as a basis for planning appropriate and effective care. The WING-AP is adaptable for use in home and residential care settings under the direction of professional nurses to benefit individuals who wander and their families.

REFERENCES

Algase, D. L. (1992a). Cognitive discriminants of wandering among nursing home residents. *Nursing Research, 41*(2), 78–81.

Algase, D. L. (1992b). A century of progress: Today's strategies for managing wandering behavior. *Journal of Gerontological Nursing, 18*(11), 28–34.

Algase, D. L. (1998). Wandering. In B. Edelstein (Ed.), *Comprehensive Clinical Psychology: Volume 7, Geropsychiatry* (pp. 371–412). London: Pergamon.

Algase, D. L. (2004). *Wandering, Adverse Outcomes, and Caregiver Strategies,* Grant application, 1 RO1 NR009244, National Institutes of Nursing Research.

Algase, D. L., Beattie, E.R.A., Bogue, E., & Yao, L. (2001). The Algase Wandering Scale: Initial psychometrics of a new caregiver reporting tool. *American Journal of Alzheimer's Disease and Other Dementias, 16*(3), 141–152.

Algase, D. L., Beattie, E.R.A., Lietsch, S. A., & Beel-Bates, C. A. (2003). Biomechanical activity devices to index wandering behavior. *American Journal of Alzheimer's Disease and Other Dementias, 18*(2), 85–92.

Algase, D. L., Beattie, E.R.A., Song, J., Milke, D., Duffield, C., & Cowan, B. (2004). Validation of the Algase wandering scale (version 2) in a cross cultural sample. *Aging & Mental Health, 8*(2), 133–142.

Algase, D. L., Beck, C., Kolanowski, A., Whall, A., Berent, S., Richards, K., & Beattie, E. (1996). Need-driven dementia-compromised behavior: An alternative view of disruptive behavior. *American Journal of Alzheimer's Disease, 11*(6), 10–19.

Algase, D. L., Son, G. R., Beattie, E., Song, J., Leitsch, S., & Yao, L. (2004). The interrelatedness of wandering and wayfinding in a community sample of persons with dementia. *Dementia and Geriatric Cognitive Disorders, 17*(3), 231–239.

Beel-Bates, C. A. (2001). *Visuospatial function in ambulatory aged women with probable Alzheimer's disease: A multiple case study.* Unpublished doctoral dissertation, University of Michigan.

Buchner, D. M., & Larson, E. B. (1987). Falls and fractures in patients with Alzheimer-type dementia. *Journal of the American Medical Association, 257,* 1492–1495.

Cancro, R. (1968). Elopements from the C. F. Menninger Memorial Hospital. *Bulletin Menninger Clinic, 32,* 228–238.

Chiu, Y., Algase, D. L., Cimprich, B., Liang, J., Whall, A., Liu, H. C., et al. (2004). Getting lost: Directed attention and executive function in early Alzheimer's disease patients. *Dementia and Geriatric Cognitive Disorders, 17*(3), 174–180.

Cohen-Mansfield, J., Werner, P., Culpepper, W. J., Wolfson, M., & Bickel, E. (1997). Assessment of ambulatory behavior in nursing home residents who pace or wander: A comparison of four commercially available devices. *Dementia & Geriatric Cognitive Disorders, 8,* 359–365.

Cohen-Mansfield, J., Werner, P., & Marx, M. S. (1991). Two studies of pacing in the nursing home. *Journal of Gerontology: Medical Sciences, 46,* M77–M83.

Costa, P. T., & McCrae, R. R. (1992). *Revised NEO personality inventory and NEO five-factor inventory: Professional manual.* Odessa, FL: Psychological Assessment Resources, Inc.

Cumming, J., Cumming E., Titus, J., Schmelzle, E., & MacDonald, J. (1982). The episodic nature of behavioral disturbances among residents of facilities for the aged. *Canadian Journal of Public Health, 73,* 319–322.

Dawson, P., & Reid D. W. (1987). Behavioral dimensions of patients at risk of wandering. *Gerontologist, 27,* 104–107.

deLeon, M., Potegal, M., & Gurland, B. (1984). Wandering and parietal lobe signs in senile dementia of Alzheimer's type. *Neuropsychobiology, 11,* 155–157.

Duffy, C. J. (1999). Visual loss and Alzheimer's disease; Out of sight, out of mind. *Neurology, 52,* 10–11.

Eustace A., Coen R., Walsh C., Cunningham J., Walsh J.B., Coakley D., Lawlor B.A. (2002). A longitudinal evaluation of behavioural and psychological symptoms of probable Alzheimer's disease. *International Journal of Geriatric Psychiatry. 17*(10), 968–973.

Folstein, M. R., Folstein, S. E., & McHugh, P. R. (1975). "Mini-mental state." A practical method for grading the cognitive state of patients for the clinician. *Journal of Psychiatric Research, 12*(3), 189–198.

Henderson, V., Mack, B., & Williams, B. W. (1989). Spatial disorientation in Alzheimer's disease. *Archives of Neurology, 46,* 391–394.

Holtzer, R., Tang, M. X., Devanand, D. P., Albert, S. M., Wegesin, D. J., Marder, K., et al. (2003). Psychopathological features in Alzheimer's disease: course and relationship with cognitive status. *Journal of the American Geriatrics Society, 51, 953–960.*

Hope, T., Keene, J., McShane, R. H., Fairburn, C. G., Gedling, K., & Jacoby, R. (2001). Wandering in dementia: A longitudinal study. *International Psychogeriatrics, 13,* 137–147.

Horgas, A. (2003). Assessing pain in persons with dementia. *Try This, 1*(2), 1–2.

Hughes, C. P., Berg, L., Danzinger, W. L., Cohen, L., & Martin, R. L. (1982). A new clinical scale for the staging of dementia. *British Journal of Psychiatry, 140, 566–572.*

Hyman, B. T., Van Horsen, G. W., Damasion, A. R., & Barnes, C. L. (1984). Alzheimer's disease: Cell-specific Pathology isolates the hippocampal formation. *Science, 225,* 1168–1170.

Katz, S., Ford, A. B., Moskowitz, R. W., Jackson, B. A., & Jaffe, M. W. (1963). Studies of illness in the aged. The index of ADL: A standardized measure of biological and psychological function. *Journal of the American Medical Association, 185, 94–98.*

Keily, D. K., Kiel, D. P., Burrows, A. B., & Lipsitz, L. A. (1998). Identifying nursing home residents at risk for falling. *Journal of the American Geriatrics Society, 46, 551–555.*

Klein, D. A., Steinberg, M., Galik, E., Steele, C., Sheppard, J., Warren, A., et al. (1999). Wandering behavior in community-residing persons with dementia. *International Journal of Geriatric Psychiatry, 14, 272–279.*

Kovach, C., Weisman, G., Chaudbury, H., & Calkins, M. (1997). Impacts of a therapeutic environment for dementia care. *American Journal of Alzheimer's Disease, 12,* 99–110.

Lam, D., Sewell, M., Bell, G., & Katona, C. (1989). Who needs psychogeriatric continuing care? *International Journal of Geriatric Psychiatry, 4,* 109–114.

Lawton, H. P., & Brody, E. M. (1969). Assessment of older people: Self-maintaining and instrumental activities of daily living. *The Gerontologist, 9,* 179.

Liu, L., Gauthier, L., & Gauthier S. (1991). Spatial disorientation in persons with early senile dementia of the Alzheimer type. *American Journal of Occupational Therapy. 45*(1), 67–74.

Madson, J. (1990). The study of wandering in person with senile dementia. *The American Journal of Alzheimer's Disease and Other Dementias, 6*(1), 21–24.

McShane, R., Gedling, K., Keene, J., Fairborn, C., Jacoby, R., & Hope, T. (1998). Getting lost in dementia: A longitudinal study of a behavioral symptom. *International Psychogeriatrics, 10,* 253–260.

Meguro, K., Yamaguchi, S., Yamazaki, H., Itoh, M., Yamaguchi, T., Matsui, H., et al. (1996). Cortical glucose metabolism in psychiatric wandering patients with vascular dementia. *Psychiatry Research, 67,* 71–80.

Moak, G. S. (1990). Characteristics of demented and nondemented geriatric admissions to a state hospital. *Hospital and Community Psychiatry, 41,* 799–801.

Monsour, N., & Robb, S. S. (1982). Wandering behavior in old age: A psychosocial study. *Social Work, 27,* 411–416.

Rheaume, Y., Riley, M. E., & Volicer, L. (1987). Meeting nutritional needs of Alzheimer's patients who pace constantly. *Journal of Nutrition for the elderly, 7,* 43–52.

Rockwood, K., Stolee, P., & Brahm, A. (1991). Outcomes of admission to a psychogeriatric service. *Canadian Journal of Psychiatry, 36,* 275–279.

Rowe, M. A., & Glover, J. C. (2001). Antecedents, descriptions, and consequences of wandering in cognitively-impaired adults and the safe return (SR) program. *American Journal of Alzheimer's Disease & Other Dementias, 16,* 344–352.

Ryan, J. P., McGowan, J., McCaffrey, N., Ryan, G. T., Zandi, T., & Brannigan, G. G. (1995). Graphomotor perseveration and wandering in Alzheimer's disease. *Journal of Geriatric Psychiatry and Neurology, 8,* 209–212.

Sanford, J. (1975). Tolerance of disability in elderly dependents by supporters at home: Its significance for hospital practice. *British Medical Journal, 3,* 471–473.

Snyder, L. H., Rupprecht, P., Pyrek, J., Breckhus, S., & Moss, T. (1978). Wandering. *The Gerontologist, 18,* 272–280.

Song, J. (2003). Relationship of premorbid personality and behavioral response to stress to wandering behavior of residents with dementia in long-term care facilities. Unpublished doctoral dissertation, University of Michigan.

Soverini, S., & Borghesi, E. (1968). On a strange case of wandering in an arteriosclerotic demented patient. *Gerontology, 16,* 846–851.

Squire, L. R. (1992). Declarative and nondeclarative memory: Multiple brain systems supporting learning and memory. *Journal of Cognitive Neuroscience, 4,* 232–243.

Thomas, D. W. (1997). Understanding the wandering patient: A continuity of personality perspective. *Journal of Gerontological Nursing, 23*(1), 16–24.

Vellas, B., Garry, P., & Guigoz, Y. (Eds.) (1999). *Mini Nutritional Assessment (MNA): Research and practice in the elderly.* Basel Switzerland: Karger.

Vieweg, V., Blair, C. E., Tucker, R., & Lewis, R. (1995). Factors precluding patients' discharge to the community: A geropsychiatric hospital survey. *Virginia Medical Quarterly, 122,* 275–278.

Ware, J. J., & Sherbourne, C. D. (1992). The MOS 36-item short-form health survey (SF-36). I. Conceptual framework and item selection. *Medical Care, 30,* 473–483.

PART III

Special Issues Associated With Wandering

CHAPTER SIX

Impact of Wandering on Functional Status

Elizabeth R. A. Beattie and Cynthia A. Beel-Bates

Wandering has been established as a "complex human activity . . . [that is] multi-faceted" (Dewing, 2005, p. 20), and as locomotion that is nondirect (Algase, Beattie, & Therrien, 2001). However, no study associating functional status loss with wandering has been reported in the literature. The purpose of this chapter is to review current research relevant to functional outcomes of wandering in the core functional domains most affected by this behavior: mobility; elimination; eating; bathing, dressing, and grooming; communication; and resting. A secondary purpose is to illustrate the characteristics of functional problems using case vignettes related to wandering and suggest clinical strategies specific to persons with dementia who wander.

Personal attributes of those most likely to display wandering behavior vary. Lai and Arthur (2003) purport that persons are likely to be older, male, with severe cognitive impairment from Alzheimer's disease (AD), on psychotropic drugs, and with an active lifestyle prior to the onset of AD. However, Algase et al. (2001) found that persons who wandered were younger and at all levels of cognitive impairment but that those with more severe cognitive impairment had a much higher percent of nondirect locomotion. Additionally, the findings of Rolland et al. (2005) found that, compared to nonwanderers, the regional cerebral blood flow to the left temporal parietal region is more severely decreased in wanderers, which suggests that wandering may have a physiological etiology (component). Conspicuously missing from the wanderer profile is any mention of the functional status of an "identified" wanderer, because there is little to no specific knowledge of individual Activities of Daily

Living (ADL) or Instrumental Activities of Daily Living (IADL) skill loss in either community-dwelling or institutionalized persons with dementia who wander. There is also a common unsubstantiated belief that wanderers lose functional skills earlier in the progression of the disease than nonwanderers.

When dementia is diagnosed the key to knowing the impact of the diagnosis on the older person and the family resides in the assessment of the person with dementia's functional status. Knowledge of functional status predicts quality of life by predicting the level of independence in self-care abilities, the degree of caregiver burden (Coen, Swanwick, Boyle, & Coakley, 1998), and the legal decisions related to guardianship of person and property (Lowenstein et al., 1989). As dementia progresses, quantifying the severity of functional disabilities assists in tracking the clinical course of the disease, determining the appropriate level of care, and assessing the effectiveness of interventions aimed at enhancing or maintaining functional abilities. The Direct Assessment of Functioning Scale (DAFS) developed by Lowenstein and colleagues has particular utility in tracking functional change in persons with dementia over time without considerable ceiling or floor effects (Gallo, 2006). Finally, functional skill limitations are predictive of long-term care admission (O'Donnell, 1992).

Wandering is specifically identified as a major problem in some functional assessment tools including the Functional Dementia Scale (Moore, Bobula, Short, & Mischel, 1983, p. 503). However, there are two standardization issues in associating functional status loss with wandering. First, although functional status is a critical concept in the measurement of disability, it lacks consistent operationalization making comparison across studies impossible (Long & Pavalko, 2004). Similarly, the phenomenon of wandering lacks a consistent consensus definition within or across disciplines, making cross study comparisons futile (Algase, 1999). Further, while knowledge about functional outcomes of wandering is mostly anecdotal, functional issues occur from early in the disease process in persons with dementia still living at home (e.g., IADLs such as wayfinding, driving, telephone use, and financial management) to severely impaired persons with dementia living in care. Even less is known about the nexus between wandering and other behavioral symptoms of dementia, such as aggression or psychosis, on function in persons with dementia.

Wandering can be an overwhelming challenge to any caregiver, but if management is approached in terms of functional capacity, there may be several obvious interventions that could improve the person with dementia's quality of life. For example, consistent foot care and comfortable well-fitting shoes may obviate foot pain and associated complications in persons with dementia who wander and are on their feet more often than their more sedentary peers. Data obtained in the conduct of functional assessments in persons with dementia who wander should be used to initiate a treatment plan that promotes a life with the most independence, fulfillment, and quality as possible.

MOBILITY AND WANDERING

Evidence suggests that wanderers are more physically robust than their less active peers and experience some physiological benefit from the exercise involved in wandering. Thus, they may appear more functionally capable of safe ambulation than is warranted by the results of functional testing of gait, balance, ambulation and transferring, and compromised visuospatial functioning and judgment. Wanderers also become fatigued from excessive walking and may continue to walk when tired and lost. Wanderers will walk in conditions that may deter other persons with dementia: in bare feet, socks, and slippers; using aids such as canes, walking chairs, and wheelchairs; carrying things in both hands; relying on unstable furniture and objects for support; following others and hanging onto other people as they walk; in poorly lit areas with debris or water on the floor; backward and sideways; and by crawling or climbing on, over, or under things, all of which increase fall and injury risk (Asaka, Morikawa, Yoshioka, & Kakuma, 1996). The three persons with dementia in the case vignettes at the end of this chapter, Gloria, Jim, and LaTonya, all clearly have quite different wandering profiles yet share the central characteristic of adept mobility.

When assessing mobility in the wanderer, the outcomes of traditional functional assessment of mobility must be evaluated in concert with a specific assessment of wandering status. Domains of wandering status include: the history of the development of wandering; the current daily distribution of wandering and the peak periods of wandering over 24 hours (temporal expression); the duration and pattern of wandering; the proportion of time spent not wandering; and critical outcomes of wandering (e.g., falling, elopement, incursion into unsafe or private domains). In functional terms, the ambulation considered wandering (pacing + lapping + random pattern ambulation) may be viewed as *dys*functional in that it does not support efficient movement between point A and point B (direct ambulation), as in Martino-Saltzman's pattern typology (Martino-Saltzman, Blasch, Morris, & McNeal, 1991). How each individual expresses wandering is likely highly idiosyncratic and changing over time, yet we have little empirical data about rate of change in wandering status over longer than a 1-week period. Thus, the functional assessment of all the domains that underpin wandering status needs to be planned to occur within an efficient time frame, such as 1 week. The following clinical tips must be considered *in addition to* the general best practice management of safe ambulation in persons with dementia.

Clinical Tips for Promoting Safe Mobility for the Wanderer

- Limit ambulation into areas of high risk for physical or emotional harm
- Ensure solid, well-fitting foot protection is worn when walking
- Encourage rest at defined low-activity periods
- Ensure correct use of sensory and walking aids
- Promote environmental legibility to support wayfinding
- Provide a clutter-free environment with well-defined paths
- Provide frequent, attractive resting spots
- Encourage walking without carrying things about
- Monitor the location of the person with dementia at regular intervals

Bathing, Dressing, and Grooming the Wanderer

The person with dementia who wanders is frequently a moving target when involved in personal care activities. Other behavioral symptoms of dementia, such as aggression and screaming, may also impact care routines, complicating the situation as in Case Vignette 2. Additionally, cognitive symptoms of dementia such as agnosia and apraxia may intimidate or upset the person with dementia when self-dressing, following dressing and grooming directions, looking in the mirror, and trying to stand still or sit.

Assessing the functional personal care skill repertoire in the person with dementia who wanders is essentially no different from doing so in the person with dementia with no wandering history. However it is a practical challenge to even consider assessment in this domain when the person with dementia is moving about a lot. It is critical to assume functionality unless it is demonstrated otherwise, for example, by the judicious use of cues and prompts at each stage of a task. Handing the person with dementia the soap and asking them to use it, prompting self-combing of the hair, and laying out clothes and prompting independent dressing all serve to balance the need for skill preservation as far into the disease process as possible, and counteract the development of excess disability (Dawson, Kline, Wiancko, & Wells, 1986; Rogers et al., 2000).

Excellent functional assessment is based on multiple views of performance over time. For the wanderer the stability of the environment (physical, social, and emotional) in which personal care occurs is particularly important, because wandering may be provoked by both stress from environmental press and unmet needs (Algase et al., 1996). In

Case Vignette 2, Jim is comfortable with his caregiver and can perform some tasks with little prompting or difficulty. His attention focus alters when his caregiver loses focus—that is the tipping point in the personal care routine where things start to go awry. A second caregiver has to be involved. Jim becomes more active and combative, and both caregivers endure minor physical resistance from Jim. Jim eventually is clean and groomed, but it all could have been easier and more pleasant. The following tips, coupled with excellent functional assessment of the preserved skills set of the person with dementia and best practice in personal care (Sloane et al., 2004), are designed to help when working with the wanderer in personal care routines.

Clinical Tips for Helping the Wandering Person With Dementia With Personal Care Routines

- Work with familiar staff in a familiar bathroom
- Work with two caregivers, if possible; have help nearby
- Support and reward remaining skills with praise
- Schedule personal care in low wandering times
- Schedule grooming tasks between pleasant events
- Be flexible in when and how often the person with dementia is bathed
- Be flexible in how many aspects of personal care can be achieved in a single care episode
- Avoid escalating the person with dementia into conflict just to undertake personal care unless the person is wet or dirty
- Ensure privacy and lock the door to prevent leaving
- Retain FOCUS on the person and the tasks at hand
- Keep the wanderer appraised of when they will be done with grooming

Elimination and Wandering

Although toileting has always been identified as a basic activity of living in most scales or assessment tools, when the task is broken down, toileting is a complex psychomotor function with associated emotional connections and social taboos. Inherent to toileting independently is the ability to search for the toilet, which requires the ability to wayfind. If the urge to toilet is recognized, the next step required involves finding a bathroom. Moving from point A to point B with purpose (leaving the dining room to go to the bathroom) is defined as direct locomotion compared to nondirect locomotion or wandering (Algase et al., 2001). Thus, those persons with dementia who wander are losing the ability to way-find and to toilet independently and spend time searching and seeking. For example in Gloria's case study, she may have been searching for the bathroom. Given the time of the day (early morning), the probability that her lapping behavior in the dining room and subsequent table leaving behavior may have been driven by her need to toilet is high.

As caregivers, learning the elimination patterns of individuals, by systematic recording and reporting of events, provides cues to unraveling the meaning of some wandering behaviors. Paying attention to the physiological intake–elimination dynamic is an obvious cue caregivers can use to prompt toileting behavior in persons with dementia. For example, Barbara, who had an irritable bowel in addition to her dementia, would often leave the table during a meal and be found defecating in a waste-basket in the utility room (the closet door down the hall from the dining room). Awareness of this pattern alerted staff to immediately accompany Barbara and redirect her to her bathroom where she could be assisted in finding the toilet, pulling down her pants and briefs adequately, sitting squarely on the toilet, sitting long enough to complete her business, wiping correctly to avoid infection, repositioning her clothes properly, and washing her hands with soap and helping her dry them. Staff recognition of Barbara's table leaving behavior as a probable toileting cue allowed them to facilitate her need to use the toilet. The outcome of this comprehensive response is threefold: Barbara's dignity is maintained, a catastrophic reaction of "finding her in the utility room with feces everywhere" is avoided, and staff time is appropriately spent directing Barbara and helping her get her need to toilet met instead of cleaning the utility room after the fact. Caregiver monitoring of the toileting activity is especially necessary when the person with dementia wanders, because steps to the task may be skipped if the person is easily distracted by anything in the environment (noise, motion, temperature changes) or by the urge to keep locomoting.

In addition to staff recognition of individual cues for toileting in persons with dementia, most dementia care units have environmental cues that assist persons with dementia in their search for the bathroom. These include brightly painted bathroom doors, striped awnings over the bathroom doors, or the word or picture of a toilet on the bathroom door. These environmental interventions are only effective for persons with dementia who retain the ability to attach meaning to these cues. Only one systematic study could be found evaluating the use of stimulus toilet cuing in persons with dementia (Hussian, 1998), but the sample is not distinguished by wandering status.

The most important intervention that assists a wanderer with toileting needs is staff monitoring and anticipation. A wanderer driven by the need to toilet will be indiscriminate about meeting the need. From the hallway, another person's room may look spatially the same to the wanderer, so the room is entered, or the wanderer reaches the end of the hall so enters the room closest to the end seeking a bathroom and potentially causing issues with other residents. It becomes the role of the staff, or family if still living at home, to come beside the resident and guide the toileting process. In the case study, it may have been more effective to guide Gloria to the bathroom 50 feet away, with the toilet as a cue right in front of her, and then suggest she use the toilet before going back to breakfast.

Clinical Tips for Helping the Wandering Person With Dementia With Elimination

- Dress wanderers in simple clothing that is easily removed
- Assess elimination patterns, toileting practices, and wandering status
- Assess legibility of cues to the person with dementia
- Assess ability to communicate elimination needs
- Provide multiple accessible toilets with clear cues
- Remove objects that resemble toilets from public places
- Identify behaviors that signal elimination needs
- Anticipate toileting needs and know where the wanderer is
- Build a toileting schedule around wandering patterns and distribution over the day, for example, after meals, before and after rest, before wandering peak periods
- Build toileting into accompanied wandering
- Reward elimination success

Communication in Wandering

Early empirical knowledge regarding impaired communication in dementia was hampered by the lack of robust measures of cognitive impairment and poor diagnostic parameters and focused on the determination of deficit rather on the identification and preservation of function. More recent studies have clearly established the magnitude of the problem for the sufferer and the caregiver (Allen, 2002; Bayles & Tomoeda, 1990; Bayles, Tomoeda, & Trosset, 1992; Glickstein & Neustadt, 1993; Gurland, Toner, Wilder, Chen, & Lantigua, 1994; Hopper, 2005). In the early stages of the disease, the functional deficits are primarily in the content area of word access and subtle conversational skills. By the midstage of the disease, persons with dementia have increased difficulty in content areas including concept formation, word finding, diminished writing abilities, the use of language rules, and reduced memory function. These difficulties become compounded in severe dementia when coupled with severe memory and intellectual deficits and by poor hearing support (Frank, 1994; Hopper, Bayles, Harris, & Holland, 2001). Assessment batteries such as the Arizona Battery of Communication Disorders (Bayles & Tomoeda, 1990) and the Functional Linguistic Communication Inventory (FLCI) have been developed to evaluate the deficit areas frequently associated with communication in dementia and have been utilized in one major study of wanderers (Algase, Beck, Whall, & the NDB Collaborative Research Group, 2003; Bayles & Tomoeda, 1990; Functional Linguistic Communication Inventory (FLCI), 2004). Since deterioration in the linguistic communication pattern of a person with dementia is inevitable, caregivers need to take active responsibility for the communication initiative.

Limited empirical data informs our understanding of the difficulties persons with dementia who wander experience in interpersonal communication functioning as their communication abilities decline and they continue to be compelled to move. Current evidence-based communication enhancing techniques for use with persons with dementia may not be relevant for use with those who move so frequently and consistently, for example, graphic and written cues and space retrieval training (Hoerster, Hickey, & Bourgeois, 2001; Hopper et al., 2005). One multiple case design intervention study testing the impact of a systematic communication intervention with identified wanderers showed promise in increasing the length of time wanderers sat while engaged in talking with another person, and decreases in some parameters of wandering, but the effects were not statistically significant across all cases (Beattie, 1997). Some evidence suggests that wanderers may be more social and extraverted than those persons with dementia who do not wander, thus more amenable to communication-based intervention (Algase et al., 1996; Thomas, 1997, 1999). However, evidence in one case study demonstrated that pressure to communicate may also produce pacing (Beattie) and that wanderers find the cognitive effort of simultaneous walking and talking difficult to sustain and therefore talk more when seated than moving (Beattie). The personality of the wanderer and the emotional tone and ambience of the communication environment as well as environmental familiarity may also serve to enhance or detract from communication readiness in wanderers (Son & Kim, 2006; Song, 2003; Yao & Algase, 2006).

In Case Vignette 1, Gloria approaches people but does not linger long enough to become engaged in communication—the attention and reciprocity essential to engagement is diminished. When approached by others she does not respond at all, seems to understand but not to respond, or makes a nonverbal response that may be difficult to interpret. The assessment of functional communication status permits the development of strategies for communication with the wanderer that may help bridge these types of issues when coupled with traditional strategies and based on respect and genuineness.

Clinical Tips for Communicating With the Person With Dementia Who Wanders

- Assess capacity for communication and usual communication behavior
- Talk while seated face to face
- Select a familiar space the wanderer seeks out often
- Gently hold the wandering person with dementia's hands to get them to stay seated
- Express only one idea at once
- Match clear nonverbal signals to show interest
- Respond positively to all attempts to communicate with you

Nutrition and Eating in Wandering

The association between weight loss and dementia is well established and is stronger in AD than in other forms of dementia (White, Pieper, Schmader, & Fillenbaum, 1996). Despite extensive research focused on systemic, metabolic factors influencing weight loss in dementia the definitive mechanisms responsible remain unclear (Wolf-Klein & Silverstone, 1994). Weight loss in dementia contributes to an increased risk of frailty, immobility, illness, and premature morbidity (White et al., 1996). Elders with dementia weigh less than those without the disease (Franklin & Karkek, 1989) and are more likely to experience a clinically significant weight loss of 10 percent or more within 6 months of admission (Ryan, Bryant, Eleazer, Rhodes, & Guest, 1995; Wang, Fukagawa, Hossain, Ooi, 1997). Evidence suggests that wanderers use more energy than nonwanderers, expending approximately 600 more calories per day than they consume (Litchford & Wakefield, 1987) and have difficulty remaining at the table during mealtimes (Beattie, Algase, & Song, 2004).

While eating is a complex task that requires planning, attention, initiation, conceptualization, and visuospatial abilities, no specific profile of functional eating skills characteristic of various levels of cognitive impairment (mild, moderate, severe) has been developed. The challenges of helping demented residents eat are well documented

(Van Ort & Phillips, 1992; Watson, 1997; Watson & Greene, 2006) yet caregivers continue to have unrealistic expectations related to a resident's functional ability during eating (Tully, Matrakas, Muir, & Musallam, 1997). Although the significant morbidity associated with weight loss in dementia has been explored, no published studies specifically examine the nexus between level of cognitive impairment, wandering, eating, and weight loss.

In persons with dementia who wander, their persistent, seemingly driven movement and reduced ability to sit at the table long enough to eat, combined with impaired functional eating skills, may result in weight loss in excess of that produced by the pathophysiology of the disease process alone. Additionally, persons with dementia may be hyper-phagic, hypo-phagic or norma-phagic; display dysphagia, dyspraxia, or pica behavior; and have issues with food recognition due to changes in the special senses and cognition (Keene & Hope, 1998; Keene, Hope, Rogers, & Elliman, 1998; Tsai, Hwang, Yang, Liu, & Kan, 1996). There is anecdotal evidence that wanderers may be hungry and some evidence they can self-report hunger with accuracy (Algase, Beattie, & Son, 2005). Empirical evidence suggests that persons with dementia eat more at mealtimes in supervised natural dining environments with highly trained feeders (Backstrom, Norberg, & Norberg, 1987; Beattie et al., 2004; Coyne & Hoskins, 1997; Lipner, Bosler, & Giles, 1990; Kayser-Jones & Schell, 1997; Morley & Silver, 1995; Young, Binns, & Greenwood, 2001). An understanding of the impact of dementia status and wandering on functional eating status is a critical factor in maintaining adequate nutrition and hydration and preventing premature weight loss.

In Case Vignette 1, Gloria receives some help from the staff to get started with the task of eating a nutritious breakfast, but not sufficient focused help to get her to begin to eat. She is quickly distracted and compelled to walk. Having been returned to the table she leaves again to resume wandering. Although she is given a cookie she crumbles it up and doesn't eat it. She leaves the fruit cup along her wandering path. In this common scenario, persons with dementia, like Gloria, may eat very little at the meal and remain hungry. While many assessment tools address some elements of eating, such as gross motor skills and food preferences, most do not include the assessment of attention, fine motor skills, and the rhythm of eating necessary to address feeding support adequately in persons with dementia, and especially in those who wander (Beattie, 2005; Watson, 1997). In addition to usual best practices in the management of food and fluid intake in persons with dementia, wanderers may benefit from additional attention to the following issues.

Clinical Tips for Supporting Food and Fluid Intake in Persons With Dementia Who Wander

- Assess usual patterns of eating, drinking, and preferred foods
- Assess wandering status and ability to sit at the table
- Assess attention to food
- Assess preferred dining company
- Assess the ability to hold and use utensils
- Assess rate of eating and ability to get food to mouth
- Schedule meals and snacks in periods of low, or no, wandering
- Provide appropriate utensils
- Use food-related cuing during eating

The Wanderer and Resting

Resting is the antithesis of wandering. It is not traditionally considered part of functional status, although it is a something that we all perform readily. We routinely rest our eyes and feet and brains. It helps us retain energy and improves quality of life. In physically overactive, elderly wanderers with poor judgment and problem solving, rest takes on new importance because the ability to self-regulate rest is diminished or absent. Rest differs from sleep because rest does not involve sleep. The characteristics of sleep disturbance in late life have been explored in numerous empirical studies demonstrating that nighttime sleep fragmentation, early morning awakening, and daytime sleep periods are all common features among the elderly, and dementia and advanced age further impact the nature of sleep (Ancoli-Israel, Parker, Sinaee, Fell, & Kripke, 1989; Bliwise, 1993; Bliwise, Yesavage, & Tinklenberg, 1992; Weinert, 2000). One study reports specific to rest and sleep issues associated with *sundowning*, or late-day agitation and pacing in persons with dementia but does not distinguish this phenomenon from wandering (Bliwise, 2000). No concept analysis differentiating rest from sleep is published. A recent intervention study (Ouslander et al., 2006) designed to improve sleep by minimizing daytime rest and increasing daytime activities showed no efficacy in improving sleep patterns in nursing home residents. In Case Vignette 3, LaTonya has an embedded sleep disturbance. She is unable to sleep during the usual hours of the night, and when she is awake she wanders. In Case Vignettes 1 and 2, Gloria and Jim show no signs of resting.

How wanderers rest, and the characteristics of their resting behavior, can be evaluated to some extent by examining time periods when the wanderer is sitting or lying of their own volition, but is awake, during periods of time when normal elders would be awake. Wanderers who do not rest sufficiently during any 24-hour period are arguably at higher risk of fatigue and dehydration than those who are able to rest (for both individual and total periods of time) more typical in normal elders and nonwanderers. In the absence of empirical evidence about the benefits of rest in wanderers, and assuming best practice in the support of night time sleep, the following clinical tips may prove helpful.

Clinical Tips for Supporting Rest in Wanderers

- Keep wanderers in well-lit areas during the day
- Minimize opportunities to lie on beds other than their own
- Develop a time-limited (30 min.) rest schedule in low wandering periods
- Encourage planned sitting down time with staff or visitors
- If the person will not sit or lie down they may sit in a chair and be pushed about, or sit in a garden swing
- Use accompanied walking to slow ambulation rate

In the continued quest to develop more reliable and valid tools for functional assessment of persons with dementia, and encourage best practices in the determination and use of functional outcomes in management, it is easy for the unique functional problems of wanderers to be marginalized. Yet, it is functional issues of this type and magnitude that mitigate against wanderers as a group, and particularly the high-risk wanderer, receiving the tailored approaches to ADL care that they clearly need. Descriptive studies of functional ability deficit in rigorously identified wanderers at different levels of cognitive impairment are a priority need in addition to the refinement of existing functional assessment tools for use with persons with dementia who wander.

Case Vignette 1

She follows the nurse closely early in the morning as he moves from room to room giving out medications. He says, "How are you Gloria? You're up early as usual.... Now don't get in my way while I'm trying to do my work." She hovers near his cart, within arms, reach of him. He has to be alert to avoid running into her. Occasionally she walks behind him into other residents' rooms, smiling and nodding at them. When the medication round is done she walks backward and forward near the nursing station, occasionally walking up to another resident and murmuring something. Eventually she follows the dietary staff into the large dining room as breakfast is being set up. In the hour before breakfast is served she circles the large room constantly, stepping quickly past the path of other nursing staff wheeling residents in, never pausing to look around or to sit and rest.

Her breakfast tray arrives at the table and it smells good—oatmeal with milk, scrambled egg, coffee, orange juice, and a fruit cup. A nurse helps her to sit down and puts a spoon in her hand saying, "Eat up now, Gloria." She stirs her oatmeal for a few minutes, tries to drink her hot coffee, tries to open the orange juice and then, open fruit cup in hand, stands up and walks away. She is 50 yards away down the long corridor by the bathroom when a nurse comes to find her and bring her back to the table. She asks, "Do you want to go to the bathroom Gloria? Here, let's go, and I'll hold your fruit and wait for you." But Gloria quietly resists the nurse's outstretched hand and keeps on moving past the bathroom, pausing by the large bay windows to look outside. She stays for several moments and then moves on, leaving the fruit cup sitting on the sill and taking with her a small lap blanket left by another resident.

A cluster of residents are by the door to the activity room waiting for Nancy, the rec. therapist. Gloria circles them, smiling and trailing the rug behind her. They smile back and she keeps on going, walking up to Nancy as she arrives and taking her hand. She is offered a cookie and takes it. Nancy says, "Hi Gloria, you need to be changed . . . your pants are falling down . . . let's find someone to help you." She walks with Gloria to find a nurse and says, "She'll bring you back when you're done." The nurse helping Gloria turns her back for a moment to pick up some bath supplies and Gloria is gone. She calls her name and gets no reply. It takes her several minutes to find her, lying on the bed in Ted's room. Ted, sitting in his wheelchair, says, "She keeps on coming in here—take her out, get her out." The nurse leads her out and finds Gloria's hand full of crumbled cookie pieces.

Case Vignette 2

Jim is not interested in going into the bathroom and taking a shower. Ed, the nurse, tells him kindly and directly several times that it's his turn. He was also offered a shower earlier in the day, and yesterday, but it has not eventuated, because none of the staff can get him into the bathroom. He keeps saying, "No . . . No . . . I don't want a bath." This happens several times a week and is an ongoing issue in his care. He has spent most of the afternoon sleeping and for the last hour has paced about in the TV room, back and forth in front of the screen while other residents are trying to watch. Celia, another resident who gets irritable with Jim, says, "Just sit down or go away!"

Ed walks up to Jim, takes his hand and leads him out of the TV room and toward the bathroom saying, "It's time for that shower, man. You'll feel great when you get clean clothes on." He has Jim's fresh clothes under his other arm. He is unable to get Jim to make the turn into the bathroom, and they walk together around the house, through the kitchen and past the bedrooms toward Jim's room. Ed gets Jim into his room and starts to undress him and put a robe on so they can walk back to the bathroom together. Jim happily helps take off his shoes, pants, and shirt. Ed pauses and looks away, and Jim slips out the door and wanders off in his undershirt. Ed sighs and goes after him, calling to a colleague, Kim, to help with Jim. Kim catches Jim just as he reaches the TV room and covers him with a robe. Kim and Ed walk on either side of Jim into the bathroom, talking about football with him. Jim says slowly, "How ... ddddid ... they win ... water?" The conversation about football continues, and Jim is led into the shower stall.

Even though he is told the water is going to go on and the room and water temperatures are warm, he kicks out at Ed as he tries to help him wash himself. He drops the soap and hangs the washcloth on the shower head over and over as Ed completes the shower. He grips Ed's arm and pushes in his nails while Ed is washing his hair. He doesn't want to sit down and have his feet washed and gives Kim a push as he tries to get him to sit. Once out of the shower Jim is anxious to be moving again and resists being fully dried. The nurses manage to dress him in the bathroom but end up putting on his socks and shoes when he sits down for dinner an hour later. He lets Sandra, the activities therapist, comb his hair as he wanders about. He carries his toothbrush around most of the evening and goes to sleep with it in his pajama pocket in the TV room around 8 P.M.

Case Vignette 3

LaTonya is all settled in bed. Her husband, Dillard, is tired after a long day at home caring for her and falls asleep quickly in the bed they have shared since their wedding 51 years ago. He never sleeps deeply anymore since she got dementia and wakes with a start to the sound of water running. The bedside clock says 12:16 A.M. He finds his wife in the kitchen making breakfast, eggs and bread out and milk waiting to be poured. He says, "LaTonya, honey, what are you doing? It's time for sleeping not for eating. Come on back to bed now." She says, "Oh, is it ... I was getting you ready for work." They lie back down and both nod off again. A lot later he hears music and realizes he is awake again and the lights on the back porch are on. La Tonya is walking about the small yard in her nightgown hanging dry laundry from the clean laundry basket on the line. The TV is on playing "I Love Lucy" re-runs. It is 4:27 A.M. He brings his wife inside, locks the door again and watches TV with her until she falls asleep just after 5 A.M. At 6:45, he wakes again, and she is not in the TV room. He finds her in their bedroom walking about like she often does when she first gets up.

REFERENCES

Algase, D. L. (1999). Wandering in dementia. In J. Fitzpatrick (Ed.), *Annual review of nursing research: Focus on complementary health and pain management* (Vol. 17, pp. 195–217). New York: Springer.

Algase, D., Beattie, E., & Son, G. (2005, November). Self-report of hunger, thirst, and pain in Persons with Dementia (PWD) in long-term care. Presentation at the 48th Annual Scientific Meeting for The Gerontological Society of America, Orlando, FL.

Algase, D. L, Beattie, E. R., & Therrien, B. (2001). Impact of cognitive impairment on wandering behavior. *Western Journal of Nursing Research, 23*(3), 283–295.

Algase, D. L., Beck, C., Kolanowski, A., Whall, A., Berent, S., Richards, K., & Beattie, E. (1996). Need-driven dementia-compromised behavior: An alternative view of disruptive behavior. *American Journal of Alzheimer's Disease, 11*(6), 10–19.

Algase, D., Beck, C., Whall, A., & the NDB Collaborative Research Group. (2003). Exploring NDB background factors as predictors of wandering, aggression and problematic vocalizations. *The Gerontologist (Program Abstracts), 43*(SI 1), 83–84.

Ancoli-Israel, S., Parker, L., Sinaee, R., Fell, R. L., & Kripke, D. F. (1989). Sleep fragmentation in patients from a nursing home. *Journal of Gerontology, 44*(1), M18–M21.

Asaka, A., Morikawa, S., Yoshioka, M., & Kakuma, T. (1996). Predictors of fall-related injuries among community-dwelling elderly people with dementia. *Age and Ageing, 25*(1), 22–28.

Backstrom, A., Norberg, A., & Norberg, B. (1987). Feeding difficulties in long-stay patients at nursing homes: Caregiver turnover and caregivers' assessments of duration and difficulty of assisted feeding and amount of food received by the patient. *International Journal of Nursing Studies, 24*(1), 69–76.

Bayles, K. A., & Tomoeda, C. K. (1990). *Arizona Battery for Communication Disorders of Dementia (ABCD)*. Tucson, AZ: Canyonlands Publishing, Inc.

Bayles, K. A., & Tomoeda, C. K. (1991). Caregiver report of prevalence and appearance order of linguistic symptoms in Alzheimer's patients. *Gerontologist, 31*(2), 210–216.

Bayles, K. A., Tomoeda, C. K., & Trosset, M. W. (1992). Relation of linguistic communication abilities of Alzheimer's patients to stage of disease. *Brain & Language, 42*(4), 454–472.

Bayles, K., & Tomoeda, C. K. (1994). *The Functional Linguistic Communication Inventory (FLCI)*. Austin, TX: Pro-Ed.

Beattie, E. R. A. (1997). The impact of nurse-patient communication style on the pattern and rhythm of wandering in severely cognitively impaired nursing home residents. Unpublished doctoral dissertation, James Cook University, Townsville, Qld, Australia.

Beattie, E. R. A. (2004). Nursing management of wandering behavior. In B. Keane (Ed.), *Practical nursing management for residential care*. Melbourne, Australia: AusMed Publications.

Beattie, E. R. A. (2005, November). Mealtime functional eating and attention deficit of table-leaving wanderers in long-term care. Presentation at the 48th Annual Scientific Meeting of The Gerontological Society of America, Orlando, FL.

Beattie E. R. A., Algase D. L., & Song J. (2004). Keeping wandering nursing home residents at the table: Improving food intake using a behavioral communication intervention. *Aging & Mental Health, 8*(2), 109–116.

Bliwise, D. L. (1993). Sleep in normal ageing and dementia. *Sleep, 16*(1), 40–81.

Bliwise, D. L. (2000). Circadian rhythms and agitation. *International. Psychogeriatrics, 12*(Suppl. 1), 143–146.

Bliwise, D. L., Yesavage, J. A., & Tinklenberg, J. R. (1992). Sundowning and rate of decline in mental function in Alzheimer's disease. *Dementia, 3*(7), 335–341.

Coen, R., Swanwick, G., Boyle, C., & Coakley, D. (1998). Behaviour disturbance and other predictors of carer burden in Alzheimer's disease. *International Journal of Geriatric Psychiatry, 12*(3), 331–336.

Coyne, M. L., & Hoskins, L. (1997). Improving eating behaviors in dementia using behavioral strategies. *Clinical Nursing Research, 6*(3), 275–290.

Dawson, P., Kline, K., Wiancko, D., & Wells, D. (1986). Preventing excess disability in patients with Alzheimer's disease. *Geriatric Nursing, 7*(6), 298–301.

Dewing, J. (2005). Screening for wandering among older persons with dementia. *Nursing Older People, 17*(3), 20–22.

Frank, E. M. (1994). Effect of Alzheimer's disease on communication function. *Journal of the South Carolina Medical Association, 90*(9), 417–423.

Franklin, C. A., & Karkek, J. (1989). Weight loss and senile dementia in an institutionalized elderly population. *Journal of the American Dietetic Association, 89*(6), 790–792.

Gallo, J. J. (2006). Activities of daily living and instrumental activities of daily living assessment. In J. Gallo, H. R. Bogner, T. Fulmer, & G. J. Pareaz (Eds.), *Handbook of geriatric assessment* (4th ed.). Sudbury: Jones & Bartlett.

Glickstein, J. K., & Neustadt, G. K. (1993). Speech-language interventions in Alzheimer's disease: a functional communication approach. *Clinics in Communication Disorders, 3*(1), 15–30.

Gurland, B. J., Toner, J. A., Wilder, D. E., Chen, J., & Lantigua, R. (1994). Impairment of communication and adaptive functioning in community-residing elders with advanced dementia: assessment methods. *Alzheimer Disease & Associated Disorders, 8*(Suppl. 1), S230–S241.

Hoerster, L., Hickey, E., & Bourgeois, M. (2001). Effects of memory aids on conversations between nursing home residents with dementia and nursing assistants. *Neuropsychological Rehabilitation, 11*(4), 399–427.

Hopper, T. (2005, Nov. 8). Assessment and treatment of cognitive-communication disorders in individuals with dementia (pp. 10–11). Retrieved December 7, 2006, from http://www.asha.org/about/publications/leader-online/archives/2005/051108/051108d.htm.

Hopper, T., Bayles, K., Harris, F., & Holland, A. (2001). The relationship between minimum data set ratings and scores on measures of communication and hearing among nursing home residents with dementia. *American Journal of Speech-Language Pathology, 10,* 370–381.

Hopper, T., Mahendra, N., Kim, E., Azuma, T., Bayles, K., Cleary, S., et al. (2005). Spaced retrieval training for individuals with dementia: Evidence-based practice recommendations for speech-language pathologists. *Journal of Medical Speech Language Pathology, 13*(2), xxvii–xxiv.

Hussian, R. (1998). Modification of behaviors in dementia via stimulus manipulation. *Journal of Aging and Mental Health, 8*(1), 37–43.

Kayser-Jones, J., & Schell, E. (1997). Mealtime experience of a cognitively impaired elder: Ineffective and effective strategies. *Journal of Gerontological Nursing, 23*(7), 33–39.

Keene, J. M., & Hope, T. (1997). Hyperphagia in dementia: 1. The use of an objective and reliable method for measuring hyperphagia in people with dementia. *Appetite, 28*(2), 151–165.

Keene, J., & Hope, T. (1998). Natural history of hyperphagia and other eating changes in dementia. *International Journal of Geriatric Psychiatry, 13*(10), 700–706.

Keene, J., Hope, T., Rogers, P. J., & Elliman, N. A. (1998). An investigation of satiety in ageing, dementia, and hyperphagia. *International Journal of Eating Disorders, 23*(4), 409–418.

Lai, C., & Arthur, D. (2003). Wandering behavior in people with dementia. *Journal of Advanced Nursing, 44*(2), 173–183.

Lipner, H. S., Bosler, J., Giles, G. (1990). Volunteer participation in feeding residents: Training and supervision in a long-term care facility. *Dysphagia, 5*(2), 89–95.

Litchford, M. D., & Wakefield, L. M. (1987). Nutrient intakes and energy expenditures of residents with senile dementia of the Alzheimer's type. *Journal of the American Dietetic Association, 2,* 211–213.

Long, J. S., & Pavalko, E. (2004). Comparing alternative measures of functional limitation. *Medical Care, 43*(1), 19–27.

Lowenstein, D. A., Amigo, E., Duara, R., Guterman, A., Hurwitz, D., Berkowitz, N., et al. (1989). A new scale for the assessment of functional status in Alzheimer's disease and related disorders. *Journal of Gerontology: Psychological Sciences, 44*(4), 114–121.

Martino-Saltzman, D., Blasch, B. B., Morris, R. D., & McNeal, L. W. (1991). Travel behavior of nursing home residents perceived as wanderers and nonwanderers. *Gerontologist, 31,* 666–672.

Moore, J. T., Bobula, J. A., Short, T. B., & Mischel, M. (1983). A functional dementia scale. *Journal of Family Practice, 16*(3), 499–503.

Morley, J. E., & Silver, A. J. (1995). Nutritional issues in nursing home care. *Ann Intern Med 123*(11), 850–859.

O'Donnell, B. F., Drachman, D. A., Barnes, H. J., Peterson, K. E, Swearer, J. M., & Lew, R. A. (1992). Incontinence and troublesome behaviors predict institutionalization in dementia. **Journal of** *Psychiatry and Neurology, 5*(1), 45–52.

Ouslander, J. G., Connell, B. R., Bliwise, D. L., Endeshaw, Y., Griffiths, P., & Schnelle, J. F. (2006). A nonpharmacological intervention to improve sleep in nursing home patients: Results of a controlled clinical trial. *Journal of the American Geriatrics Society, 54*(1), 38–47.

Rogers, J. C., Holm, M. B., Burgio, L. D., Hsu, C., Hardin, J. M., & McDowell, B. J. (2000). Excess disability during morning care in nursing home residents with dementia. *International Psychogeriatrics, 12*(2), 267–282.

Rolland, Y., Payoux, P., Lauwers-Cances, P., Voisin, T., Esquerre, J. P., & Vellas, B. (2005). A SPECT study of wandering behavior in Alzheimer's disease. *International Journal of Geriatric Psychiatry, 20*(9), 816–820.

Ryan, C., Bryant, E., Eleazer, P., Rhodes, A., & Guest, K. (1995). Unintentional weight loss in long-term care: Predictor of mortality in the elderly. *South Med J, 88*(6), 721–724.

Sloane, P. D., Hoeffer, B., Mitchell, C. M., McKenzie, D. A., Barrick, A. L., Rader, J., et al. (2004). Effect of person-centered showing and the towel bath on bathing-associated aggression, agitation, and discomfort in nursing home residents with dementia: A randomized, control trial. *Journal of the American Geriatric Society, 52*(11), 1795–1804.

Son, G. R., & Kim, H. R. (2006). Culturally familiar environment among immigrant Korean elders. *Research and Theory for Nursing Practice, 20*(2), 159–171.

Song, J. A. (2003). Relationship of premorbid personality and behavioral responses to stress to wandering behavior of residents with dementia in long term care facilities (Doctoral dissertation, University of Michigan, 2003). *Proquest Dissertations and Theses 2003.* Section 0127, Part 0569 209 pages. Publication Number: AAT 3096205.

Thomas, D. (1997). Understanding the wandering patient: A continuity of personality perspective. *Journal of Gerontological Nursing, 23*(1), 16–24.

Thomas, D. (1999). Evaluating the relationship between pre-morbid personality characteristics and wandering among patients with dementia. *Activities, Adaptation and Aging, 23*(4), 33–48.

Thompson, M. P., & Morris, L. K. (1991). Unexplained weight loss in the ambulatory elderly. *Journal of the American Geriatric Society, 39*(5), 497–500.

Tsai, S. J., Hwang, J. P., Yang, C. B., Liu, K. M., & Kan, Y. S. (1996). Characteristics of dementia patients with hyperphagia. *Kaohsiung Journal of Medical Science, 12*(3), 197–201.

Tully, M., Matrakas, K., Muir, J., & Musallam, K. (1997). The eating behavior scale: A simple method of assessing functional ability in patients with Alzheimer's disease. *Journal of Gerontological Nursing, 23*(7), 9–15.

Van Ort, S., & Phillips, L. (1992). Feeding nursing home residents with Alzheimer's disease. *Geriatric Nursing, 13*(5), 249–253.

Wang, S. J., Fukagawa, N., Hossain, N., & Ooi, W. L. (1997). Longitudinal weight changes, length of survival, and energy requirements of long-term care residents with dementia. *Journal of the American Geriatrics Society, 45*(10), 1189–1195.

Watson, R. (1993). Feeding difficulty in elderly patients with dementia: Confirmatory factor analysis. *Journal of Advanced Nursing, 18*(1), 25–31.

Watson, R. (1997). Measuring feeding difficulty in patients with dementia: Perspectives and problems. *International Journal of Nursing Studies, 34*(6), 405–414.

Watson, R., & Green, S. (2006). Feeding and dementia: A systematic literature review. *Journal of Advanced Nursing, 54*(1), 86–93.

Weinert, D. (2000). Age-dependent changes of the circadian system. *Chronobiolica. International, 17*(3), 261–283.

Whall, A., Black, M., Groh, C., Kupferschmidt, B., & Foster, N. (1997). The effect of natural environments upon agitation and aggression in late stage dementia patients. *American Journal of Alzheimer's Disease and Other Dementias, 12*(5), 216–220.

White, H., Pieper, C., Schmader, K., & Fillenbaum, G. (1996). Weight change in Alzheimer's disease. *Journal of the American Geriatrics Society, 44*(3), 265–372.

Wolf-Klein, G., & Silverstone, F. (1994). Weight loss in Alzheimer's Disease: An international review of the literature. *International Psychogeriatrics, 6*(2), 135–142.

Yao, L., & Algase, D. (2006). Environmental ambiance as a new window on wandering. *Western Journal of Nursing Research, 28*(1), 89–104.

Young, K., Binns, M., & Greenwood, C. (2001). Meal delivery practices do not meet needs of Alzheimer patients with increased cognitive and behavioral difficulties in a long-term care facility. *Journals of Gerontology, Series A, Biological Sciences and Medical Sciences, 56*(10), M656–M661.

CHAPTER SEVEN

Caregiver Issues Associated With Wandering

Elizabeth A. Perkins, Nancy Lynn, and William E. Haley

As described in detail in other chapters in this book, wandering is a common and problematic behavior among individuals with Alzheimer's disease (AD) and other dementias. However, while most research conducted on wandering has been conducted in nursing homes and other institutional settings, the vast majority of individuals with AD live in the community, under the care of their family members. These family members face special challenges in managing wandering, as well as the multitude of other problems that occur in the course of dementia and the long-term job of being a caregiver.

In order to understand how wandering affects family caregivers and issues in the implementation of wandering interventions that can be used by family caregivers, it is important to understand the broader context of family caregiving and what is known about evidence-based interventions for caregivers. The present chapter will provide a general overview of caregiving, including the particular demands of dementia caregiving and the application of the stress and coping paradigm to the study of caregiving. A second section addresses why wandering is a concern for family caregivers, what is known about the occurrence of wandering in community settings, and what impact wandering behaviors have on caregivers. The third section discusses what is known about the effectiveness of caregiving interventions and wandering interventions specific to in-home caregiving. The chapter concludes with a discussion of conceptual and methodological challenges in implementing effective wandering interventions in community settings and suggestions for future practice innovations and research.

CAREGIVING—AN OVERVIEW

There is no doubt that family caregivers are increasingly acknowledged as providers of a widespread activity of paramount importance at both the individual and societal level. At the individual level, family caregivers allow a care recipient to remain in their own or their family caregiver's home and receive the individualized attention of a loved one. At the societal level, though it is difficult to quantify the precise economic impact of caregiving; it has been estimated to save $288 billion annually in the United States (Arno, Levine, & Memmott, 1999). This is over double for the combined cost of home health care ($32 billion) and nursing home care ($83 billion) annually (Arno et al., 1999). It is apparent that were it not for this army of volunteer caregivers, the health care system in the United States would rapidly be overwhelmed, due to the lack of capacity to serve the levels of need that currently exists. Current estimates suggest that 21 percent (approximately 44 million) of the U.S. population undertake informal unpaid caregiving to a friend or relative aged 18 and above (National Alliance for Caregiving [NAC] & AARP, 2004). More than three-quarters of all caregiving is directed toward the provision of care to older adults aged 50 and above, and currently engages 16 percent (i.e., 33 million) of the U.S. population (NAC & AARP, 2004). Family caregivers are the major work force (78%) of long-term care provision within home settings, despite their informal and unpaid status (Thompson, 2004). Only a small percentage (4.5%) of older adults aged 65 and above actually reside in a nursing home setting, a figure that has actually decreased from 5.1 percent in 1990, and further establishes the fact that most older adults stay at home, with the support of family caregivers for as long as possible (U.S. Census Bureau, 2000).

The particular health conditions that precipitate caregiving duties can vary. Examples include caregiving for those with cancer (e.g., Vanderwerker, Laff, Kadan-Lottick, McColl, & Prigerson, 2005), those who have sustained major strokes (McCullagh, Brigstocke, Donaldson, & Kalra, 2005), and those with Parkinson's disease (Martínez-Martín et al., 2005). Furthermore, subpopulations of caregivers can care for those with lifelong chronic impairments such as severe mental health issues (e.g., McDonell, Short, Berry, & Dyck, 2003), or intellectual, developmental, and physical disabilities (e.g., Haley & Perkins, 2004).

Overall, caregiving can be summarized as providing a pivotal role for health care provision in its role within in-home health care and delaying placement of loved ones into institutionalized care. Every single day, a largely unacknowledged army of caregivers willingly report for duty, fulfilling a variety of tasks, for people with vastly different needs. Their contribution is both extraordinary and humbling at the same time.

Demands of Dementia Caregiving

Dementia caregiving has been recognized as being particularly stressful for a number of reasons. AD is generally slowly progressive, has a long deteriorating course, and typically includes marked deteriorations in multiple aspects of cognition, self-care (e.g., Activities of Daily Living (ADL) and Instrumental Activities of Daily Living (IADL)), and changes in personality and behavior. In addition to wandering, common and highly distressing behavioral problems in AD include dangerous behavior, embarrassing behavior, waking the caregiver, agitation, anger, and depression. Pearlin, Mullan, Semple, and Skaff (1990) describe the actual daily care responsibilities of caregivers (e.g., bathing the patient, managing wandering) as primary stressors. Pearlin et al. also note that caregivers may experience secondary stressors, or spillover effects, from caregiving, including negative effects and heightened stress in marital and family relationships, as well as occupational roles.

Impact on Personal Time

A common feature of caregiving is the time-consuming nature of the endeavor. Though early involvement of caregiving tasks may not involve anything more than a manageable weekly visit to help with finances, groceries, and sorting medications, with time and the progression of dementia, the supervision required by the care-recipient can effectively be all-encompassing. From figures derived from the National Caregiving Study, it was reported that 36.8 percent of the dementia caregivers provide care for 8 hours a week or less, however 16.1 percent of dementia caregivers reported providing constant care depending on the severity of the dementia (Ory, Hoffman, Yee, Tennstedt, & Schulz, 1999). Goode, Haley, Roth, and Ford (1998) found that, in a longitudinal study of AD families, caregivers reported about 62 hours per week spent on caregiving at a baseline assessment, but that caregivers who still had their family member at home a year later reported an average of 83 hours per week in caregiving. A study to determine the characteristics of caregiving in the final year of life of the care recipient with dementia found that for 50 percent of the sample, a minimum of 46 hours are spent on caregiving tasks, and more than half of caregivers described themselves as being "on duty" 24 hours a day (Schulz et al., 2003).

In many instances, caregiving essentially becomes a career that can span many years. The average period of time that a caregiver provides assistance to a spouse or older family member with a chronic illness is 4.3 years, with approximately 30 percent reporting a caregiving career in excess of 5 years (NAC & AARP, 2004). However, AD with its insidious onset and gradual progression can be one of the most arduous for a caregiver, and it is not uncommon for family caregivers to provide in-home care for a relative with AD for 10 years or more.

Physical, Psychological, Social, and Financial Impacts of Dementia Caregiving

The unique stresses and considerable demands of caregiving can adversely impact the physical and psychological health of a caregiver, as well as having social and financial ramifications. Negative physical health effects of caregiving have long been noted specifically in dementia caregiving and in broader studies of general caregiving stress. Such intensive caregiving can result in compromised immune system functioning (Kiecolt-Glaser, Dura, Speicher, Trask, & Glaser, 1991), greater time needed for wound healing (Kiecolt-Glaser, Marucha, Malarkey, Mercado, & Glaser, 1995), and blood pressure elevations (King, Oka, & Young, 1994). Even more alarming is that just the status of being a highly strained caregiver can significantly elevate mortality rate over several years (Schulz & Beach, 1999). The impacts on psychological health are no less disturbing. Caregivers have an increased risk of developing a depressive disorder (approximately 30%) or suffering from significant depressive symptoms (55%), when compared to population norms and matched control groups (Haley & Bailey, 1999; Schulz, O'Brien, Bookwala, & Fleissner, 1995). They also report increased feelings of stress, lower levels of subjective well-being, and lower levels of self-efficacy compared with both noncaregiving controls, and other nondementia caregivers (Pinquart & Sörensen, 2003).

Caregiving has been noted to have serious social ramifications for the social life of both the caregiver and the caregiver's own family. Reduced time to spend with their own family and friends is often reported (NAC & AARP, 2004). Increased supervision of a care recipient often leads to reductions in vacations, hobbies, and leisure activities that a caregiver can independently undertake (NAC & AARP, 2004). Due to reduced participation in general social activities, caregivers are at greater risk for increasing social isolation, which often results in a decline in social support over time (Haley & Bailey, 1999; Robinson-Whelen, Tada, MacCallum, McGuire, & Kiecolt-Glaser, 2001). It is a sad irony that social support can decline at a time when caregiving duties are becoming ever more overwhelming, and more help rather than less is required.

Finally, the unpaid status of caregiving can result in substantial economic hardship for both the caregiver and their family (Langa et al., 2001). This is due in part to the primary caregiver becoming increasingly unable to work outside of the home, due to increased levels of supervision and the escalating demands of caregiving duties (e.g., Schulz et al., 2003). As previously stated, the "career" of a dementia caregiver can span several years and can therefore adversely affect the ability of caregivers to save for their own retirement needs and may force the caregiver to abandon their own retirement plans.

Application of the Stress and Coping Paradigm to Study Caregiving

The caregiving experience has often been studied by incorporating aspects of Lazarus and Folkman's (1984) model of stress and coping (e.g., Haley, Levine, Brown, & Bartolucci, 1987; Harwood, Ownby, Burnett, Barker, & Duara, 2000; Pearlin et al., 1990). Lazarus and Folkman define stress as "a particular relationship between the person and the environment that is appraised by the person as taxing or exceeding his or her resources and endangering his or her well-being" (p. 19). An individual may perceive a situation or event (i.e., potential stressors; e.g., caregiving duties) as irrelevant, benign, or stressful. If perceived as stressful, an individual may appraise the situation as either harmful, threatening, or challenging. These subjective appraisals and individual responses to stress explain why people can and do react very differently when faced with the same set of circumstances.

How a stressful situation is appraised is only part of the stress-coping model. People can overcome stress by effectively adopting strategies that manage potential stressors, that is, coping. According to Lazarus and Folkman (1984), there are two major types of coping. Coping can be emotion-focused (e.g., finding empathy in a support group to alleviate frustration) or problem-focused (e.g., utilizing behavioral techniques to address particular challenging behaviors such as wandering). However, if there is either no resolution or an unfavorable resolution, then psychological distress can ensue, and stress can proliferate. The unrelenting nature of the chronic strains and stress that can accompany dementia caregiving may not always be ameliorated using problem-focused or emotion-focused coping. There remain particular circumstances where there is no possibility of satisfactory outcomes in terms of final resolution (e.g., the knowledge of the progressive nature and increasing severity of dementia). Despite intractable situations, it was recognized that some caregivers are still able to effectively combat stress. This prompted the addition of meaning-based coping to the Stress and Coping model (Folkman, 1997). Examples of meaning-based coping include revising one's goal to regain purpose and control, using one's spiritual beliefs, or reevaluating the caregiving experience as a period of great personal growth. It has been suggested that caregivers may sustain their quality of life by deriving self-esteem in their caregiving role (Nijboer, Triemstra, Tempelaar, Sanderman, & van den Bos, 1999). The critical aspect of Lazarus and Folkman's (1984) model is the emphasis on how the individual personally appraises a situation rather than the occurrence or severity of the potential stressor per se.

In addition, stress and coping models emphasize that the ability to successfully handle caregiving stressors is largely dependent on the coping resources of the caregiver, compared with the vulnerability of the caregiver (Vitaliano, Zhang, & Scanlan, 2003). Lazarus and Folkman (1984) categorized coping resources as being either internal (e.g., personality, sense of meaning, problem solving skills, use of benign appraisals, previous experience) or external (e.g., money, social support, or an appropriately modified environment).

One can view stress and coping with caregiving as a balancing act with high levels of stressors being factors that increase the likelihood of negative caregiver outcomes, while high levels of resources tend to decrease the likelihood of caregiver distress. As noted in Figure 7.1, caregivers can face both primary and secondary caregiving stressors (as described previously), but also other life stressors and strains (e.g., bereavement, poverty, and crime). Interventions for family caregivers, which will be described in greater detail later, can enhance caregiver well-being by reducing stressors (e.g., decreasing wandering), improving internal resources (e.g., teaching caregivers

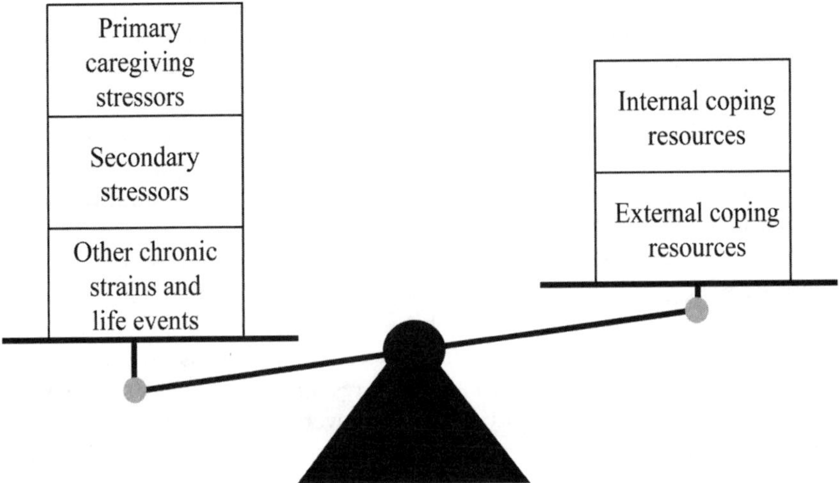

FIGURE 7.1 Caregiving: A balancing act of stress and coping.

coping skills, or altering appraisals), or enhancing external resources (e.g., improving social support, or improving the physical environment).

Thus, when assessing stressors that can impact caregiver well-being, it is important to assess not only primary stressors, but also other stressors, how caregivers appraise stressors (e.g., how stressful and controllable the caregiver views these problems as), and caregivers' internal and external resources. The remainder of this chapter will concentrate specifically on the complex behavior of wandering, with particular regard to issues that manifest for caregivers.

How Does Wandering Impact Caregivers?

According to Silverstein, Flaherty, and Tobin (2002), the first consequence of wandering is emotional, both for the person with dementia who wanders from home and for their family, who are under a great deal of stress. Behavioral problems, including wandering, can be extremely difficult for family members to manage (Haley, Wadley, West, & Vetzel, 1994). Caregivers in one study (Ford, Goode, Barrett, Harrell, & Haley, 1997) reported wandering and getting lost as the second most stressful behavioral problem (after dangerous behaviors). Caregivers consistently rated behavioral problems as more stressful than deficiencies in instrumental activities of daily living or activities of daily living, although wandering occurred much less frequently. Caregivers are all too aware of the dangers of wandering. Tragic consequences can befall a wanderer including serious injury (Colon-Emeric, Biggs, Schenck, & Lyles, 2003) and, if unable to be located in a timely manner, death (Rowe & Glover, 2001).

According to Hope and colleagues (2001), the variety of ways wandering behaviors can manifest can vary dramatically and therefore, caregivers will have different stresses to contend with. In a study by Logsdon and colleagues (1998), over half of the sample of caregivers reported at least moderate levels of distress about wandering. The level of distress also increased significantly as the frequency of wandering increased. Caregivers indicated that one of their biggest worries is that the person with dementia will wander and become lost in the community. As established by studies that have utilized stress and coping models, caregivers' subjective appraisals of problem behaviors can be better predictors of caregiver well-being than the actual severity or frequency of those behaviors (Haley et al., 1987).

Research has demonstrated that wandering often occurs within a cluster of other behavioral, cognitive, and functional impairments (Logsdon et al., 1998). This may serve to compound the amount of distress felt by caregivers. In some cases, all areas of impairment need to be addressed in order to provide stress relief, and in other cases only particularly troublesome areas warrant attention. Each case should be approached individually. Additionally, the vigilance required by caregivers can be very stressful—near constant monitoring, regardless of the potential function of the behavior, is necessary (Feliciano, Vore, LeBlanc, & Baker, 2004). This can become particularly fatiguing not only on a day to day basis, but due to the intermittent nature of wandering, over the course of months and years. Furthermore, the situation can be further exacerbated if a caregiver has limited social support and little or no access to respite care, to have adequate "off-time" where they are free from their supervisory function.

Nighttime wandering can be particularly stressful for caregivers because of the disruption of their own sleep. Wandering itself, along with excessive nighttime activity that includes wandering, are significant predictors of future institutionalization (Gaugler et al., 2000; Hope, Keene, Gedling, Fairburn, & Jacoby, 1998). Neistein and Siegal (1996) blame the constant vigilance necessary of caregivers of dementia patients as contributing to this finding. Caregivers may find this level of supervision and management simply too stressful or may feel they are unable to provide constant supervision for their loved one, leading to placement in a long-term care facility. A surprising finding recently noted in the literature is that if frequent behavior problems (including wandering) occur very early in the caregivers' career, then caregivers are more likely to suffer from increased burden, depressive symptomatology, and to institutionalize their care recipients sooner (Gaugler, Kane, Kane, & Newcomer, 2005). A proposed explanation given by Gaugler and colleagues is that new caregivers who are quickly exposed to problematic behaviors, have insufficient time to adjust and master the demands of their new role, and quickly become overwhelmed.

Finally, caregivers have to grapple with the ethical issues regarding the use of restraints, locks, and monitoring devices to manage wandering behaviors. Furthermore, restriction of freedom can be particularly difficult in earlier stages of dementia, when the care recipient has extensive periods of lucidity. In fact, many people who have become lost on a previous occasion continue to go out unaccompanied by a caregiver (McShane, Gedling, Keene, et al., 1998). In such circumstances one can see the difficulty the caregiver may encounter when trying to curtail possible activities that would make wandering potentially more hazardous.

CAREGIVING INTERVENTIONS

General Information Regarding Caregiving Interventions

The primary goal of caregiving research is not just to describe how the caregiving experience impacts health and well-being, or to identify what aspects cause particular distress, but to provide a sound evidence-base from which interventions can be designed and implemented to alleviate the considerable burden of caregiving and promote better outcomes in caregiver well-being. Sörensen, Pinquart, and Duberstein (2002) conducted a meta-analysis of the efficacy of 78 caregiver intervention studies. Overall, the best results were found when using structured and individualized interventions. Of the six types of intervention studies that were compared, psychotherapy and psychoeducational interventions were the two most effective, consistently reporting positive improvements for caregivers in five clinically relevant domains. These were burden, depression, well-being, ability or knowledge, as well as improvement in care recipients' symptoms. A similar pattern was reported when the meta-analysis was confined to randomized studies, except no improvement was noted for psychoeducational interventions on caregiver well-being and care recipients' symptoms.

According to Sörensen and colleagues (2002), psychotherapy required a therapeutic relationship to be established between the trained professional and the caregiver. Cognitive-Behavioral Therapy was the most common type of psychotherapy and used elements such as challenging negative thinking and assumptions, engagement of pleasant activities, and teaching effective time management strategies. Psychoeducational interventions provided information in group settings about the care recipient's disease process and training and resources for the caregiver to manage disease-related problems. The information was delivered in a structured format, in lectures, group discussions, and supplied written materials. Both types of interventions have a large educational component. In psychotherapy it is directed toward increasing self-knowledge of the caregiver, whereas the psychoeducational approach is directed toward increasing the knowledge of the care recipient's disease and symptoms.

One important finding was that although interventions were effective for all types of caregiving contexts, nevertheless, for dementia caregivers the effects were not as pronounced. Sörensen et al. (2002) attribute this to the unpredictable nature of behavior problems and personality changes. Birkel and Jones (1989) suggest behavior problems may be less modifiable than physical aspects of care, leading Sörensen and colleagues to conclude that dementia caregivers may be a difficult population to effect change.

Despite dementia caregivers seemingly being at a disadvantage for reduced magnitude of effects compared with other caregivers, there is still every reason to be optimistic regarding the ability of caregiving interventions to improve well-being. A notable example of a structured dementia caregiver intervention study used individualized, family, and support group sessions, as well as unlimited ad hoc counseling to their intervention group (Mittelman, Roth, Coon, & Haley, 2004). This study found sustained benefits in reducing caregiver depressive symptoms, and the intervention group showed less depressive symptoms for a 3-year period compared with a randomized control group.

Caregiving Interventions That Address Wandering Behaviors

There is ample literature regarding the relative success of general caregiving interventions to improve well-being in caregivers, as reviewed in the previous section. However, there are fewer examples of studies that have specifically targeted wandering as an outcome measure for improvement in the care recipient and for the reduction of stress and burden in the caregiver. Often, as illustrated in the following three studies, caregiver interventions include wandering under the rubric of "problem behaviors." Interventions that address wandering can be categorized into three design types—(a) those concerned with reducing caregiver burden and reactivity to promote positive outcomes while not addressing problem behaviors in the care recipient; (b) those designed to effectively manage, modify, or reduce wandering behavior in the care recipient by educating the caregiver on management strategies and techniques, again with the goal of promoting positive caregiver outcomes; and (c) interventions that target both problem occurrence and reaction. The following studies are notable examples of these designs.

Mittelman, Roth, Haley, and Zarit (2004) investigated the efficacy of a targeted caregiver intervention to reduce negative appraisals of behavior problems in dementia caregiving, including wandering behaviors. This is another example of a study that used the stress and coping paradigm as a theoretical framework. There was no significant difference between the intervention group and the "usual care" control group in reported frequency of behavior problems in their respective care recipients. In both groups, the frequency of behavior problems increased for the duration of the 4-year study period. However, there was significant reduction in caregiver reaction scores to behavioral problems that continued to decline over the 4-year period, whereas reaction scores continued to increase in the control group. Therefore, as predicted by the stress and coping models, despite increasing frequency of problem behaviors, the caregivers were no longer appraising them negatively and could effectively cope despite increasing behavioral demands.

Teri, McCurry, Logsdon, and Gibbons (2005) studied the impact of an individualized psychoeducational intervention, that included educating caregivers on behavior modification techniques, communication techniques, increasing pleasant events, and development of strategies to improve caregiver support. A novel aspect regarding this study was that each caregiver was required to choose the three most problematic behaviors exhibited by their care recipient, and their subsequent intervention was individually tailored to address them. Wandering was one of the behaviors that the authors listed as being targeted by caregivers. Overall, when considering the success across all three target behaviors, 62 percent of caregivers had significant improvement in their caregiver-reactivity scores, 57 percent reported a reduction in the frequency of the problem behaviors, and 52 percent reported reduction in problem severity. Furthermore, significant reductions occurred for depressive symptoms, subjective burden, and reactivity to all potential problem behaviors, and these benefits were maintained at a 6-month follow-up. Although the results are encouraging, it is not known whether these effects were particularly salient to certain problem behaviors above others as they were not independently analyzed by behavior type.

Burgio, Stevens, Guy, Roth, and Haley (2003) conducted a study comparing in-home caregiver behavioral training with a telephone support control group. This intervention attempted to give caregivers improved behavioral management skills, as well as addressing caregiver appraisals and attempting to improve caregiver mastery. The in-home training program was effective both in reducing behavioral problems and in reducing stressfulness appraisals, although the control group also showed similar benefits over time.

General Strategies Used by Caregivers to Manage Wandering

There are a number of management techniques that specifically target wandering behaviors, not necessarily with the primary intent to either reduce the behavior or promote well-being in the care recipient—rather they contain the wandering behavior, alert the caregiver that it is happening, or provide vital information in the event that the wanderer successfully evades the caregiver.

Identification Information and Tracking Devices

Mace and Rabins (1999) advise caregivers to write simple instructions on a card the person carries and can refer to if lost. Regardless of the severity of the dementia, the authors suggest the impaired person wear an identification bracelet or necklace identifying them as a person with dementia and containing the person's contact information. This information can be a life saver for a person if they get lost.

Furthermore, a more formalized program is provided by the Alzheimer's Association called Safe Return®, which offers invaluable information for preventing someone from becoming lost and also aids in the search to find a lost person. Registration in the program includes identification bracelets, necklaces, or clothing tags to facilitate the return of the lost person. When a person becomes lost, the caregiver can call a toll-free telephone number in order to activate a search for the person. Safe Return® staff work with local law enforcement and first responders to locate the lost individual. See Chapter 13 for more information on the Safe Return® project.

McShane, Gedling, Kenward, and colleagues (1998) evaluated an electronic tracking device for use with older adults with dementia at risk of wandering and becoming lost. The device consists of a small transmitter worn by the person with dementia and a hand-held direction-finding receiver used by the person searching for the wanderer. The device was moderately successful in the few cases in which a person became lost while wearing the transmitter. Caregivers who needed the least amount of training for the device used it most successfully, while others were reluctant or unable to use the tracking system. However, as technology in this area improves, tracking devices may be a viable option for caregivers in use with care recipients who are at risk for wandering. See Chapter 15 for more information on technology solutions to manage wandering.

Exercise

Mace and Rabins (1999) also suggest caregivers take the person with dementia on long, vigorous walks each day in an effort to curtail wandering. They remind caregivers that it may take several weeks before any improvement is noticeable. It is also important to notice if the wandering behavior has a particular pattern and to tie-in walks to coincide with such a pattern. For example—nighttime wandering may be helped by taking a long walk before bedtime, or if wandering occurs in the morning hours, then a long walk after breakfast may be beneficial. Teri et al. (2003) have demonstrated that a combined patient exercise/caregiver training program improves the quality of life and daily functioning of patients with AD, but did not focus specifically on wandering in their study.

Home Modifications

Modifying the home environment can be as simple as installing alarms and locks on the doors. Mace and Rabins (1999) note that for some individuals, spring-operated latches or other similar devices may be effective, because the person cannot learn how to operate them. Windows, even on the second story of a home, must also be secured. Caregivers need to be aware of outside hazards in the area such as wooded areas, dangerous roads, swimming pools, and other bodies of water. See Chapter 16 for more information on environmental modifications as well as Chapter 14, which describes a home safety program for community-based wanderers.

Physical Restraints

For some individuals who wander, infrequent use of physical restraints may be warranted. Mace and Rabins (1999) suggest the use of soft restraints such as Posey restraints, or a Gerichair, a recliner with a locking tray, which prevents the person from getting up. These devices should be used only as a last resort in a small number of cases when there are serious safety and health risks associated with persistant wandering. There are significant risks associated with using these devices inappropriately or incorrectly, which caregivers must be made aware.

Management Techniques Tested in Nursing Homes and Long-Term Care Settings

There are a number of management techniques that have been utilized in long-term care settings and reviewed in detail in other chapters in this book. Many of these show great promise for implementation in home settings though some would require considerable modification. These interventions may include sensory stimulation (Lucero, Pearson, Hutchinson, Leger-Krall, & Rinalducci, 2001), visual barriers and redirection (Feliciano et al., 2004), music (Siders et al., 2004), cloth barriers (Roberts, 1999), and improved environmental ambiance (Yao & Algase, 2006).

There are obviously management techniques used in long-term care facilities that can be applied very easily to the home setting, but there are also situations when such approaches are too expensive, unfeasible in terms of supervision, and are not readily transferable to home settings. Burgio et al. (2003) utilized a variety of such interventions in their in-home caregiver training program, such as behavioral analysis (e.g., examining circumstances that heighten wandering), environmental modifications (e.g., mirrors on doors), reducing excessive stimulation (such as television), use of distraction, and differential reward of other behavior. These interventions are described in a treatment manual available from Burgio and colleagues and are addressed in more detail in Chapter 11.

METHODOLOGICAL CHALLENGES AND FUTURE DIRECTIONS

There are still many unanswered questions that need to be addressed to guide appropriate interventions for caregivers who must cope with wandering behaviors in their home. Part of the difficulty that researchers face is to decide what to prioritize in their research design. Is it better for wandering specific interventions to be employed, or is the best approach to incorporate it as a component of a comprehensive package of interventions?

It is possible that specific interventions may have limited success in improving caregiving well-being in general. As Lai and Arthur (2003) conclude, interventions that have used medications, activity programs, behavioral modification, or environmental manipulation to combat wandering behaviors are still questionable in their overall efficacy. It is clear that wandering specific interventions are still not optimal, and research is needed to further refine them.

A salient issue with wandering is, because of its intermittent nature, positive results of intervention studies may be profoundly underestimated, not because the intervention is ineffective, merely because the duration of the study may not be enough to determine a clinically meaningful change. Another measurement issue is if the caregiver intervention is first and foremost intended to improve caregiver well-being, reactivity to the wandering, and to lessen their feelings of burden, then the measures chosen must be relevant to capture that change. The importance of selecting specific outcome measures appropriate to the intervention has been highlighted by Zarit, Stephens, Townsend, and Greene (1998). Though their comments were in relation to how daycare facilities can be studied for their ability to promote psychological well-being in dementia caregivers, they are also relevant in the context of any caregiver intervention. In this situation, for example, monitoring caregiving burden as an outcome on a wandering specific intervention may be too crude to detect an effect, whereas if a measure of caregiving burden only with regard to wandering was measured, then a more positive outcome may very well be detected.

Zarit et al. (1998) also argued that multiple time points, both proximal and distal, are required in case some measures of outcomes take longer to detect change than others. For example, measures of depressive symptomatology may not register an immediate change post intervention but could manifest several months later. Given that the dementia caregiver will rarely be so lucky as to only have wandering as an issue, the question remains as to what is the best way to support dementia caregivers? How is success in an intervention to be judged? A researcher must determine if improvement on wandering specific measures only is desired, or if improvement of more global measures of caregiver well-being is the goal. Ultimately, interventions should be beneficial to the caregiver. Given the time constraints a caregiver endures, it is imperative that interventions are easy to undertake and that the beneficial effects are of a duration that far outweighs the time over which the intervention was implemented.

Although meta-analyses have compared the efficacy of various types of intervention designs (e.g., Sörensen et al., 2002), caregiver interventions have rarely been decomposed to ascertain the necessary and sufficient active ingredients in intervention. There may be types of caregivers who respond better to one approach above others. Furthermore, if combined approaches do not result in demonstrably better outcomes, future interventions could be considerably cheaper, ultimately leading to greater number of caregivers receiving assistance.

Lai and Arthur (2003) state that the reasons why wandering behavior manifests are still not understood. Due to lack of theories regarding etiology of wandering, researchers and clinicians have been hindered in what to target in interventions (Kiely, Morris, & Algase, 2000). Other theoretical frameworks (e.g., stress and coping models) have been adopted to guide intervention design, but etiologically-based interventions may be more effective in behavior management, with the potential of bolstering caregiver outcomes.

It is evident that research that examines wandering behavior within community-dwelling older adults still lags behind that conducted with their counterparts who reside in long-term care facilities. This is despite the fact that more adults with dementia are cared for at home rather than in residential long-term care. Furthermore, most studies of the effectiveness of management techniques are also conducted in nursing homes. Future research needs to address the feasibility of translating these techniques from the nursing home environment to a usable form for informal caregivers.

Clinicians, researchers, and policy makers are urged to recognize that family caregivers are at risk for adverse outcomes psychologically and physically due to stresses they face in their role. It is crucial to address the needs of family caregivers as part of comprehensive care for the person with dementia. Research needs to ascertain under what circumstances to implement wandering specific or general caregiver interventions to optimize outcomes. Caregivers make many sacrifices in emotional, financial, health, and social terms to provide this care. We should do everything possible to ensure that they receive the appropriate levels of support and professional guidance needed to maintain their essential role for as long as they desire to. Family caregivers have many different issues to contend with, but the stressful and potentially dangerous, and sadly sometimes fatal results of a wandering care recipient, requires urgent attention to address the evident gaps in our current knowledge of this phenomenon.

REFERENCES

Arno, P. S., Levine, C., & Memmott, M. M. (1999). The economic value of informal caregiving. *Health Affairs, 18*(2), 182–188.

Birkel, R. C., & Jones, C. J. (1989). A comparison of the caregiving networks of dependent elderly individuals who are lucid and those who are demented. *The Gerontologist, 29*(1), 114–119.

Burgio, L., Stevens, A. B., Guy, D., Roth, D. L., & Haley, W. E. (2003). Impact of two interventions on White and African-American family caregivers of individuals with dementia. *The Gerontologist, 43*(4), 568–579.

Colon-Emeric, C. S., Biggs, D. P., Schenck, A. P., & Lyles, K. W. (2003). Risk factors for hip fracture in skilled nursing facilities: Who should be evaluated? *Osteoporosis International, 14*(6), 484–489.

Feliciano, L., Vore, J., LeBlanc, L. A., & Baker, J. C. (2004). Decreasing entry into a restricted area using a visual barrier. *Journal of Applied Behavior Analysis, 37*(1), 107–110.

Folkman, S. (1997). Positive psychological states and coping with severe stress. *Social Science & Medicine, 45*(8), 1207–1221.

Ford, G. R., Goode, K. T., Barrett, J. J., Harrell, L. E., & Haley, W. E. (1997). Gender roles and caregiving stress: An examination of subjective appraisals of specific primary stressors in Alzheimer's caregivers. *Aging and Mental Health, 1*(2), 158–165.

Gaugler, J. E., Edwards, A. B., Femia, E. E., Zarit, S. H., Stephens, M. P., Townsend, A., et al. (2000). Predictors of institutionalization of cognitively impaired elders: Family help and the timing of placement. *Journal of Gerontology Series B: Psychological Sciences, 55*(4), P247–P255.

Gaugler, J. E., Kane, R. L., Kane, R. S., & Newcomer, R. (2005). The longitudinal effects of early behavior problems in the dementia caregiving career. *Psychology and Aging, 20*(1), 100–116.

Goode, K. T., Haley, W. E., Roth, D. L., & Ford, G. R. (1998). Predicting longitudinal changes in caregiver physical and mental health: A stress process model. *Health Psychology, 17*(2), 190–198.

Haley, W. E., & Bailey, S. (1999). Research on family caregiving in Alzheimer's disease: Implications for practice and policy. In B. Vellas & J. L. Fitten (Eds.), *Research and practice in Alzheimer's disease: Vol. 2* (pp. 321–332). Paris: Serdi.

Haley, W. E., Levine, E. G., Brown, S. L., & Bartolucci, A. A. (1987). Stress, appraisal, coping and social support as predictors of adaptational outcomes among dementia caregivers. *Psychology and Aging, 2*(4), 323–330.

Haley, W. E., & Perkins, E. A. (2004). Current status and future directions in family caregiving and aging people with intellectual disabilities. *Journal of Policy and Practice in Intellectual Disabilities, 1*(1), 24–30.

Haley, W. E., Wadley, V. G., West, C. A. C., & Vetzel, L. L. (1994). How caregiving stressors change with severity of dementia. *Seminars in Speech and Language, 15*(3), 195–205.

Harwood, D. G., Ownby, R. L., Burnett, K., Barker, W. W., & Duara, R. (2000). Predictors of appraisal and psychological well-being in Alzheimer's disease family caregivers. *Journal of Clinical Geropsychology, 6*(4), 279–297.

Hope, T., Keene, J., Gedling, K., Fairburn, C. G., & Jacoby, R. (1998). Predictors of institutionalization for people with dementia living at home with a carer. *International Journal of Geriatric Psychiatry, 13*(10), 682–690.

Hope, T., Keene, J., McShane, R. H., Fairburn, C. G., Gedling, K., & Jacoby, R. (2001). Wandering in dementia: A longitudinal study. *International Psychogeriatrics, 13*(2), 137–147.

Kiecolt-Glaser, J. K., Dura, J. R., Speicher, C.E., Trask, O. J., & Glaser, R. (1991). Spousal caregivers of dementia victims: Longitudinal changes in immunity and health. *Psychosomatic Medicine, 53*(4), 345–362.

Kiecolt-Glaser, J. K., Marucha, P. T., Malarkey, W. B., Mercado, A.M., & Glaser, R. (1995). Slowing of wound healing by psychological stress. *The Lancet, 346*(8984), 1194–1196.

Kiely, D. K., Morris, J. N., & Algase, D. L. (2000). Resident characteristics associated with wandering in nursing homes. *International Journal of Geriatric Psychiatry, 15*(11), 1013–1020.

King, A. C., Oka, R. K., & Young, D. R. (1994). Ambulatory blood pressure and heart rate responses to the stress of work and caregiving in older women. *Journal of Gerontology: Medical Sciences, 49*(6), M239–M245.

Lai, C. K. Y., & Arthur, D. G. (2003). Wandering behaviour in people with dementia. *Journal of Advanced Nursing, 44,* 173–182.

Langa, K. M., Chernew, M. E., Kabeto, M. U., Herzog, A. R., Ofstedal, M. B., Willis R. J., et al. (2001). National estimates of the quantity and cost of informal caregiving for the elderly with dementia. *Journal of General Internal Medicine, 16*(11), 770–778.

Lazarus, R. S., & Folkman, S. (1984). *Stress, Appraisal and Coping.* New York: Springer.

Logsdon, R. G., Teri, L., McCurry, S. M., Gibbons, L. E., Kukull, W. A., & Larson, E. B. (1998). Wandering: A significant problem among community-residing individuals with Alzheimer's disease. *Journal of Gerontology, Series B: Psychological Sciences, 53*(5), P294–P299.

Lucero, M., Pearson, R., Hutchinson, S., Leger-Krall, S., & Rinalducci, E. (2001). Products for Alzheimer's self-stimulatory wanderers. *American Journal of Alzheimer's Disease and Other Dementias, 16*(1), 43–50.

Mace, N. L., & Rabins, P. V. (1999). *The 36-Hour Day.* New York: Warner.

Martínez-Martín, P., Benito-León, J., Alonso, F., Catalán, M. J., Pondal, M., Zamarbide, I., et al. (2005). Quality of life of caregivers in Parkinson's disease. *Quality of Life Research, 4*(2), 463–472.

McCullagh, E., Brigstocke, G., Donaldson, N., & Kalra, L. (2005). Determinants of caregiving burden and quality of life in caregivers of stroke patients. *Stroke, 36*(10), 2181–2186.

McDonell, M.G., Short, R. A., Berry, C. B., & Dyck, D. G. (2003). Burden in schizophrenia caregivers: Impact of family psychoeducation and awareness of patient suicidality. *Family Process, 42*(1), 91–103.

McShane, R., Gedling, K., Keene, J., Fairburn, C., Jacoby, R., & Hope, T. (1998). Getting lost in dementia: A longitudinal study of a behavioral symptom. *International Psychogeriatrics, 10*(3), 253–260.

McShane, R., Gedling, K., Kenward, B., Kenward, R., Hope, T., & Jacoby, R. (1998). The feasibility of electronic tracking devices in dementia: A telephone survey and case series. *International Journal of Geriatric Psychiatry, 13*(8), 556–563.

Mittelman, M., Roth, D., Coon, D., & Haley, W. E. (2004). Sustained benefit of supportive intervention for depressive symptoms in Alzheimer's caregivers. *American Journal of Psychiatry, 161*(5), 850–856.

Mittelman, M. S., Roth, D. L., Haley, W. E., & Zarit, S. (2004). Effects of a caregiver intervention on negative caregiver appraisals of behavior problems in patients with

Alzheimer's disease: Results of a randomized trial. *Journal of Gerontology, Series B: Psychological Sciences, 59*(1), P27–P34.

National Alliance for Caregiving & AARP. (2004). *Caregiving in the US*. Retrieved May 9, 2006, from http://www.caregiving.org/data/04finalreport.pdf.

Neistein, S., & Siegal, A. P. (1996). Agitation, wandering, pacing, restlessness, and repetitive mannerisms. *International Psychogeriatrics, 8*(Suppl. 3), 399–402.

Nijboer, C., Triemstra, M., Tempelaar, R., Sanderman, R., & van den Bos, G. A. (1999). Determinants of caregiving experiences and mental health of partners of cancer patients. *Cancer, 86*(4), 577–588.

Ory, M. G., Hoffman, R. R., Yee, J. L., Tennstedt, S., & Schulz, R. (1999). Prevalence and impact of caregiving: A detailed comparison between dementia and nondementia caregivers. *The Gerontologist, 39,* 177–185.

Pearlin, L. I., Mullan, J. T., Semple, S. J., & Skaff, M. M. (1990). Caregiving and the stress process: An overview of concepts and their measures. *The Gerontologist, 30*(5), 583–594.

Pinquart, M., & Sörensen, S. (2003). Differences between caregivers and noncaregivers in psychological health and physical health: a meta-analysis. *Psychology and Aging, 18*(2), 250–267.

Roberts, C. (1999). The management of wandering in older people with dementia. *Journal of Clinical Nursing, 8*(3), 322–324.

Robinson-Whelen, S. R., Tada, Y., MacCallum, R. C., McGuire, L., & Kiecolt-Glaser, J. K. (2001). Long-term caregiving: What happens when it ends? *Journal of Abnormal Psychology, 110*(4), 573–584.

Rowe, M. A., & Glover, J. C. (2001). Antecedents, descriptions, and consequences of wandering in cognitively-impaired adults and the Safe Return (SR) program. *American Journal of Alzheimer's Disease and Other Dementias, 16*(6), 344–352.

Schulz, R., & Beach, S. R. (1999). Caregiving as a risk for mortality. The Caregiver Health Effects Study. *Journal of the American Medical Association, 282*(23), 2215–2219.

Schulz, R., Mendelsohn, A. B., Haley, W. E., Mahoney, D., Allen, R. S., Zhang, S., et al. (2003). End-of-life care and the effects of bereavement on family caregivers of persons with dementia. *The New England Journal of Medicine, 349*(20), 1936–1942.

Schulz, R., O'Brien, A. T., Bookwala, J., & Fleissner, K. (1995). Psychiatric and physical morbidity effects of dementia caregiving: Prevalence, correlates, and causes. *The Gerontologist, 35*(6), 771–791.

Siders, C., Nelson, A., Brown, L. M., Joseph, I., Algase, D., Beattie, E., et al. (2004). Evidence for implementing nonpharmacological interventions for wandering. *Rehabilitation Nursing, 29*(6), 195–206.

Silverstein, N. M., Flaherty, G., & Tobin, T. S. (2002). *Dementia and wandering behavior: Concern for the lost elder.* New York: Springer.

Sörensen, S., Pinquart, M., & Duberstein, P. (2002). How effective are interventions with caregivers? An updated meta-analysis. *The Gerontologist, 42*(3), 356–372.

Teri, L., Gibbons, L. E., McCurry, S. M., Logsdon, R. G., Buchner, D. M., Barlow, W. E., et al. (2003). Exercise plus behavioral management in patients with Alzheimer disease: A randomized controlled trial. *Journal of the American Medical Association, 290*(15), 2015–2022.

Teri, L., McCurry, S. M., Logsdon, R., & Gibbons, L. E. (2005). Training community consultants to help family members improve dementia care: A randomized controlled trial. *The Gerontologist, 45*(6), 802–811.

Thompson, L. (2004, March). *Long-term care: Support for family caregivers.* Long Term Care Financing Project, Georgetown University. Issue Brief. Retrieved May 8, 2006, from http://ltc.georgetown.edu/pdfs/caregivers.pdf.

U.S. Census Bureau. (2000). *The 65 years and over population: 2000.* Retrieved May 8, 2006, from http://www.nationalatlas.gov/articles/people/a_age65pop.html.
Vanderwerker, L. C., Laff, R. E., Kadan-Lottick, N. S., McColl, S., & Prigerson, H. G. (2005). Psychiatric disorders and mental health service use among caregivers of advanced cancer patients. *Journal of Clinical Oncology, 23*(28), 6899–6907.
Vitaliano, P. P., Zhang, J., & Scanlan, J. M. (2003). Is caregiving hazardous to one's physical health? A meta-analysis. *Psychological Bulletin, 129*(6), 946–972.
Yao, L., & Algase, D. (2006). Environmental ambiance as a new window on wandering. *Western Journal of Nursing Research, 28*(1), 89–104.
Zarit, S. H., Stephens, M. A. P., Townsend, A., & Greene, R. (1998). Stress reduction for family caregivers: Effects of adult day care use. *Journal of Gerontology, Series B: Social Sciences, 53*(5), S267–S277.

CHAPTER EIGHT

Cultural Issues Associated With Wandering

Inez Joseph and Gwi-Ryung Son Hong

INTRODUCTION

There are some unique cultural issues associated with wandering. *Culture* is usually defined as a community in which individuals value and respect one another and help each other, much like family members might do (Galanti, 2005). A culture emerges regardless of the care setting, including a home within a community, an assisted living facility, or a long-term care facility. Dependency and deterioration that often accompanies aging and disease, dementia and Alzheimer's, is supported by growth, creativity, and regenerativity in a vastly improved quality of life through community support.

There is a great deal of discussion in literature around the issues of wandering and the potential adverse outcomes to patients, such as falls, fractures, fatigue, weight loss, sleep disturbances, abuse by those they encounter along the way, and even untimely death (Aud, 2004; Rowe & Bennett, 2003; Algase, Beattie, Leitsch, & Beel-Bates, 2003; Lucero, 2002; Goldsmith, Hoeffer, & Rader, 1995; Thomas, 1995; Cohen-Mansfield, Werner, Culpepper, & Barkley, 1997). There are also numerous cultural issues associated with wandering, which unfortunately have not been addressed adequately in literature (Cohen & Day, 2000; Galanti, 2005).

Extensive research has mentioned the differences in Asian and Western culture, demonstrating that Asian culture is described as valuing harmony and accepting passively, while Western culture presumably places greater value on individualism and assertiveness. Thus, a person's behavior is vastly influenced by not only the macro level of culture such as health care system, language, social value, and the relationship between caregiver and care recipient, but also by the micro level of a person's own experiences such as personal preference, familiarity, and activities. In Eastern cultures, wandering behavior may be viewed as part of the normal aging processes, while it is considered as abnormal behavior in Western culture.

There is some evidence that rates of wandering behaviors vary by ethnicity. The prevalence of wandering/purposeless or inappropriate activities was reported to be as high as 89 percent in all ethnic minority populations including African Americans, Asian Americans, Hispanics, and Native Americans at the clinical dementia rating (CDR) stage of 2 or 3 (Chen, Borson, & Scanlan, 2000), as opposed to the rates for pacing and wandering, which ranged from 3 percent (Rabins, Mace, & Lucas, 1982) to 59 percent (Teri, Larson, & Reifler, 1988) in persons with dementia (PWDs) who were mostly white. In addition, Sink, Covinsky, Newcomer, and Yaff (2004) found that blacks showed more wandering behavior than whites. In our search, only three studies (Algase, Son, et al., 2004; Song et al., 2003; Son, Song, & Lim, 2006) were conducted specifically on wandering behavior among persons with dementia/AD in different cultures. Given the trends for differences found in earlier studies, this points to a strong need for researchers to examine these differences more fully in future research.

The very first cross-cultural comparison study (Song et al., 2003) examining wandering behavior in residents of long-term care settings in the United States, Canada, and Australia noted that U.S. residents (mean age = 86.1) were significantly older than Canadians (mean age = 82.8), and Australians (80.2). Overall, nurses in Canada reported significantly lower ratings on wandering than nurses in either the United States or Australia, where rates were similar. Although the nature of wandering behavior of PWDs in these three countries was not significantly different, the issues of staff training and cultural tolerance for various behaviors may contribute to differences.

A comparison study with both American and Japanese nursing home residents found the same trend of wandering behaviors decreasing at night (Schreiner, Yamamoto, & Shiotani, 2000). The Japanese sample showed higher means for exit seeking, inappropriate disrobing, and inappropriate handling, whereas the American sample showed higher negativism and repetitious mannerisms. In both samples, wandering, general restlessness, and repetitive questioning were the most frequent behaviors. Wandering was noted as the highest mean score among the behaviors in the Japanese sample, and it was highly correlated with general restlessness (r = .63), exit seeking (r = .69), and inappropriate handling (r = .46). Among nursing home residents, wandering behavior was the highly prevalent behavior regardless of ethnic group.

Using the same instruments, Revised-Algase Wandering Scale for wandering behavior of community-residing PWDs in both the United States and Korea, Son et al. (2006) found that PWDs in Korea (n = 69) demonstrated lower wandering scores in all subscales of measurement than those in the United States (n = 266) (Algase, Beattie, et al., 2004), although the difference between the two samples was not statistically confirmed (Algase et al., 2004; Son et al., 2006). Of the 69 PWDs studied in Korea, 36 (52.1%) were identified by family caregivers as wanderers ranging from wanderers at times to a problematic wanderer. A total of 155 (57.8%) community-residing PWDs out of 266 in the U.S. study were identified into three categories based on the level of wandering: wanderer at times (n = 68); wanderer but not a problem (n = 34); and wanderer and a problem (n = 36). PWDs in Korea showed the highest score of eloping behavior subscale (mean = 2.04) and PWDs in the United States showed the highest score of persistent walking (mean = 2.28) among wandering subscales. The cognitive functional level, as measured by the Mini Mental State Examination (MMSE), was moderately impaired (mean score = 14.85, SD = 5.97) in the Korean population, and the mean age of Korean PWDs (mean age = 75.9 years) was younger than that in the United States (mean age = 78.6 years). Overall, about half of the study sample from either Korea or the United States demonstrated wandering behavior among community residing PWDs.

Culture and Caregiving

As the elderly population increases, the experiences of caring and providing care for a family member who wanders is expected to increase (Rust & Strothers, 2000). Health care professionals cannot ignore the importance of cultural factors such as beliefs and practices in diverse cultures, specifically when managing the care of elderly wanderers. Caregivers must recognize the impact of a multicultural society in the clinical area on such things as communication and health care practices.

African American and Caucasian families of dementia are faced with numerous challenges when their loved one wanders. They eventually loose their freedom, jobs, and their social contacts. However, African American caregivers reported lower stress and higher levels of family support, while Caucasian caregivers reported the opposite. In addition,

African American caregivers did not obtain information or attend support groups as frequently as Caucasian caregivers did.

Wandering is one of several significant predictors of community-residing caregivers' stress and burden. However, cultural differences and the caregiver's perception of wandering behavior may work as mediating or buffering factors on stress and burden. For example, many studies found that black caregivers report less burden than whites (Connell & Gibson, 1997; Haley et al., 1996), and more black caregivers used prayer and faith conviction as coping strategies than whites (Haleyet al., 1995). A black caregiver responsible for a person with a wandering behavior, perceives and accepts wandering behavior differently than white caregivers.

Cohen and Day (2000) stated that cultural heritage is an essential enduring aspect of self-identity for older adults, including those with Alzheimer's disease and other dementias. They further stated that health care workers needed to be cognizant of life experiences, assets, beliefs and values, and caregiving practices associated with a particular culture. For example, Hinrichsen and Ramirez (1992) found that black elderly developed ties with their family members and relied on them for social, emotional, and practical support, which might predispose them to wandering. Elderly residents in long-term care facilities with close family ties are more likely to try to return to those families when they are confused, unhappy, or in pain.

Despite the large numbers of clients with dementia who wander, caregivers of African Americans and Caucasians expressed concern about their financial well-being (Connell & Gibson, 1997). They are faced with limited insurance coverage and severe financial strain, because they have been paying out-of-pocket expenses for care. Caregivers consider paying a better alternative so that they may have some time for themselves.

CULTURAL ISSUES IN WANDERING BEHAVIOR

Regardless of ethnicity, caring for a patient who wanders requires tenacity and dedication (Galanti, 2005). Because wanderers come from different backgrounds, there is a risk of stereotyping cultural groups. Health care providers must be familiar with cultural issues related to wandering before they can make appropriate and healthy interventions for persons they are treating. Galanti (2000) outlined several issues that may be associated with wandering:

Wake-up Time and Bedtime

If an individual who is accustomed to getting up early is not allowed to continue their routine, they might become confused and experience feelings of discomfort. Health care professionals must remember that patients differ in many ways. Some of these differences are due to a patient's illness, personality, socioeconomic class, or education, but the most profound differences may be cultural. For example, blue-collar workers often wake up earlier than white-collar workers because of different demands in job responsibilities. Having a good knowledge of cultural customs can help avoid misunderstanding and enable practitioners to provide better care. This is a significant issue with all groups, because the beginning of the day establishes the manner in which a routine will be carried out. Some ethnic groups pride themselves in being industrious and responsible. Hence, even when physical and mental limitations present themselves, members of these groups will resist having to change a routine and go to great lengths to preserve the manner in which they have lived their lives. The best indicator of quality care is the practitioner's acceptance of an individual's value system (e.g., the importance of industry) and then demonstrating a willingness to provide a care plan that allows for the patient's predisposition. Such an approach is likely to reduce the amount of confusion and conflict that results from trying to impose common expectations on all patients.

Personal Care Scheduling

Different cultures have routines that they are accustomed to. Some individuals need to be fully bathed and dressed before starting their day. If this routine is broken with an individual who wanders, they may become confused and begin looking for their clothing. This could lead them away from meals or activities if they feel their needs have not been met. In some instances, the importance of personal hygiene and dress is so prevalent that to exercise control, patients will demand to put on layers and layers of clothing, feeling that a delay in dressing them means that they are not appropriately clothed to carry on their routines. While consideration must be given to the patient load in a given facility, the range of habits and preferences are such that, with a little planning, most needs can be met. For example, those who wish to rise and dress early can be accommodated, and those who are more casual about beginning a hygiene routine can be left for last. The practitioner who is willing to be creative in terms of the time and manner in which care is given will likely have happier, better adjusted patients.

Food Preferences

In the Chinese culture, people will only accept food on the third offer. To accept earlier would be considered rude. This is not true in America; Americans generally accept food on the first offer. A group of nurses from mainland China described having great difficulty in the United States, because when they turned down food on the first offer, a second offer was not extended. Many Chinese nurses reported that they were constantly hungry until they learned the custom. Iranians expect food to be offered twice, the first out of politeness and the second offer demonstrated sincerity. This allows one to maintain social traditions, even when there is no extra food to share. When one considers the importance of diet and nutrition, it is essential that practitioners and caregivers become aware of each patient's personal preferences when it comes to food consumption. First, the food must be palatable, and efforts must be made to give a patient some of what they desire—taking into consideration the dietary restrictions in place. The individual with dementia needs as much consistency as possible. So, they must recognize the food, and it should be presented on a timetable with which the person is accustomed. Strong variation in mealtimes can increase the opportunities for decreased or depressed appetite and a tendency to "wander" because of the frustration associated with either a too early or too late meal schedule.

Eye Contact

In the Asian culture, direct eye contact with a superior (i.e., physician/nurse superior to patients; male superior to female) shows lack of respect. For example, in the Korean culture, people focus their eyes around the neck area, otherwise it is considered disrespectful. Among many Middle Eastern cultures, eye contact is avoided between men and women, because direct eye contact is considered to be sexually suggestive. In many Native American cultures, the eyes are believed to be the window of the soul. It is believed that one who looks directly into the eyes of another can steal the soul. When an individual feels uncomfortable or confused about what message the caregivers are sending, they may wander to avoid conflict or inappropriate interactions and feelings of discomfort. Therefore, while a professional may think that the issue of eye contact is a simple one, it is, in fact, fairly complex. Hence, both when attempting to send a message and "decode" the patient's response, the culture of the individual being "treated" must be given paramount consideration. A lack of familiarity with cultural customs can burden the organization and put the patient at risk. Remember, again, patients will avoid conflict at all costs. There is evidence of this in the number of reported "wanderings" each year—unfortunately often with fatal consequences.

Language

Most cultural misunderstandings result from failure to acknowledge the differences in language barriers. If a patient does not understand directions they may wander about until they find someone else to assist them. The Asian culture is extremely hierarchical, and it is viewed as inappropriate for a young person to tell an older person what to do or say. Instructions to a patient may have to be conveyed through an older family member. In the West Indies, for example, the oldest siblings give the instructions. It is well understood that health care providers must make sure that when they are communicating, the receiver understands what is being conveyed. Furthermore, one of the most important things that a practitioner can do is to show respect by acknowledging how communication occurs within a given culture. As noted, there is no one best way. Patient values represent the determinant in how a message should be communicated. It pays to remember that communication has not taken place until the message is received and acted on as intended. As a consequence, patients who feel violated and disrespected may go to great lengths to avoid conflict and "wander" initially to "teach a lesson," but eventually find themselves "lost" in the process.

Gender

Sexual segregation is a part of many Middle Eastern cultures. It can be a source of conflict or discomfort if patients are placed in a mixed-gender environment, particularly because it is suggested that an individual of the same sex give care. In this culture, it is also forbidden for a male to look at the body of a female if they are not married. Husbands are expected to protect their wives and act as conciliators. Unfortunately, a number of misconceptions abound with regard to the African American community and gender issues. The fact is that older men and women in this ethnic group tend to be very conservative and demand respect and privacy when it comes to sexual issues. As a result, it seems prudent for health care providers to err on the side of caution. That is, care must be taken to allow for gender separation except in the rare instances where husbands and wives are residing in the same facility. In this case, the couple may provide support for each other. But again, one must be careful so the wife does not feel the need to seek her husband's protection, and the husband should not be put in the position of having to provide it. Such behavior could result in the unfortunate circumstance of both parties "wandering" to avoid an uncomfortable situation.

Touching

In Middle Eastern, Orthodox, and Jewish cultures, touching between members of the opposite sex must be avoided, especially touching of females by males. Many Asians may not like being touched, and they avoid any physical contact. Although health care individuals emphasize the importance of touch, health care workers must realize that this practice was developed in the context of Western nursing and may not be appropriate for all cultures. A corollary concern is "social distance." In other words, some patients may be offended if health care workers "invade their personal space." It is a good idea to take cues from the recipient of the care as to what they are comfortable with. Unless it is absolutely necessary in the dispensing of quality care, discretionary touching should be avoided—unless the patient in some way initiates or indicates that they are comfortable with the contact.

Psychosocial (Nurses, Medical Staff, and Patients)

According to literature, many foreign-born nurses are trained only for technical nursing care. Ideally, health care workers trained in other cultures should be given guidance and training as to what is expected of someone in their position. When caregivers enter the room of a patient, they are stepping into an entire social world. When that patient is from a culture with different customs from those of the caregiver, the potential for problems increases dramatically. A classic example is that of an 86-year-old female patient who requested the nursing agency not send her a foreign-born caregiver, because it made her have feelings of anxiety and discomfort. After interviewing the patient, she stated that foreign caregivers were cold and reserved. The following case study exemplifies this point, and you will note that without proper understanding of the culture of a patient, outcomes can be devastating.

Case Study I: Mr. Tibbs

Mr. Tibbs is a 77-year-old African American male recently diagnosed with wandering behaviors related to progressing dementia. He has been a resident at a small, long-term care facility for 9 months. He was placed there after the death of his wife of 61 years. He has no surviving family. His only son was killed in an automobile accident just after arriving in Iran during Desert Storm. Mr. Tibbs is a veteran of two wars and lost his hearing during an air evacuation during his last tour of duty. The wandering began soon after his admission. He states that he is searching for his wife and his son. He is near his home and says that he wants to return to his family very much. He has progressive difficulty remembering where he is or what his activities were during the preceding 24 hours.

The challenges apparent in this case relate primarily to values in the African American culture. Foremost is the importance of family. Most elderly persons in this culture would prefer to remain with family members even when only marginal care may be available, as opposed to being in a facility with highly skilled care available. In the black community, family members who are sent to a facility, even for good reason, are regarded as being "discarded" or "warehoused." So patients with even limited abilities of discernment fight to be reunited with family members to protect the image of the family as much as to find personal comfort and security.

Another issue has to do with the ability to assume leadership. Again, in African American culture, the oldest male in the family is considered the leader—regardless of his physical or mental circumstances. And, the female is considered a "queen" (comparable to the African designation "Queen Mother"). In this regard, adult children who themselves have children or grandchildren have been known to visit a nursing home facility to ask permission of their father or get his opinion about some family issue. By the same token, matriarchs are given so much respect that a woman (a senior citizen herself) remarked, "I don't buy a loaf of bread without asking Mama what kind she wants." (Note: the speaker was in her early 70s and "Mama" was in her 90s.) So, returning to home and this culture is paramount, and often wandering results in the patient's overwhelming desire to reclaim their role in the family.

The interdisciplinary care team met to discuss Mr. Tibbs's growing restlessness and wandering behaviors. The staff found him a mile from the facility the night before. He became combative when they brought him back but responded to a light sedative and has been sleeping for the past three hours. The team looked at a number of strategies to help Mr. Tibbs adjust to his new surroundings. They began by looking at the problems associated with Mr. Tibbs's wandering:

1. *Predisposing factors*—personality traits, previous work and family roles, previous behavior patterns and habits, and morbidities (i.e., dementia, cognition problems, deafness, pain management, unresolved bereavement).
2. Nonpharmacological interventions:
    a. To manage the problem of wandering and its immediate adverse outcomes;
    b. To change the meaning of the problem, thereby redefining demands of caregiving; and,
    c. To manage symptoms of stress resulting from the problem and the adverse outcomes for caregivers.
3. Interventions/strategies identified by team:

a. DO NOT attempt to prevent or stop the wandering behavior unless the environment is unsafe. Allow wandering in safe place, for example, outside in sheltered walkways or gardens. Avoid crowded areas.
b. Observe when, where, and why the wandering behavior occurs. Try to accommodate Mr. Tibbs—he may be trying to find the bathroom.
c. Consider personal and cultural values related to working with the following, for example, in Mr. Tibbs's case: the elderly, confused or demented, ethnically different persons, veterans, males, and wanderers.
d. Facilitate clear and accurate communication through verbal and nonverbal methods. Remember that Mr. Tibbs is deaf. Use nonverbal cues. Since staff cannot effectively engage in conversation with Mr. Tibbs while he is pacing, they may just walk quietly beside him.
e. Recognize and accept Mr. Tibbs's need for closeness or distance.
f. Acknowledge Mr. Tibbs's decisions about cultural preferences or needs. Be flexible with providing personal care.
g. Recognize Mr. Tibbs's need to have contact with his family members and friends, even though they are gone.
h. Be available whenever Mr. Tibbs is moving to intervene quickly to help him remain safe and present. Maintain a calm environment.
i. Avoid restraints.
j. Make sure Mr. Tibbs has a coded identification bracelet in case he slips away from the facility and staff. It may also be an alarm-triggering bracelet or band.
k. Place pictures of Mr. Tibbs at the reception desk and other exits where others may see him as he attempts to leave the facility when wandering.

Case Study II: Javanese Culture (Sakit Jiwa Ng, 2001)

Javanese is the term used to describe a native of the Indonesian island of Java and is the largest ethnic group in Indonesia. In the Javanese culture, individuals pride themselves for being refined with regard to emotional expression and outward demeanor. Many of these individuals' symptoms, such as anger, suspicion, sadness, and confusion, are viewed as pathological in the community at large by clinical personnel. These individuals felt that the perception of the Javanese culture did influence their illness, especially regarding emotion, aggression, and social connection. When an individual in this culture is offended or angry, they try to cope by being quiet. Though social withdrawal is also socially disapproved of, it is less stigmatized than anger or violence. In this culture, strong expressions of sadness and resentment do not conform to the cultural ideal of a smooth affect. In this case, if a physician was aware of the Javanese culture, the patient could have been treated for her symptoms. Having a thorough knowledge of one's culture can avoid misunderstanding and enable the physician to render better holistic care.

An elderly Javanese woman 82 years of age was sent to the emergency room and was later admitted and scheduled for surgery three days post-admission due to the fact the doctors needed to do an extensive work up. Twelve hours after admission, she complained to her daughter that she was in pain but did not tell the nurses or her doctor. The nurses and the medical team were unaware that in the Javanese culture, women are taught to be refined and not to show emotions or complaint. The family was very upset with the physician, because her mother was in great pain and neither the nurses nor the physician paid her any attention. The nurses and doctor had ignored the daughter's request, because the patient did not seem to be in much pain. Within 24 hours she became increasingly confused and began wandering and pacing within the nursing unit she was admitted to without a destination in mind. The nurses simply redirected her back to her room and addressed ADL needs only. She maintained her silence and didn't verbally express complaints of her pain. The next day the patient became very ill and was sent to surgery immediately. The patient died while in surgery. The family member blamed the doctor, because she felt that if the doctor had operated sooner while her mother was in pain, she might have lived.

CLINICAL TIPS

- Nurture carefully the diversity in your team and in your patient care.
- Use integrity at all times.
- Learn how to express respect for people of another culture as a first step in dealing with a diverse population.
- Enhance your cultural competence by understanding the language, beliefs, and customs.
- Combine a medical and cultural history when assessing an individual, such as choice of religion, beliefs, and customs that are used daily by the family member.

- Use validation therapy in your practice and good eye contact when speaking with the patient.
- Employ individuals who are bilingual for the population being served.

PRACTICE IMPLICATIONS

Wandering is a significant problem in health care for the elderly. Cultural diversity associated with wandering is a topic with limited exploration in literature. Transcultural health care is a formal area of study that includes holistic cultural care and health and illness patterns of individuals and groups. There are many differences and similarities in cultural values and beliefs of the health care consumer (Leininger, 1995). In today's world, health care professionals can no longer ignore the importance of cultural factors, such as beliefs and practices in their respective culture. According to Rust and Strothers (2000), America will continue to experience a growth in a diverse society. This growth adds to the life and richness of our culture today. Thirteen percent of America's population is black. About 11 percent of today's population in America is Hispanic and Latino, and is estimated to expand to 50 percent of the U.S. population by 2050 (Rust & Strothers, 2000). In the health care setting, health professionals must recognize the multicultural society in the clinical area. As the population of the elderly increases, the experiences of caring and providing care for a family member who wanders is expected to increase.

Kagawa-Singer (1994) believes that the elderly of different cultures will teach others their traditions, beliefs, and practices. This expansion will help cultures survive. Life stages and social function define elders in most cultures as more than chronological age. In the Native American culture, one can be considered an elder at age 45. On the other hand, in the Japanese culture, the 60th, birthday is marked with an elaborate celebration.

To fully understand diversity, Mr. Tom (June 1960) in a personal communication stated that an elderly Hispanic man was critically ill, comatose, and had little chance of recovering from his illness. Nevertheless, his family traveled from their hometown (approximately 150 miles away) three times a week to sit at the patient's bedside.

One physician who observed this was puzzled. So he asked a colleague who happened to be Hispanic, "Can you explain something to me? How is it that this family will drive here three days a week, sit at the bedside of their loved one for 10 to 12 hours, and then get in their cars and drive home? After all, the patient doesn't know that they're here. Do you understand this culture?" An African American was present and stated, "This isn't too far from the truth and beliefs of my culture. The fact is that if it had been an African American family, chances are that a 24 hour vigil would have been kept by at least one individual until the patient 'went home'—and the family would regard 'home' both figuratively and literally. The patient would either return to their residence or go home to 'The Maker.' "

This story illustrates two important points:

a. It is important to have a diverse population of health care providers, and
b. It is equally important to have some knowledge of the cultural values that patients from diverse populations bring to the health care setting.

Porter (2000) stated that communicating with a diverse population can be hampered both professionally as well as personally unless significant emphasis is stressed on cultural differences. It is essential that health care providers become educated and oriented to cultural differences to survive in an increasingly competitive health care arena. She further stated that upgrading one's cultural awareness is important because doing so will:

a. Decrease health care disparities among a diverse population,
b. Enhance the quality of health care and outcomes,
c. Help health care providers gain a competitive edge in the marketplace, and
d. Decrease their liability and malpractice claims.

Cohen and Day (2000) stated that cultural heritage is an essential enduring aspect of self-identify for older adults, including those with Alzheimer's disease and other dementias. They further stated that health care workers need to be cognizant of life experiences, assets, beliefs and values, and caregiving practices associated with a particular culture.

CLINICAL APPROACHES TO WANDERING

FACT: What the family considers normal and abnormal health behavior may be based on cultural perceptions (Leininger, 1995). Learning about different cultures helps health care workers appreciate the diverse cultures and gain valuable insight into a specific culture. Leininger defined culture as the beliefs and life patterns of a particular group.

CLINICAL APPROACH: Assess for the influence of cultural beliefs, norms, and values on the family's understanding of wandering behavior. Inform the client's family about the meaning of and reasons for wandering behavior. An understanding of wandering behavior will enable the client's family to provide the client with a safe environment.

FACT: African American caregivers of persons with dementia may evidence less desire than other caregivers to institutionalize their family members and are more likely to report unmet service needs (Hinrichsen & Ramirez, 1992).

CLINICAL APPROACH: Provide supportive counseling to assist families in determining if and when institutionalization of the person with dementia who wanders is appropriate.

FACT: African American and Caucasian families of dementia clients may report restricted social activity (Haley et al., 1995).

CLINICAL APPROACH: Refer the family to social services or other supportive services to assist with the impact of caregiving for the person who wanders. Provide the caregiver with a list of support programs in their area.

FACT: Studies indicate that minority families of clients with dementia use few support programs even though these programs could have a positive impact on caregiver well-being (Loukissa, Farran, & Graham, 1999). African American families are less likely to see illness as a burden and will view the illness as a family illness.

CLINICAL APPROACH: Encourage the family to use support groups or other service programs (respite care) to assist them in caring for their loved one.

FACT: Validation lets the client know that the nurse has heard and understands what was said (Stuart & Laraia, 2002).

CLINICAL APPROACH: Validate the family's feelings regarding the impact of the client's wandering on the family's lifestyle.

FACT: Acknowledgments of race and ethnicity issues will enhance communication, establish rapport, and promote treatment outcomes (D'Avanzo, 2001).

CLINICAL APPROACH: Acknowledge racial and ethnic differences at the onset of care. Be conscious of the dynamics when people from different cultures interact. Ethnic issues can cause conflict and force individuals out of their comfort zones.

CONCLUSION

Because there are limited comparison studies on wandering behavior by race and ethnic group, the prevalence rate of wandering behavior by race is not available in literature. However, the overall wandering behavior as one dementia-related behavior is prevalent among PWDs regardless of culture or ethnic background. Furthermore, regardless of culture or ethnic groups, many studies on the predictors of caregiver burden and stress consistently demonstrated that dementia-related behaviors, including wandering behavior, were the most significant factors on burden and institutionalization among caregivers of PWDs (Coen, Swanwick, O'Boyle, & Coakley, 1997; Dunkin & Anderson-Hanley, 1998; Kramer, 1997; Kwon, 1995; Picot, 1995; Son, Wykle, & Zauszniewski, 2003; Steele, Rovner, Chase, & Folstein, 1990). Crosscultural comparison using a common valid measurement of wandering would be important in determining the aspects of wandering, whether it is based on pathological, cultural, or environmental factors (Song et al., 2003). So far, Cohen and Magai (1999) found the differences in the neuropsychiatric symptoms between U.S.-born African Americans and African Caribbeans suggesting the possibility of an underlying biological process, instead of cultural differences. Interventions targeting improving behavioral symptoms in persons with dementia will be based on whether cultural and environmental or biological or genetic factors have a greater influence on dementia-related behaviors. Caregiving to PWDs who exhibit wandering behavior is a stress and burden to family caregivers. A support system from local and national levels is always needed. Educational materials and resources written in different ethnic languages are also very necessary for minority populations.

Health care providers must be familiar with cultural issues related to wandering behavior before they can make appropriate and healthy interventions for people they are treating. They also have to understand that culture is a community in which members value and respect each other. Throughout history, ethnic and cultural issues of the population continue to expand. Health care professionals will continue to face a patient population that requires skills for negotiating cultural differences.

REFERENCES

Algase, D. L., Beattie, E.R.A., Leitsch, S. A., & Beel-Bates, C. A. (2003). Biomechanical activity devices to index wandering behavior in dementia. *American Journal of Alzheimer's Disease and Other Dementias, 18*(2), 85–92.

Algase, D. L., Beattie, E. R., Song, J. A., Milke, D., Duffield, C., & Cowan, B. (2004). Validation of the Algase Wandering Scale (Version 2) in a cross cultural sample. *Aging & Mental Health, 8*(2), 133–142.

Algase, D., Son, G-R., Beattie, E., Song, J., Leitsch, S., &. Yao, L. (2004). The interrelatedness of wandering and wayfinding in a community sample of persons with dementia. *Dementia and Geriatric Cognitive Disorder, 17*(3), 231–239.

Aud, M. A. (2004). Dangerous wandering: Elopements of older adults with dementia from long-term care facilities. *American Journal of Alzheimer's Disease and Other Dementias, 19*(6), 361–368.

Chen, J. C., Borson, S., & Scanlan, J. M. (2000). Stage-specific prevalence of behavioral symptoms in Alzheimer's disease in a multi-ethnic community sample. *American Journal of Geriatric Psychiatry, 8*(2), 123–133.

Coen, R. F., Swanwick, G. R, O'Boyle, C. A., & Coakley, D. (1997). Behavior disturbance and other predictors of caregiver burden in Alzheimer's disease. *International Journal of Geriatric Psychiatry, 12*(3), 331–336.

Cohen, C. I., & Magai, C. (1999). Racial differences in neuropsychiatric symptoms among dementia outpatients. *American Journal of Geriatric Psychiatry, 7*(1), 57–63.

Cohen, U., & Day, K. (2000). The potential role of cultural heritage in environments for people with dementia. In D. Holems, J. Teresi, & M. G. Ory (Eds.), *Special care units (Research & practice in Alzheimer's disease, 4)*. New York: Springer.

Cohen-Mansfield, J., Werner, P., Culpepper, W. J., & Barkley, D. (1997). Evaluation of an in-service training program on dementia and wandering. *Journal of Gerontological Nursing, 23*(10), 40–47.

Connell, C. M., & Gibson, G. D. (1997). Racial, ethnic, and cultural differences in dementia caregiving: review and analysis. *The Gerontologist, 37*(3), 355–364.

D'Avanzo, C. E. (2001). Developing culturally informed strategies for substance related interventions. In M. A. Naegle, & C.E. D'Avanzo (Eds.), *Addictions and substance abuse, strategies for advanced practice nursing* (pp. 59–104). St. Louis: Mosby.

Dunkin, J. J., & Anderson-Hanley, C. (1998). Dementia caregiver burden: A review of the literature and guidelines for assessment and intervention. *Neurology, 51*(1), S53–S60.

Galanti, G-A. (2000). An introduction to cultural differences. *Western Journal of Medicine, 172*(5), 335–336.

Galanti, G-A. (2005). Caring for culturally diverse patients at home. Retrieved July 6, 2006, from http://ggalanti.com/articles/articles_home_health.html.

Goldsmith, S. M., Hoeffer, B., & Rader, J. (1995). Problematic wandering behavior in the cognitively impaired elderly. *Journal of Psychosocial Nursing, 33*(2), 6–12.

Haley, W. E., Roth, D. L., Coleton, M. I., Ford, G. R., West, C. A., Collins, R. P., et al. (1996). Appraisal, coping, and social support as mediators of well-being in black and white family caregivers of patients with Alzheimer's disease. *Journal of Consulting & Clinical Psychology, 64*(1), 121–129.

Haley, W. E., West, C. A., Wadley, V. G., Ford, G. R., White, F. A., Barrett, J. J., et al. (1995). Psychological, social, and health impact of caregiving: A comparison of Black and White dementia family caregivers and noncaregivers. *Psychology and Aging, 10*(4), 540–552.

Hinrichsen, G. A., & Ramirez, M. (1992). Black and white dementia caregivers: A comparison of their adaptation, adjustment, and social utilization. *The Gerontologist, 32*(3), 375–381.

Kagawa-Singer, M. (1994). Diverse cultural beliefs and practices about death and dying in the elderly. *Gerontology & Geriatrics Education, 15*(1), 101–116.

Kramer, B. J. (1997). Differential predictors of strain and gain among husbands caring for wives with dementia. *The Gerontologist, 37*(2), 239–249.

Kwon, J-D. (1995). *The research of Korean dementia family: Development of the measurement tool and model for the caregiving*. Seoul: Hong Ik Jae.

Leininger, M. (1995). *Transcultural nursing: Concepts, theories, research & practices.* New York: McGraw-Hill, Inc.

Loukissa, D., Farran, C. J., & Graham, K. L. (1999). Caring for a relative with Alzheimer's disease: The experience of African-American and Caucasian caregivers. *American Journal of Alzheimer's Disease, 14*(4), 207–216.

Lucero, M. (2002). Intervention strategies for exit-seeking wandering behavior in dementia residents. *American Journal of Alzheimer's Disease and Other Dementias, 17*(5), 277–280.

Picot, S. J. (1995). Rewards, cost, and coping of African American caregivers. *Nursing Research, 44*(3), 147–152.

Porter, S. (2000). *Contemplating cultural competency.* American Academy of Family Physicians, FP Report, August, Volume 6, Number 8. Retrieved August 9, 2006, from http://www.aafp.org/fpr/20000800/04.html.

Rabins, P. V., Mace, N. L., & Lucas, M. J. (1982). The impact of dementia on the family. *JAMA, 248*(3), 333–335.

Rowe, M. A., & Bennett, V. (2003). A look at deaths occurring in persons with dementia lost in the community. *American Journal of Alzheimer's Disease and Other Dementias, 18*(6), 343–348.

Rust, G., & Strothers, H. (2000). Strategies for expanding your patient base in diverse communities. Retrieved July 6, 2006, from http://www.aafp.org/fpm/20000500/31stra.html.

Sakit Jiwa Ng (amuk) (2001). *Cultural formulation of psychiatric diagnosis. Culture medicine and psychiatry* (Chapter 25, pp. 411–425). The Netherlands: Kluwer Publishers.

Schreiner, A. S., Yamamoto, E., & Shiotani, H. (2000). Agitated behavior in elderly nursing home residents with dementia in Japan. *Journals of Gerontology Series B: Psychological Sciences & Social Sciences. 55*(3), P180–P186.

Sink, K. M., Covinsky, K. E., Newcomer, R., & Yaffe, K. (2004). Ethnic differences in the prevalence and pattern of dementia-related behaviors. *JAGS, 52*(8), 1277–1283.

Son, G-R., Song, J. A., & Lim, Y. M. (2006). Translation and validation of the Revised-Algase Wandering Scale (Community Version) among Korean elders with dementia. *Aging & Mental Health, 10*(2), 143–150.

Son, G-R., Wykle, M. L., & Zauszniewski, J. A. (2003). Korean adult child caregivers of older adults with dementia: Predictors of burden and satisfaction. *Journal of Gerontological Nursing, 29*(1), 19–28.

Song, J. A., Algase, D. L., Beattie, E. R., Milke, D. L., Duffield, C., & Cowan, B. (2003). Comparison of U.S., Canadian, and Australian participants' performance on the Algase Wandering Scale-Version 2 (AWS-V2). *Research & Theory for Nursing Practice, 17*(3), 241–256.

Steele, C., Rovner, B., Chase, G. A., & Folstein, M. (1990). Psychiatric symptoms and nursing home replacement of patients with Alzheimer's disease. *American Journal of Psychiatry, 147*(8), 1049–1051.

Stuart, G. W., & Laraia, M. T. (2002). Therapeutic nurse-patient relationships. In G. W. Stuart & M. T. Laraia (Eds.), *Principles and practice of psychiatric nursing* (pp. 30). St. Louis: Mosby.

Teri, L., Larson, E. B., & Reifler, B. V. (1988). Behavioral disturbance in dementia of the Alzheimer's type. *Journal of American Geriatric Society, 36*(1), 1–6.

Thomas, D. W. (1995). Wandering: A proposed definition. *Journal of Gerontological Nursing, 21*(9), 35–41.

CHAPTER NINE

Root Cause Analysis of Reported Wandering Adverse Events in the Veterans Health Administration

Joseph M. DeRosier, Lesley Taylor, James Turner, and James P. Bagian

INTRODUCTION

This chapter provides information on missing patient events contained in the Veterans Health Administration Patient Safety Information Database. The database contains Root Cause Analysis (RCA) and Aggregated Review reports completed by Veterans Health Administration RCA teams on missing patient events and close calls. The data was reviewed to determine when and where patients are reported missing and the root cause/contributing factors and actions teams identified to address identified system vulnerabilities.

BACKGROUND

Veterans Health Administration policy (Department of Veterans Affairs, 2002a) mandates that individual Root Cause Analysis reports and semiannual Aggregated Review reports (Sidebar 1) be completed on adverse events, including missing patient events and close calls, and submitted to the National Center for Patient Safety (NCPS). Missing patient events and close calls reported at the 154 VA medical centers and approximately 875 outpatient clinics are triaged by the facility Patient Safety Manager using the Safety Assessment Code (SAC) developed by NCPS (Bagian et al., 2001). All reports from the outpatient clinics are submitted by the host VA medical center. The SAC is a risk assessment tool that uses probability of occurrence and outcome severity to determine both an actual score and the most likely worst case score, also known as the potential score within Veterans Health Administration. Reported events are triaged using a Safety Assessment Code which includes a severity and probability scoring matrix. Events that receive an actual score of "3" (highest score) receive an individual RCA. Reported events that receive an actual score of "1 or 2" and a potential score of "3" may be either aggregated and collectively reviewed every 6 months by Aggregate Review teams or receive an immediate RCA at the direction of the facility Patient Safety Manager (PSM).

ABOUT THE VETERANS HEALTH ADMINISTRATION INDIVIDUAL RCA AND AGGREGATE REVIEW REPORTS

Root Cause Analysis (RCA) reports are completed to determine what happened, why it happened, and what can be done to prevent it from happening again. RCA reports are completed on a wide variety of topics including missing patient events. There are two types of patient safety reports completed within the Veterans Health Administration that are submitted to NCPS: individual RCAs and aggregated. Both report forms have been designed to serve as a cognitive aid for the team conducting the analysis. The questions in the reports, when answered sequentially, help the team gather information and conduct interviews to reach the ultimate goal of identifying root cause/contributing factors, actions, and outcome measures.

The individual RCA form consists of 22 questions. The first 9 questions are completed by the facility patient safety manager, and they provide demographic and background information about the event. The team begins their work at question 10 with the development of an initial flow diagram and completion of a brief narrative description of what happened. Questions 11, 12, and 13 help the team organize and identify the internal documents and records needed for review, identify who they need to interview, and list external sources of information (books, articles, etc.) that need to be reviewed. Question 14 ties together what is learned during the analysis in a final flow diagram and final narrative description of the event. Root cause/contributing factors are entered into question 15. Questions 16, 17, and 18 require the team to review previously implemented interventions, consult with the original reporter to verify that the team's understanding of the event is correct, and list any lessons learned that need to be shared. Actions and outcome measures to address the root cause/contributing factors are identified in question 19. Questions 20, 21, and 22 capture costs associated with the RCA and additional analytical tools and methods used by the team, attachments to the report, and team and top management concurrence.

Missing patient Aggregated Reviews are used to analyze multiple close call events that have been reported over the previous six months. Review teams are tasked with looking for one or more shared systems issues (common threads) present in the majority of the events. A process flow diagram is developed in place of the individual RCA event flow diagram. Teams look for variations between what should have happened and what did happen to identify system vulnerabilities and to develop root cause/contributing factor statements and corresponding actions and outcome measures.

Root Cause Analysis evaluations of adverse events are not unique to the Veterans Health Administration and are used throughout health care to improve patient safety. As of June 1, 2006, there were approximately 380 individual missing patient Root Cause Analysis reports and 340 missing patient Aggregated Reviews entered into the Veterans Health Administration Patient Safety Information database. These analyses were submitted from 131 Veterans Health Administration facilities.

As individual RCAs are received at the National Center for Patient Safety (NCPS) they are coded by analysts using the NCPS developed Primary Analysis and Categorization (PAC) process (Sidebar 2). Codes have been developed to categorize the location, the activity or process at the time of the event, the type of action(s), and outcome measures. The PAC data does not provide the level of detail needed to present a complete picture of missing patient events, so additional analysis was conducted. To supplement the PAC data 100 of the most recent (as of June 1, 2006) individual Root Cause Analysis event reports were selected for further analysis. Ninety-one (91) of these 100 individual RCA reports were found to address missing patient events as defined by Veterans Health Administration national policy; the remaining nine events addressed absent patient events and were not included. All of the 91 individual Root Cause Analysis reports used in this analysis were submitted to the Veterans Health Administration Patient Safety Information database between October 1, 2004 and June 1, 2006.

PRIMARY ANALYSIS AND CATEGORIZATION

The Primary Analysis and Categorization (PAC) process was developed internally at NCPS through a team led by the Director of Patient Safety Information Systems. Over the course of several years of testing and refinement this classification system evolved into an operational taxonomy that is applied to all individual Patient Safety Root Cause Analysis Reports that are submitted to the national database. The taxonomy includes the following categories: Selected Event type (32 categories), Location of Event (48 categories), Activities or Processes connected with the Event (27 categories), Action type (39 categories), and Outcome Measure type (10 categories). Aggregated Reviews are not categorized at this time due to the breadth and nature of these reports, which encompass many events into one report making it impossible to code a single location, for example. PAC allows a variety of ways to mine the RCA data and helps to better understand the data.

This analysis and the data presented in this chapter are based upon a review of approximately 25 percent, or 100 reports (reduced to 91 reports), of the individual missing patient RCA reports and approximately 50 percent, or 170, of the missing patient Aggregated Reviews in the Patient Safety Information database as of June 1, 2006. More Aggregated Reviews were analyzed, because by design they contain aggregate information and less detail than individual reports, therefore a larger sample size was needed.

The definition of a Missing Patient used in Veterans Health Administration (VHA) is provided in the VHA Directive 2002–013 "Management of Wandering and Missing Patient Events" (Department of Veterans Affairs, 2002b). Directives are used to establish national policy within Veterans Health Administration. Directive 2002–013 defines a *Missing Patient* as "a high-risk patient who disappears from an inpatient or outpatient treatment area or while under the control of VA, such as during transport." A *high-risk patient* is defined as a patient "who is incapacitated because of frailty, or physical or mental impairment." The Directive further defines incapacitated patients as patients who:

- Are legally committed;
- Have a court-appointed legal guardian;
- Are considered to be dangerous to themselves or others;
- Have a lack of cognitive ability (either permanently or temporarily) to make relevant decisions; OR
- Have a physical or mental impairment that increases their risk of harm to themselves or others.

A patient who leaves a treatment or care area without the knowledge or permission of staff but does not meet the definition of a high-risk patient is considered to be an Absent Patient.

ANALYSIS QUESTIONS

This analysis was completed with the following questions in mind.

- What services/departments participate in missing patient individual RCAs and Aggregated Reviews?
- How long does the average missing patient individual RCA and Aggregated Report take to complete?
- Is there a day of the week and time of day when patients are more likely to be reported as missing?
- What services/departments report missing patient events?
- What activities are patients involved in prior to being declared missing?
- What root cause/contributing factors are identified for missing patient events?
- What types of actions have been identified by RCA and aggregate teams to address missing patient events, and have they been effective?

ANALYSIS RESULTS

Services/Departments Participating in Missing Patient RCA Activities

Nursing service/department participants accounted for approximately 23 percent of the 2,792 team members who investigated missing patient events (Figure 9.1) followed by Police and Security Service (12%) and Other Administrative Services (11%).

Average Time Spent on Root Cause Analysis and Aggregated Review Investigation

On average individual Root Cause Analysis teams spent 49.3 team hours to complete their investigation and develop their report. Aggregate Review teams spent an average of 34.5 hours to complete their analysis and report.

When Patients Are More Likely to Be Reported as Missing

Patients are more likely to be reported as missing on Tuesday (21%), Wednesday (25%), and Thursday (21%). Saturday (13%) and Monday (10%) were the next most frequent days. Sunday and Friday each had 5 percent of the reported events.

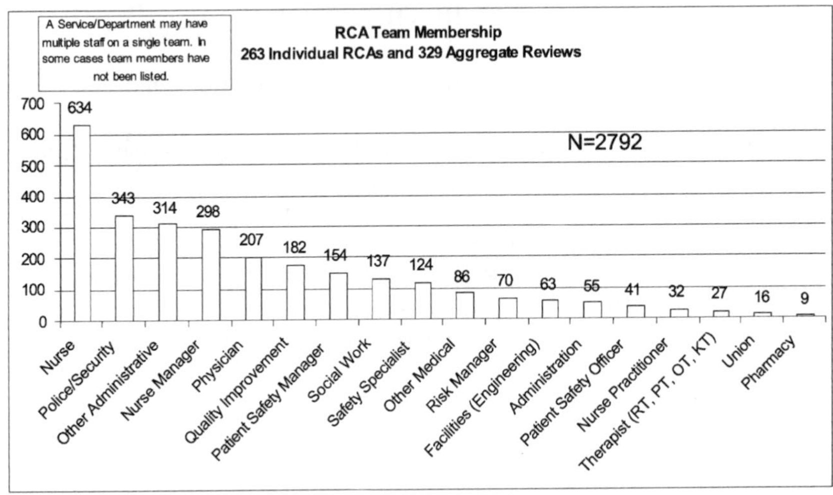

FIGURE 9.1 RCA team membership.

First shift was the most frequent time of day for missing patient events to be reported (Figure 9.2). For the purposes of this analysis the shifts are defined to be: first shift 7 A.M. to 3 P.M., second shift 3 P.M. to 11 P.M., and third shift 11 P.M. to 7 A.M.. Approximately 30 percent of the missing patient events were associated with the admitting and assessment/reassessment processes. These activities primarily occur during first shift, which may account for approximately 65 percent of the events being reported during this time frame.

Services/Departments Reporting Missing Patient Events

Based upon the 91 individual RCAs analyzed, acute care units (Figure 9.3) reported the most missing patient events (17.6%), followed closely by long-term care units (16.5%), and locked behavioral health (locked psych) units (16.5%). However, it should be noted that during this time period (October 1, 2004 to June 1, 2006) there were approximately 8 times more acute care patients than long-term care patients, and 6 times more acute care patients than behavioral health patients. Therefore, long-term care and behavioral health units are represented at a disproportionately greater level than acute care settings with respect to missing patients.

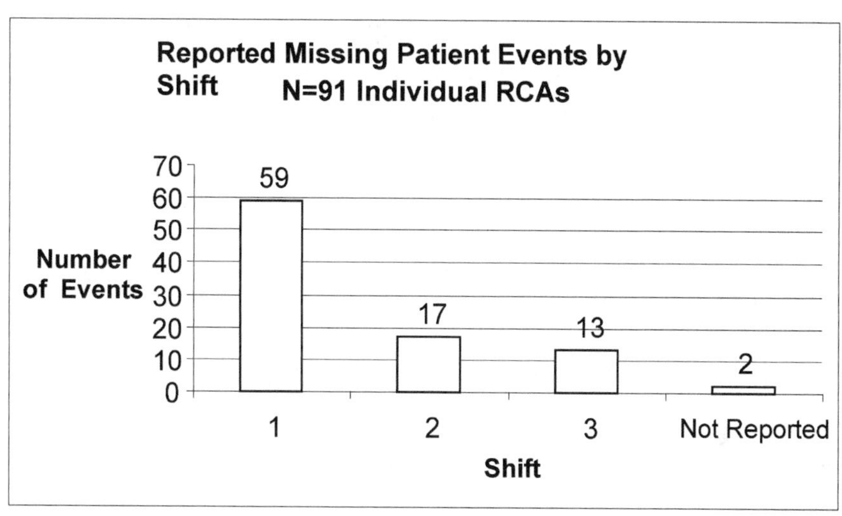

FIGURE 9.2 Reported missing patient events by shift.

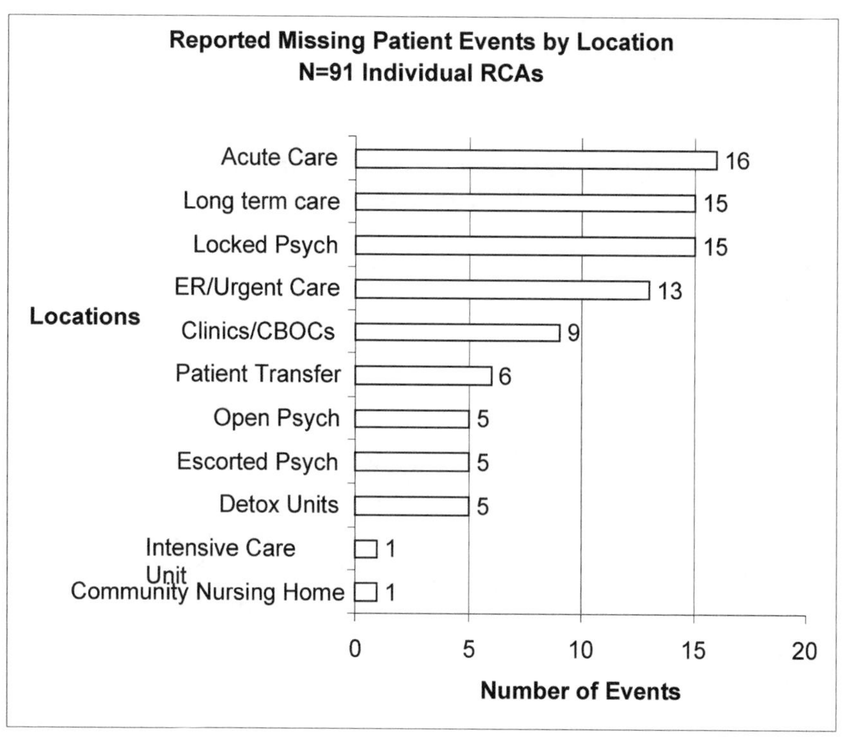

FIGURE 9.3 Reported missing patient events by location.

Patient Activities Prior to Being Reported Missing

From the PAC data (Figure 9.4) the majority of the patients were reported missing when routine care was being provided. In some cases the patients had monitoring equipment being used including bracelets and alarms or door locking systems. Patient transports, both within the hospital and to and from the hospital, were a vulnerable activity. Some patients left or became missing during Activities of Daily Life (ADLs), which by the PAC definition includes explicit mention of, or reference to, eating, washing, showering, bathing, brushing teeth, dressing, sleeping, toileting, and smoking.

Missing Patient Event Root Cause/Contributing Factors

RCA teams identified a myriad of root cause/contributing factors for missing patient events (Figure 9.5). Approximately 530 root cause/contributing factors were identified in the 263 individual and Aggregated Reviews. These root cause/contributing factors have been grouped into the following general categories or processes:

1. Assessment/reassessment (23%),
2. Admitting (7%),

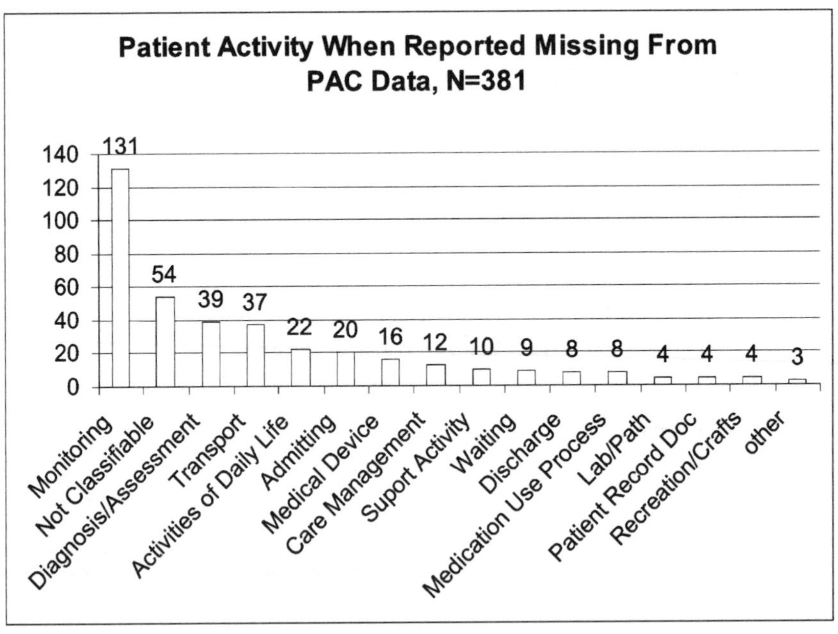

FIGURE 9.4 Patient activity when reported missing from PAC.

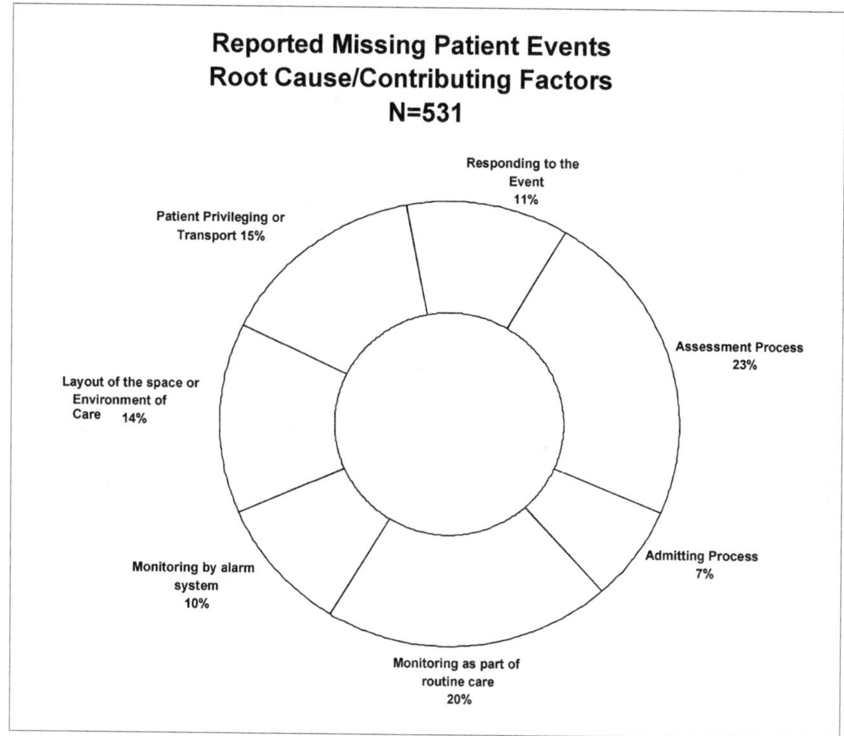

FIGURE 9.5 Reported missing patient events: Root cause/contributing factors.

3. Monitoring patients by observation during routine care (20%),
4. Monitoring patients by alarm system (10%),
5. The layout and design of the care area or environment of care issues (14%),
6. Patient privileging or transport (15%), and
7. Initiating/conducting the search (Responding to the Event) for the missing patient (11%).

Table 9.1 provides a summary of the root cause/contributing factors identified by missing patient RCA teams.

Actions

Of the 768 actions reviewed (from the 263 RCAs) over 50 percent were categorized as weak actions (Sidebar 3) addressing policy/procedures, training, or requiring further analysis by process experts (Figure 9.6).

TABLE 9.1 Root Case/Contributing Factors Identified by Missing Patient RCA Teams

Category	Root cause/contributing factors relating to:
Assessment Process (23%)	• Use of an elopement risk assessment or the lack of staff education on how to use the assessment. • No documentation or little communication of missing patient risk assessments between staff and between staff and patient/family. • Missing patient risk assessments were not used consistently, or when used, the assessment criteria were inconsistently applied. • Not implementing preventative measures identified in the missing patient assessment.
Monitoring During Routine Care (20%)	• Staffing levels are lower than required to monitor high-risk patients. • The level of observation that is ordered is not sufficient. • Staff were not educated about treating high-risk patients. • Policies for handling high-risk patients did not exist. • Observations of the patient did not occur as needed or indicated.
Providing Privileges or Transporting the Patient (15%)	• Patient privileging or transport policies were unclear or inconsistent. • The absence of a tracking system for patients leaving units (i.e., sign-out log or wander alert system). • Written privileging orders were not completed. • Patients were not supervised during transport or during long clinic/urgent care waiting times. • Facility smoking policies allowed patients to walk to the smoking area unsupervised.

(Continued)

TABLE 9.1 Root Case/Contributing Factors Identified by Missing Patient RCA Teams

Category	Root cause/contributing factors relating to:
Physical Plant Layout and Environment of Care Issues (14%)	• The layout of area or environment was not conducive to treating high-risk elopement patients. • The lack of or failure of physical barriers (e.g., secured doors). • Area where outpatients are seen prior to admission to locked ward is not secured.
Responding to the Event (11%)	• The procedures addressing how to respond to a missing patient event were complex or hard to understand. • The procedure on how to respond to a missing patient event was not available to staff when it was needed. • There were significant delays in communication between services about a missing patient. • The most effective methods of communication were not used during a missing patient event. • There was no system in place to document areas that had been searched resulting in rework and delays in locating the patient.
Monitoring the Patient Using an Alarm (10%)	• Monitoring equipment was absent, not used, or failed to function properly. • Monitoring equipment failed to operate due to criteria not being established regarding maintenance and staff education. • There was a slow, and in some cases no response to monitoring system audible alarms. • Monitoring systems were not standardized in the facility, and the differences in operation between the systems led to staff confusion and improper operation or response.

(Continued)

TABLE 9.1 Root Case/Contributing Factors Identified by Missing Patient RCA Teams (Continued)

Category	Root cause/contributing factors relating to:
Admitting Process (7%)	• Contraband searches were not consistently done when patients were admitted. • Staff were not educated on admitting duties regarding elopement/wandering risk. • The high-risk (for elopement or wandering) status of a patient was not communicated to staff following the patients admission. • The lack of a formal check-in process for patients entering the Emergency Department/Urgent Care permitted patients to leave without detection.

Approximately 31 percent of the actions were classified as intermediate strength actions. These actions address communication issues or the need to enhance documentation in the patient medical record, changing staffing rations or assignments, improving patient assessment and reassessment methods, improving collaboration among caregivers, and developing cognitive aids for staff. Approximately 15 percent of the actions were classified as strong actions. Strong actions included making changes to the physical plant or layout of the physical space, and replacing or installing equipment. Examples of physical layout changes included the creation of a secured unit for high-risk patients; constructing smoking areas for inpatient psychiatric patient use; changing the layout in nursing units to provide a visitor check-in area; changing secondary entry doors to be exit only; and, installing new observation mirrors, surveillance cameras, and door locking systems.

NCPS ACTION STRENGTH RATINGS

The action strength ratings used in the Veterans Health Administration were developed by the National Center for Patient Safety following the roll out of the root cause analysis process. When RCA reports were reviewed it was found that teams primarily identified training and policy/procedure changes to address root cause/contributing factors, which by themselves are generally less effective. The hierarchy of actions (strong, intermediate, weak) was created to help teams think

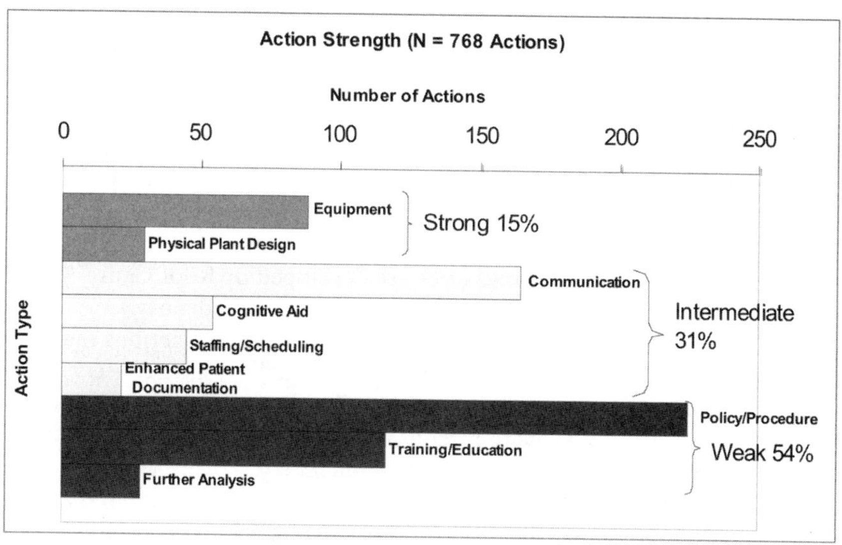

FIGURE 9.6 Action strength.

about additional actions other than relying solely upon training and policy and procedure changes. Actions that eliminate vulnerabilities by making it impossible to do the task incorrectly are strong actions; actions that support individuals by helping them remember to do their tasks correctly are intermediate actions; and those actions that require the individual to perform the task based upon their knowledge and memory without additional support are weak actions. Strong actions include making changes to the building, purchasing new equipment, implementing engineering controls such as a forcing function, removing steps from the process, and standardizing on equipment. Intermediate actions include increasing staff or decreasing workload, enhancing software, reducing distractions, using cognitive aids and checklists, and enhancing communication (e.g., read back). Weak actions include implementing double checks, adding warning labels or signs, implementing a new policy, and training. This list is not intended to be all encompassing and does not preclude teams from identifying actions classified as weak in RCA reports. Signage, training, and policies and procedures are important and should not be ignored, but they should not stand alone and be the only actions taken. This hierarchy is intended to serve as a cognitive aid to help RCA teams think of actions that incorporate human factors principles to modify systems in lieu of placing all responsibility upon staff to always remember to do things correctly.

After an RCA action has been implemented the facility Patient Safety Manager (PSM) has the ability to enter the patient safety information database and rate how effective it was at eliminating or reducing the system vulnerabilities identified in the root cause/contributing factor statement. The effectiveness rating scale that is used is based on the Likert Scale of 1 to 5: 1 = much worse; 2 = worse; 3 = unchanged; 4 = better; and 5 = much better. Action effectiveness is subjectively scored by the PSM against previously developed outcome measures in the Root Cause Analysis report. Outcome measures are developed by Root Cause Analysis and Aggregate Review teams for each action they identify.

Of the 91 individual RCAs analyzed there were 202 actions that had their effectiveness assessment reported by the facility Patient Safety Manager following implementation (Figure 9.7). No action effectiveness was rated a "1" or "2"; 43 were rated "3" (unchanged); and the remaining 159 were rated as "4" (better) or "5" (much better).

Table 9.2 shows the relationship between action strength and action effectiveness. Note that the odds ratio if a strong action is developed and implemented being rated as "much better" is 2.5.

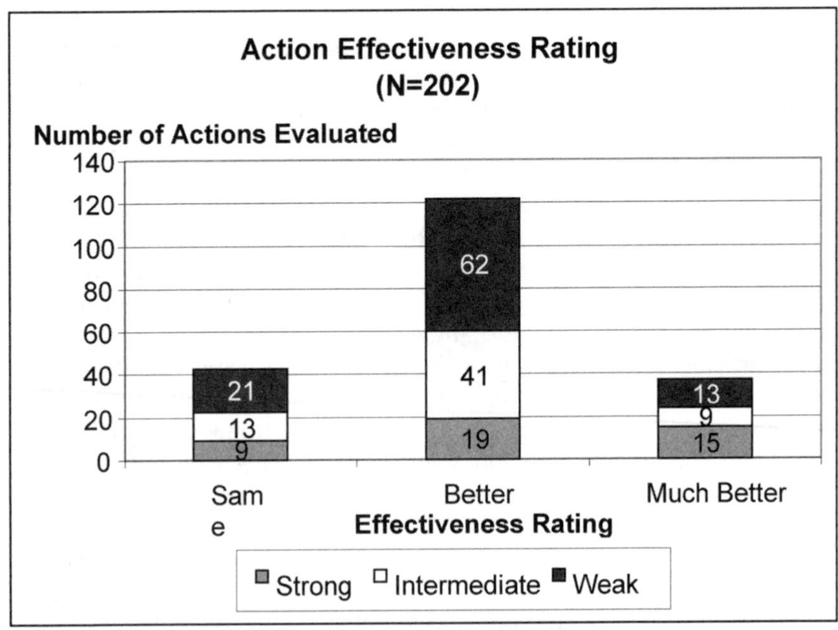

FIGURE 9.7 Action effectiveness rating.

TABLE 9.2 Action Strength vs. Effectiveness Table

	Effectiveness Rating		
Action Strength	Same	Better	Much Better
Strong	21% (N = 9)	44% (N = 19)	35% (N = 15)
Intermediate & Weak	21% (N = 34)	65% (N = 103)	14% (N = 22)

Table 9.3 provides examples of actions taken from individual RCA reports where PSMs have reported the action effectiveness as better (4) or much better (5).

PRACTICE IMPLICATIONS

The Veterans Health Administration patient safety data revealed two areas of focus for practical consideration and implementation. The highest percentage of challenges is found within two system-wide processes; assessment/reassessment and patient monitoring during routine care.

Assessment process vulnerabilities accounted for 23 percent of the root cause/contributing factors identified by RCA and Aggregate Review teams. These included standardized escape and elopement assessment process and forms for use by staff in all services within the facility. For example, urgent care departments did not have the same escape and elopement assessment as the one used in long-term care. This led to patients being placed in the inappropriate unit (open vs. secured). Increased communication between these departments may have averted this missing patient event. Another example is where the wandering and elopement assessment existed but was not applied consistently or was not effectively communicated. This led to preventative measures not being implemented resulting in the missing patient event. Additional examples include events where an observation level was not ordered (i.e., one-on-one), or patients were given inappropriate privileges (i.e., were allowed to visit the smoking area unattended).

Secondly, the data indicates that during routine care of the patient policies and procedures did not support clinical staff. The root cause/contributing factors reviewed in this category revealed issues with inadequate staffing levels to care for patients at high-risk for wandering or elopement, the absence of policies and procedures for the handling high-risk patients, and staff not being trained on policies and procedures.

TABLE 9.3 Actions Taken From RCA Reports (Activeness Effectiveness [4] or [5])

Root Cause/Contributing Factor Addressed	Effective Actions
Strong Action Examples	
Unlocking the door to allow some patients to go to the dining room for meals may have increased the likelihood that a patient would have the opportunity to elope.	On locked units, all meals should be provided on the unit rather than sending/escorting some patients off the unit for meals.
Timeliness related to the missing patient process may be compromised due to the frequency of false alarms, confusion about policy, and current lack of practice, increased the likelihood that a patient could be off property before a search has been initiated.	Install alarm system to sound after patient enters the double barrier/buffer zone (Sally port). Once in this zone, the present outer door will automatically lock to prevent the patient from leaving the unit.
Lack of adequate door alarms in the Adult Day Healthcare area increased the likelihood that a patient could leave the area without being detected.	Purchase a wander alert system for Adult Day Care Center for its four doors.
The environment was not secure because the door alarm was not always active (turned on). This allowed disoriented patients to wander off the unit.	Order new doors for fire escape exits located on the medical unit with alarms that cannot be disconnected by staff.
The number of obvious exit points increases the likelihood of a high-risk patient getting through first line barriers.	(1) Direct dietary staff to the central elevator to prevent patients from activating the alarm near the east elevators; (2) Disguise new door with mural, so high-risk patient will be less likely to go through it [*note:* this may violate fire safety regulations and should be approved by the local fire marshal before implementation]; (3) Place black floor tiles in front of each door area leaving a perception of a dark hole.
Intermediate Action Strength Examples	
Level III privileges for a noncompliant, committed patient allowed the patient 2 hours of unsupervised time that provided an opportunity for him to elope unnoticed.	Nursing staff will contact station police to escort patients back to unit who refuse to return to unit for sign-in.

(Continued)

TABLE 9.3 (Continued)

Root Cause/Contributing Factor Addressed	Effective Actions
Lack of communication between staff may have led to untimely reporting that a patient was missing.	Develop a cognitive aid for the hourly count sheet to remind the checker to inform the charge nurse immediately when a patient is missing.
Due to inconsistency in the hand-off communication between staff, the existing process of maintaining 1:1 observation of suicidal and homicidal patients did not occur.	The ER admission template will provide secondary checks for behavioral health patients who are present at change of shift. The template will specify and document if the patient is currently suicidal, homicidal, has weapons, plan for suicide, etc.; and, that he/she cannot be left alone during medical clearance and must be escorted to the inpatient psych unit if admitted.
Awarding off-ward privileges to committed patients increased the risk for elopement.	Committed patients will not be allowed to have off-ward privileges (remain Level I) unless approved by the Chief of Staff for the Mental Health Program.
Clinical staff working outside of behavioral health unit were not familiar with the suicide risk procedures or the increased risk for patient elopement. This led to the elopement of a high-risk patient who committed suicide following elopement.	Develop a process for the after hours psychiatric physician to communicate with the psychiatric team/provider regarding behavioral health patients placed on suicide precautions who are admitted to nonpsychiatric services and require follow-up.
Weaker Action Strength Examples	
Public transportation bus drivers servicing the hospital did not have any method to identify eloping or wandering patients, which led to a patient using the bus to elope without detection.	A memo has been sent to the bus company informing them of the problem and the solution.
Double doors leading to the tunnel were not locked, which allowed the patient to elope.	Prior to each meal, the doors to the hallway/tunnel will be checked for proper lockage.

(Continued)

TABLE 9.3 Actions Taken From RCA Reports (Activeness Effectiveness [4] or [5]) (Continued)

Root Cause/Contributing Factor Addressed	Effective Actions
A policy/procedure did not exist requiring that the hospital policy/security office be notified when committed patients were admitted. This increased the likelihood a committed patient could leave the station without being noticed.	Revise and implement Missing Patient Policy that is compliant with the National Directive.

These two categories include over 40 percent of the root cause/contributing factors identified by Missing Patient RCA and Aggregate Review teams. Targeting efforts on putting a standardized wandering assessment is in place, and ensuring that it is consistently applied and communicated will address many of the identified system vulnerabilities. Writing policies and procedures will not, by themselves, prevent missing patient events from occurring, however, they are one of several barriers that will help to avoid escape and elopement events.

METHODOLOGICAL ISSUES

Individual RCAs and Aggregated Reviews used in this analysis provide varying levels of specificity in the event description. Thus, tables and graphs provided have varying denominators due to the degree of information supplied. This variation impacts the reliability of data due to the categorization that must be performed. The Individual Root Cause Analysis Reports submitted by Veterans Health Administration (VHA) facilities to the VHA National Center for Patient Safety (NCPS) are reviewed by one or more of six different NCPS Analysts using a standardized NCPS patient safety taxonomy with established guidelines and definitions. For the focused analysis on the individual Missing Patient RCAs and Aggregated Reviews reports inconsistencies in categorizing the reports are possible, however, there were only two individuals working on these data sets, and established definitions were also used.

GAPS IN RESEARCH

The Veterans Health Administration patient safety database does not provide information on costs associated with implementation of actions specified in the RCA or Aggregated Review, nor are costs incurred in conducting grid searches conducted to find missing patients; including the costs associated with taking staff away from their normal care duties. It is also difficult to place a dollar value on those rare missing patient events that end in fatality. Without knowing these costs it is difficult to develop a business case to justify interventions such as a wander alarm/alerting system or use of a global positioning tracking system.

Due to the nature of the free text reporting of the RCA and Aggregated Review data in the Veterans Health Administration patient safety database a wide variation exists in what information is entered into the narrative questions. The narrative format offers a wealth of information, but the information provided can be inconsistent based upon what the individual RCA or Aggregate teams feel is pertinent for their event. This can make analyzing the data more difficult when mining for particular content such as the patient outcome as a result of the event (e.g., found and returned, injury, or death) and the cause that precipitated the event.

CONCLUSION

Aggregating and analyzing missing patient RCA reports helps to provide a basic understanding of when and where missing patient events occur so that interventions and resources may be directed toward prevention. The RCA and Aggregated Review data show that assessing patients for elopement and wandering risk and then communicating the assessment results are critical steps to help prevent patients from becoming missing patients. It also shows that missing patients are reported from acute care units as frequently as from locked behavioral health and long-term care units and that the emergency department is also vulnerable. Patients are more likely to be reported as missing during the middle of the work week (Tuesday to Thursday) on first shift (7 A.M. to 3 P.M.). A large range of actions have been reported as being effective in controlling or eliminating missing patient events. These have included physical plant changes such as installing Sally ports at the entrance to locked behavioral health units, installing door alarms and locking systems, enhancing patient escort and patient privileging procedures, and communicating with external transportation services (bus and taxi) on elopement and wandering dangers.

REFERENCES

Bagian, J., Lee, C., Gosbee, J., DeRosier, J., Stalhandske, E., Eldridge, N., et al. (2001). Developing and deploying a patient safety program in a large health care delivery system: You can't fix what you don't know about. *The Joint Commission Journal on Quality Improvement, 27*(10), 522–532.

Department of Veterans Affairs (VHA) (2002a). *VHA handbook 1050.1 national patient safety improvement handbook* (January 30, 2002). Washington, DC: Author.

Department of Veterans Affairs (VHA) (2002b). *VHA directive 2002–13 management of wandering and missing patients* (March 4, 2002). Washington, DC: Author.

CHAPTER TEN

Getting Lost: Antecedents, Wandering Behavior, and Search Strategies

Meredeth A. Rowe and Andrea J. Pe Benito

INTRODUCTION

For individuals and their families, a dementia diagnosis commences a very challenging and often difficult period of life. Persons with Alzheimer's disease, the most common form of dementia, generally survive between 8–20 years from the time of diagnosis. As the disease progresses, individuals require an increasing amount of assistance with personal care tasks as well as supervision to ensure safety (Rowe & Bennett, 2003). Impairments in memory, executive function, abstract thinking, and judgment may contribute to individuals becoming lost inside or outside of the home. The consequences of becoming lost can be as severe as death, and numerous cases of deaths have been reported in the news media after individuals became lost (Rowe, Feinglass, & Wiss, 2004). In this chapter, we summarize previous research on the antecedents and outcomes of getting lost in the community. We also review interventions designed to prevent such episodes as well as search strategies that can be effectively used by law enforcement agencies and officials to find wanderers lost in the community.

REVIEW OF LITERATURE/CASE STUDIES

Wandering Versus Getting and Becoming Lost

It is estimated 60 percent of persons with Alzheimer's disease will, at some point over the course of their illness, become separated from their caregiver, instigated when they are alone and unsupervised in the community for some interval of time (http://www.alz.org/Care/Behaviors/wandering.asp). A number of terms are currently applied, both accurately and inaccurately, in reference to these scenarios, including wandering, elopement, and getting lost. However, because distinct meanings accrue to these terms, it is important to clarify the differences among them. Wandering as empirically defined in Chapter 1 is "a syndrome of dementia-related locomotion behavior having a frequent, repetitive, temporally disordered, and/or spatially disoriented nature that is manifested in lapping, random, and/or pacing patterns, some of which are associated with eloping, eloping attempts, or getting lost unless accompanied." Elopement is generally applied to an unattended exit from a care setting. Getting lost means that the individual involved cannot find his or her way, implying a *state* of spatial disorientation, that can occur either inside or outside the boundaries of the care setting, and either in proximity to a residential setting or out in the community. In contrast, *becoming lost* is an isolated (sometimes repeated) *event* whereby the person with dementia enters the community without assistance or supervision and becomes unable to find the way back to their residence or caregiver.

This distinction of terms can be important when assessing the risk of a person with dementia becoming lost in the community. Two points are relevant in this regard: (1) some cognitively impaired individuals who engage in wandering behavior as previously defined may never become lost, and (2) persons with no previous history of wandering behavior may, indeed, become lost (Rowe et al., 2004). These distinctions are further important, because they clarify the often held but mistaken belief that wandering behavior is the single or preeminent risk factor for individuals becoming lost. In contrast, the research findings reviewed in this chapter demonstrate that wandering is only *one* of many possible antecedents of a becoming lost episode.

Antecedents for Becoming Lost in the Community

The majority of becoming lost events begin with a departure from home. However, a sizeable proportion of these events occur when a cognitively impaired individual departs from an institutional setting. Episodes of becoming lost in the community are preceded by an array of behaviors and circumstances, as illustrated in Table 10.1 (Rowe & Glover, 2001).

The information in Table 10.1 was compiled from files recorded in the Safe Return® Program's missing and discovery database; a selection of illustrative cases will be briefly described here (see Chapter 13 for more information).

Another class of still poorly understood antecedents of becoming lost in the community is those that occur not in conjunction with departures from residential settings, but from departures that occur out into the community, either when care recipients are in the company of a caregiver or when they are alone. For example, one Safe Return® account documents the retrieval of a woman who was wandering around the parking lot (fortunately wearing an information bracelet) by a department store employee. Using the bracelet information, employees paged the husband on the store intercom, and he quickly came for her. Even long-established and routine patterns of activity that occur in the community pose a risk to unattended persons with dementia. Missing person searches are not infrequently initiated when such a person becomes unable to return home in conjunction with, for example, a walk to and from church. In another Safe Return® case, a police officer found an older, Spanish-speaking woman roaming the streets, extremely confused and not knowing her name. She had become lost, because she was in an unfamiliar place. As described in another Safe Return® report, a care recipient left and became lost in the community, during the instant that her caregiver dropped and recovered a set of keys. Because multiple and diverse factors are often involved in becoming lost, pinpointing the antecedent can be difficult. Because our current state of knowledge on antecedents does not allow

TABLE 10.1 Antecedent Situations in Which Persons With Dementia Began the Unattended Wandering

Context	% (n = 146)
At daycare, nursing home, or other caregiving facility	17.9
Outside home with caregiver	14.3
Agitated/difficult behavior of CI individual in the home setting	13.1
Caregiver distracted	13.1
Normal outing alone and didn't return	13.1
Home alone	10.7
Caregiver asleep	7.1
Out driving alone	6.0
Being transported by professional services	4.8

Case 1

In one case of home departure, the caregiver, a daughter, last sighted the care recipient, her mother, as she helped her into bed. The caregiver awoke to find her mother missing and her mother's pajama bottoms wet and lying on the floor. In this instance, the antecedent to the event of becoming lost in the community was the cognitively impaired person's unattended exit while the caregiver slept.

Case 2

In another case, a person with dementia left the house and was unable to return, having earlier informed her husband that she wished to visit her (in reality deceased) mother and sister. Thus, an agitated state served as the antecedent for becoming lost.

Case 3

Similarly, impulsivity can precede a becoming lost event. For example, a mother's wandering out of the kitchen door was the precipitant of a missing person report, illustrating the point that something as seemingly innocuous as unsupervised movements around the home can also precede an event of becoming lost.

Case 4

More surprising, perhaps, are cases in which care recipients became lost in the vicinity of the institutional care setting in which they reside. One man walked out of his facility wearing a code alert bracelet designed to alert staff to his departure from facility grounds, the alarm failing to detonate for unknown reasons (Rowe & Glover, 2001).

the establishment of causality and thus prediction, prevention of community-based getting lost behavior is key.

Prevention Strategies

Prevention strategies on several levels, ranging from caregiver to community involvement, can be implemented in order to reduce the possibility that an at-risk person with dementia becomes lost. It is imperative that health practitioners educate family caregivers not to rely on the care recipient's past behaviors as a predictor of current or future conduct, particularly becoming lost (Rowe & Glover, 2001). A primary preventive strategy is to avoid leaving the care recipient alone and unattended, as much as possible. As illustrated in the previous section, a care recipient can wander off and become lost during the few seconds that it takes a caregiver to pick up a set of keys. The unpredictable nature of the behavior of the at-risk, cognitively impaired individual necessitates 24-hour supervision, although constant vigilance intensifies caregiver burden and stress (Rowe & Glover, 2001). Yet, health practitioners can assist by helping caregivers understand and plan ahead for the possible problems associated with caring for a cognitively impaired individual, as well as by providing them with appropriate resources (Rowe et al., 2004).

SIDEBAR 1

Clinical Tips

Health practitioners should encourage caregivers to:

- understand that wandering and becoming lost in the community are different problems;
- realize that all persons with dementia are at risk of becoming lost in the community regardless of age, physical condition, level of care, or wandering proclivity;
- ensure adequate home safety (locks, a home security system, or the installation of CareWatch©);
- regularly update the care recipient's photographs to be readily available to the police, searchers, or media in case they become lost;
- inform trusted neighbors about the care recipient's dementia, and possibly ask them to escort them home if the person with dementia is found alone;
- avoid leaving the care recipients by themselves (24-hour supervision, respite care services, or a way to keep in regular touch if the care recipient lives independently);
- report if the person with dementia is expressing increased agitation or frustration to health care practitioners;
- have a step-by-step search plan (hasty search, call 911, and Safe Return®);
- have initial 5-mile residential search as part of search plan (public buildings, residential yards, stores, and streets), followed by a nonresidential search (wooded areas, fields, or near bodies of water) after 6–12 hours if care recipient is not found; and
- use the media (television, news, or radio) as a component of a search plan, to increase public awareness in case the person with dementia becomes missing.

Aside from supervision, practitioners can guide the caregiver in techniques for establishing adequate home safety and security for the care recipient. If a caregiver is asleep or distracted in some other way, securing the home environment so the care recipient cannot leave without assistance provides the needed level of additional security. Caregivers can make sure all doors leading outside are locked, have locks installed out of care recipients' reach, or have the lock changed to a type the care recipient cannot operate. Motion sensors that produce a tone when motion is detected can be found in hardware stores and placed on doors to warn caregivers of a potential unattended exit. To take home safety to another level, a home security system that monitors the care recipient around the house and alerts the caregiver should a door to the outside open, is also available (Rowe, Lane, & Phipps, 2007). But these are not the only measures that can be taken.

Updating photographs of the cognitively impaired individual regularly would be ideal, for these can be ready for distribution to search teams, police officers, hospitals, and the media, in case the care recipient should go missing. Also, caregivers can notify trusted neighbors that a person with dementia lives in the immediate area and can ask them to guide him or her home if seen outside unaccompanied. If available, the caregiver can utilize respite services to avoid leaving the care recipient alone. For persons with dementia who live independently, ensuring they are in regular contact with someone able to accurately assess their safety is another preventive approach. As aforementioned, one possible precipitating event leading to becoming lost in the community is a care recipient getting agitated and hastily departing from a site, familiar or not. Health care practitioners can suggest that caregivers report increased agitation and belligerence, so nonpharmacologic or pharmacologic strategies may be recommended. Such a solution may lessen the chance that care recipients will manifest behaviors resulting in leaving the safety of their homes or facilities. Other helpful community resources that caregivers need to know about include: experts in the community who may be able to offer guidance, caregiver support groups, and most significantly, the Safe Return® program (see Chapter 13).

Successful Search Strategies

If, however, a care recipient does become lost, the caregiver should have a predetermined search plan to follow. The first step in such a plan should include a hasty search (Rowe, 2003; Rowe et al., 2004), in which the caregiver takes 5 to 10 minutes to look through the house and then the yard. After this, the caregiver should call 911 to notify the local law enforcement agency, and then contact Safe Return® if the person with dementia has been previously enrolled in this program. Following this, it is a good idea to enlist friends and neighbors in the search, assigning sections of the immediate area to each person. The caregiver should be easily reachable by phone at all times. Because the care recipient might return home on his or her own, someone (preferably, the caregiver so as not to alarm the care recipient) should stay home while the search is being conducted.

If law enforcement personnel are needed, it is recommended that a concentrated search begin within a 5-mile radius from where the individual was last seen (Rowe & Glover, 2001), because this constitutes the parameter where most individuals are found alive. Residential yards, public buildings, stores, highways, and streets are all places that might be accessible to the care recipient and should be searched. If necessary, the search should continue throughout the night, because cognitively impaired individuals usually keep walking and may be easier to identify at this time.

If 6 to 12 hours have passed and the missing individual is still not found, the search should be refocused on areas in which persons who become lost are more often found dead than alive. Research has established that those found dead generally have secluded themselves in natural places such as woods, fields, ditches, near or in bodies of water, or heavily treed areas (Rowe & Bennett, 2003; Rowe et al., 2004). Not only are these individuals very difficult to find because they are in areas not normally occupied, they will often make additional attempts to seclude themselves by hiding in the bushes or under leaves or branches. It is very rare that lost individuals seek help or respond to calls from families or searchers. It seems that once they seclude themselves, they remain there until found. Thus, search and rescue teams need to maintain an aggressive approach to find a well-secluded individual. Those who choose to seclude themselves do so fairly close to the place last seen, with almost 50 percent being found within half a mile (Rowe & Bennett, 2003). In this area, searchers need to conduct a very intensive search of the natural areas, literally searching every square foot. Searchers can space themselves 2–3 feet apart to make a horizontal search line, and move forward slowly searching every square foot. Bodies of water, thick shrubbery, deserted structures, and bottoms of cliffs should all be scrutinized. If this is not successful, the radius should be increased to one mile. If still not successful, the same area should be re-searched as most individuals are eventually found in an area that was previously searched.

The two most common causes of death are exposure (about 75%) and drowning (about 20%) (Rowe et al., 2004). In order to prevent death by exposure, searchers need to be aware of air temperatures. There is much less time when conditions of extreme heat or cold prevail outside, sometimes less than 24 hours. In these situations, it is recommended that an intensive search be conducted as soon as possible, because individuals most likely to die are those who have secluded themselves, not those who are walking in the community.

Of note, persons with dementia who reside in residential care facilities have a very high incidence of death after becoming lost. Twenty-three percent of deaths occurred in individuals from these facilities while only 2–5 percent of this population is housed in this type of facility (Rowe et al., 2004).

Of course all available search resources, such as scent-sniffing dogs, aircraft, or heat-sensing radar should be utilized, but the vast majority of care recipients were found by searchers on foot or Good Samaritans. Reverse 911 can also be of great assistance as sometimes individuals will wander into strangers' yards or might be seen walking in the neighborhood. Reverse 911 is a program established by law enforcement in which homes in the area are called with a prerecorded message indicating assistance is needed in searching for an individual.

If someone becomes lost while driving, the search must first be directed toward locating the vehicle (Rowe & Bennett, 2003). The radius for a vehicle search should be the approximate miles that could be driven on the gas available in the car. It is unusual for someone with dementia to have the ability to put additional gas in the car. Once the car is found, the individual may have wandered away. The focus then should start within a 0.5–1 mile radius of where the car was found.

Local chapters of the Alzheimer's Association should follow-up each missing (or found) person report in order to inform caregivers of available community resources and services (Rowe & Glover, 2001). At this point, the public awareness media campaigns, such as described in Chapter 13, are most beneficial, because they facilitate communication between the public and the missing individual. Letting the general public know how to identify cognitively impaired individuals who may have become lost can increase the chances they will be found (Rowe, 2003).

For individuals who have previously become lost in the community, caregivers may want to consider obtaining a tracking device. The most common one available in some communities is Project Lifesaver (www.projectlifesaver.org). This uses a radio frequency emitting transmitter worn on the wrist like a watch. Local law enforcement agencies purchase three receiver antennas tuned to the transmitters radio frequency setting and can then move them through the community by foot, car, or air to locate the transmitter worn by the individual with dementia. To ascertain the availability of such a service in a particular community, the local law enforcement agency should be contacted. There are also privately purchased tracking devices that can be useful. Global Positioning System tracking devices are less helpful because of the difficulty in identifying a transmitter without good exposure to the sky. This is critical since individuals most at risk of dying have secluded themselves in wooded areas.

PRACTICE IMPLICATIONS

Educating the public on how to identify persons with dementia who may have become lost, as well as how to aid them in returning safely, are additional ways in which the community can be of assistance. Through media campaigns or presentations to public service organizations, the public can be enlightened about this program and can learn to recognize whether a person with dementia may be lost (and how to communicate with them). These types of preemptive strikes can be taken, not only by caregivers, but by community leaders as well.

Likewise, professional caregivers, such as physicians and other health care practitioners, have a responsibility to educate support personnel in formal care settings in the preparation and implementation of sufficient safety plans for clients or residents who go missing (Rowe et al., 2004). Administrators of such facilities should review all safety plans and assess their effectiveness. To reduce a delay in starting a search when the case arises, professional caregivers should have a clear, formal policy and plan for reporting missing individuals, including timely contact with law enforcement. Because the level of security in residential care settings varies, practitioners serving in advisory roles to institutions in establishing the strongest available safety policies can serve as advisors, provide models, and set standards for appraising policies in other institutions. In this way, practitioners provide assistance to caregivers who are contemplating institutional placement. Wherever the care recipient may live, either at a formal care setting or at home, communication and teamwork among health care practitioners, caregivers, and the community creates a strong prevention plan (Rowe & Glover, 2001).

GAPS IN RESEARCH

It is interesting that a person with dementia makes a very distinct choice after they become lost in the community (e.g., continuing to walk in populated areas versus secluding themselves in natural areas). This fact is very informative for planning searches. However, we know little about under what circumstances this choice is made. Are the important factors inherent to the disease state, previous life patterns, weather, geographic chance, or other clinical or demographic variables? We also know little about the specifics of the seclusion behavior. What are the characteristics of the locations that are chosen? For instance, if a wooded area is entered, how far into the area will the individual travel? This information is critical in order to better focus search efforts resulting in a more rapid discovery and lower costs. Do the recommended search techniques result in a more rapid discovery of those who become secluded after becoming lost?

Other than general care principles, we know little about prevention strategies. Does camouflage of the home or institution exits prevent unattended exits? What technologies can be employed when the individual must be left alone? It is unknown why persons from residential facilities have a very high death rate after becoming lost.

There is also a gap in basic knowledge on becoming lost in the community. We do not have an empirically-based incidence rate. It is unclear what clinical, demographic, or disease factors place an individual at greater risk of becoming lost.

Finally, health care practitioners have inadequate knowledge of this problem and do not assist families in implementing prevention strategies. The Safe Return® program is grossly underutilized. Tracking technology currently is also underused, perhaps because it is bulky, expensive, and serves only a single purpose. Because caregivers typically think that the risk of becoming lost is nonexistent, they are not inclined to use a technology that serves only this purpose.

CONCLUSION

It is critical for caregivers and health care personnel to remember that *any* person with dementia is at risk of becoming lost in the community. Prevention strategies are essential, because it is not uncommon for a care recipient to be found only after death has occurred, or in some instances, never found. Starting a search immediately is crucial, and neighbors can be of great assistance, especially if they have been informed ahead of time about the possibility of such an occurrence. Law enforcement support should be enlisted as early in the search as possible, depending on the situation. For example, if it is cold outside and the surrounding area provides optimal places for a person to hide, the need for timely rescue escalates rapidly as death often occurs as a result of exposure. The most prudent strategies, obviously, will be those preventive in nature. Education and training, however, are often necessary precursors to these strategies, since informal and formal caretakers, as well as a majority of community law enforcement personnel have received little, if any, preparation for managing this kind of dementia-related crisis.

RESOURCES

Alzheimer's Association: www.alz.org; 1-800-272-3900
Project Lifesaver International: www.projectlifesaver.org; 1-877-580-5433
Safe Return®: www.alz.org/safereturn/; 1-888-572-8566
Resources for finding lost individuals: www.nursing.ufl.edu/dementia/

REFERENCES

Algase, D. L., Son, G. R., Beattie, E., Song, J. A., Leitsch, S., & Yao, L. (2004). The interrelatedness of wandering and wayfinding in a community sample of persons with dementia. *Dementia and Geriatric Cognitive Disorders, 17*(3), 231–239.

Rowe, M. A. (2003). People with dementia who become lost. *American Journal of Nursing, 103*(7), 32–39.

Rowe, M. A., & Bennett, V. (2003). A look at deaths occurring in persons with dementia lost in the community. *American Journal of Alzheimer's Disease and Other Dementias, 18*(6), 343–348.

Rowe, M. A., Feinglass, N. G., & Wiss, M. E. (2004). Persons with dementia who become lost in the community: A case study, current research, and recommendations. *Mayo Clinic Proceedings, 79*(11), 1417–1422.

Rowe, M. A., & Glover, J. C. (2001). Antecedents, descriptions and consequences of wandering in cognitively-impaired adults and the Safe Return (SR) program. *American Journal of Alzheimer's Disease and Other Dementias, 16*(6), 344–352.

Rowe, M. A., Lane, S., & Phipps, C. (2007). CareWatch: A home monitoring system for use in homes of persons with cognitive impairment. *Topics in Geriatric Research, 23*, 3–8.

PART IV

Interventions

CHAPTER ELEVEN

Behavior Management of Wandering Behavior: Staff Training Issues

Lawrence Schonfeld, Lisa M. Brown, and Victor A. Molinari

INTRODUCTION

Wandering among residents in nursing homes (NHs) and assisted living facilities (ALFs) is a frequently reported behavior problem. While there have been improvements in training requirements over the years, certified nursing assistants (CNAs) and other direct care staff in comparison to supervisory staff and administrators receive the least amount of training on knowledge about dementia, modifying the environment, and identifying and managing problem behaviors (Schonfeld et al., 1999). A number of curricula, training tapes, and train-the-trainer approaches have been described in the literature, but usually the focus is on behavior problems in general, not wandering specifically. In this chapter, we focus on training issues relative to implementation of behavior modification procedures for wandering behavior by staff members in long-term care facilities and applications.

REVIEW OF THE LITERATURE

Staff training in behavior modification usually is broad-based. In NHs, Kramer and Smith (2000) have noted that while 75 hours of training is required to become a CNA, much of the training addresses the residents' basic care needs, while little is specifically devoted to care of people with dementia. Kramer and Smith (2000) identify several characteristics that might facilitate successful implementation of behavior management skills. These include: a strong administrative support system, training staff on management issues, experiential learning rather than merely attending and listening to lectures, a peer-oriented approach with videotapes of CNAs implementing techniques for residents with dementia, and problem solving and support groups for the NH staff to discuss difficulties they are experiencing.

Research on behavior problems in ALFs is still relatively recent. Wandering may be of greater concern for ALFs, because these facilities rely on a home-like environment and philosophy of maintaining residents' independence. Although increasing numbers of ALFs are developing dementia-specific units, when an ALF resident wanders it may lead to a transfer out of the facility, often to a more restrictive unit or to a NH.

In a survey of 612 ALF administrators and supervisory staff in Florida, Schonfeld (2003) found that wandering or trying to leave the ALF was among the most frequently reported and among the most difficult behavior problems facing the staff and occurred an average of about 2.5 times per week. Not surprisingly, training in behavior management techniques was noted as a priority by the respondents.

The consequences of wandering not only affect residents through falls, injuries, weight loss, fatigue, sleep disturbance, getting lost, or death, but also affect caregivers through increased stress and job dissatisfaction, as they attempt to deal with intrusions into others' rooms and safety concerns. Staff training is the key to improved care, management of behavior problems, and hopefully, reduced caregiver stress and job turnover.

Requirements for NHs and ALFs regarding dementia education and methods for managing disruptive behaviors differ from state to state. In a six-state survey of directors of nursing from 899 NHs, less than half of the nursing staff (49%) and only about a third (32%) of nurses' aides had expertise in managing disruptive behaviors (Borson, Reichman, Coyne, Rovner, & Sakauye, 2000).

It is no surprise that wandering is not singled out for specialized staff training. It is typically associated with other behavior problems such as nonaggressive agitation (Cohen-Mansfield, Werner, Marx, & Freedman, 1991; Colombo et al., 2001), screaming and calling out (Snyder, Rupprecht, Pyrek, Brekhus, & Moss, 1978), physical aggression (Dawson & Reid, 1987), depression (Hope et al., 2001; Kiely, Morris, & Algase, 2000; Klein et al., 1999), and disturbed nighttime sleep (Hope et al.; Klein et al.). Our recent research on male, NH residents within the Veterans Health Administration system of the Department of Veterans Affairs (VA) also revealed a strong association between the presence of wandering and all other behavior problems recorded on using the Minimum Data Set (MDS; Schonfeld et al., in press).

Although the literature on wandering has been part of the general research on behavioral issues, a few studies were specific to the problem. Among the earliest studies on behavior modification of wandering were those conducted by Hussian and colleagues, primarily within a geropsychiatric inpatient population. Hussian (1981) noted that wandering was influenced by environmental and other stimulus conditions, and observed that wandering tended to occur where much of the stimulation and reinforcement was located on the unit (areas where others were present, as well as windows, water fountains, food trays). Hussian and Davis (1985) classified four variables associated with wandering: akathisia (restlessness that is often associated with the use of antipsychotic medications), exit-seeking behavior (requests to leave as well as attempts to use exit doors), modeling or following another person who is walking, or self-stimulation such as touching and turning doorknobs.

Effectiveness of Staff Training

Numerous studies over the past 30 years have demonstrated the effectiveness of training staff in the use of behavior modification procedures. Behavior modification involves definition of the target behavior, collecting baseline data, setting short and long-term behavioral goals, identifying the reinforcement principles and plans to modify the behavior, and specifying the method for evaluating effectiveness of the plan. Outcomes are typically measured not only in the suppression of unwanted behaviors, such as physical and verbal aggression, resistance to delivery of personal care, and wandering, but also in increases in adaptive behavior such as independence in performing activities of daily living (ADL) skills, positive social interactions, and orientation or adaptation to their environment (Burgio & Burgio, 1990; Hussian, 1986, 1987). Despite numerous studies demonstrating improvement in residents' function as the result of implementation of behavior modification techniques, long-term retention by the staff in the use of these skills remains an issue (Burgio et al., 2002).

Training CNAs, nurses, and other direct care staff often involves lecture format with curricula written at a simple level (e.g., eighth grade reading level), either by expert instruction or train-the-trainer approaches (Burgio et al., 2002; Cohen-Mansfield, Werner, Culpepper, & Barkley, 1997; Schonfeld et al., 1999). Successful applications by the staff are evaluated by direct observation or videotaped sessions with their interactions with residents (Wood, Cummings, Schnelle, & Stephens, 2002).

PRINCIPLES OF BEHAVIOR MODIFICATION

Training staff in the use of behavior modification techniques requires that several principles be adopted. The first principle is that the behavior must be sufficiently maladaptive or problematic to warrant the use of a behavioral intervention. Frequent wandering in the halls of a facility may be tolerated as long as the resident is safe and no harm is coming to the resident or to other residents. To make such judgments concerning whether to address behavior problems, interdisciplinary treatment teams should be utilized. Treatment teams may consist of direct care staff, nursing supervisors, physicians, social workers, and other paid caregivers. In addition, family members should be involved and assuming competency, the resident as well. If the treatment team decides that the behavior is both high frequency and problematic, then a plan should be implemented.

The second principle is that the resident, even if diagnosed with cognitive impairment or dementia, should be assumed to have some capacity for learning through the appropriate use of reinforcement techniques until proven otherwise. The literature is replete with examples of successful implementation of behavior modification that involve suppression of behavior problems while leading to increased positive, adaptive behaviors. A few key examples borrowed from the literature can motivate staff to practice the techniques with their residents. Videotapes of staff applying shaping and reinforcement techniques, using simple prompts, verbal cues, and so forth, are appropriate methods to help convince the staff members being trained that the techniques are both simple and effective.

A third is the principle of parsimony. In behavior modification, the principle of parsimony refers to reliance on observations of the antecedents (i.e., those events that reliably precede the target behavior) to help predict the onset of the target behavior, and not to hypothesize or make assumptions about unobservable motivations for engaging in the behavior. To accomplish this, staff members will identify antecedent conditions to behavior problems as well as the consequences that maintain those behaviors. Staff members must not jump to conclusions about a resident's motivation for exhibiting the behavior, but instead observe the antecedent conditions to repeated behaviors, attempt to discern the pattern of events, and then reinforce adaptive, incompatible behaviors while extinguishing the maladaptive behavior.

A fourth principle NH and ALF staff members must adopt is that while behavior modification techniques require some effort or labor in the early stages of implementation, they will provide substantial benefits or "payoffs" if conducted properly, such as less time spent in trying to suppress unwanted behaviors and actually encouraging more independence in ADLs. Staff members are often skeptical about their ability to implement behavioral techniques, because their busy schedules will not permit them to observe baseline behavior or employ reinforcements.

Finally, it is necessary for staff members to learn what successful implementation of a treatment plan means. Often, staff tends to believe that if the behavior problem has not been completely eliminated, the plan has failed. Staff must accept that small decreases in wandering represent some degree of success and that the plan for modifying the behavior should be maintained or altered somewhat to achieve further improvements.

Teaching the Steps for Conducting Behavior Modification

Once the training addresses the aforementioned principles, trainees are taught the skills necessary to modify maladaptive behaviors. The following steps describe the method by which long-term staff can be trained to address wandering in their facilities.

1. Identifying and Defining the Behavior Problem

A definition of a target behavior must be objective, specific, and parsimonious, in that the behavior can be verified by observations of one or more individuals over a specified period of time and doesn't involve unfounded assumptions such as guessing about the resident's motivation for wandering.

In this example, neither staff member is using the principle of parsimony, and each assumes a motive without observing the behavior of

Case Vignette

On a typical day, Mr. Green walks for hours around the hallways of his NH. He approaches all closed doors in the facility and touches or turns each doorknob. He never seems to go through the door, but occasionally opens the door and stares at the opening for a few minutes before closing it and continuing walking. On several occasions, he has set off the alarm connected to the exit door.

A staff member labels the behavior as "attempting to elope from the NH" and asks the supervisor to implement precautionary measures to prevent elopement, such as locking all the exit doors and residents' rooms when they are not in them. An evening staff member recalls that Mr. Green was once a security guard at a warehouse and believes that Mr. Green is checking the doors to make sure the facility was safe just as he did for his work. He believes Mr. Green should be allowed to roam freely about the NH.

elopement. However, neither assumption may be accurate and is likely irrelevant to implementing behavioral techniques. The problem definition should be clear to all staff members involved in the process. Having at least two staff members observe and define the behavior should facilitate the definition so that as the plan evolves, the staff can easily determine whether the behavior is changing or not. In the example of Mr. Green, one might define the problem as "Wandering the halls and opening doors to residents' rooms or to exits."

Appropriate training of staff allows a more scientific approach for defining the behavior. Through observations of the resident the behavior problem is identified and labeled in simple terms. Staff are trained to identify "antecedents" that precede the high frequency behavior problem as well as the consequences that are reinforcing the behavior. These constitute the A-B-C behavior chain (antecedents-behavior-consequences).

To assist staff with the recording of the A-B-C chain, various forms have been developed. For example, Jackson and Patterson (1980) describe the Behavior Analysis Form (BAF) that provides one column for each of the three parts of the chain. When an unusual behavior occurs, a staff member uses the BAF to record the occurrence and break down the components of the chain of events. Should that behavior occur again, any staff member will be able to compare notes on the behavior using the behavior chain. As shown in Figure 11.1, to use the BAF, the staff member begins by writing down in the second column (Behavior) a brief and simple description of the behavior and its duration. Referring to the case vignette, the behavior as recorded would be: "Walked around the hallways near the television lounge then walked toward the fire exit door and turned the knob." Then in the first column, the staff member records the antecedent conditions observed: date and time, location on the unit, persons in the vicinity, the specifics of the interaction, and other events that preceded the behavior. The third column describes the consequences. In particular staff should be aware of and record any stimulus that might "strengthen" the behavior problem, that is, the positive reinforcers such as attention from staff members. Also shown in Figure 11.1, under observed behavior for the first event it is noted that Mr. Green's attempt to leave the unit through an exit door set off an alarm. This was preceded by a request from a CNA, Ms. Martin, that Mr. Green join the other residents in the television lounge (i.e., the antecedent to the behavior). The consequences included staff rushing to that location and Ms. Martin yelling at him not to use that door again. In the second instance, later in the day, Mr. Green began wandering the hallways and trying door knobs. He entered another resident's room and went in, causing her to become upset and yell. The antecedents were recorded as "no one around" and Mr. Green stating that he was bored. The consequences were that the resident affected by the intrusion became upset and screamed. He asked her what she was doing in his room, then fell while trying to leave.

The recording of these two incidents of wandering and their antecedents and consequences does not constitute a treatment plan. It only provides the foundation for staff members to report behavior problems to the treatment team and use the information to devise a plan to change the behavior.

Behavior Analysis Form (BAF) (modified by)

Resident's Name: John Green SS# 999-99-9999 Unit: East Wing

ANTECEDENT(S)	BEHAVIOR(S)	CONSEQUENCE(S)
Date: 6/25/06 Time: 10:15 a.m Location: Television lounge. Persons in Vicinity: CNA Martin and 3 residents: Mrs. Jackson, Ms. Miller, and Mr. Allen Specifics of Interaction: CNA Martin asked him to join others in the TV lounge. Other Events: Mr. Green said he did not want to join the others.	Observed Behavior: Walked up and down hallways near the television lounge then walked towards the fire exit door and turned the knob. Duration of Behavior: 3 minutes	Interpersonal Interaction: Mr. Green told the residents in TV lounge he was going home. Mr. Allen said "see you tomorrow!" Other Environmental Interactions: Security alarm went off. All staff ran to the exit door. CNA Martin yelled at him to not use that door again. Recorder: Wilma Smith,

FIGURE 11.1 A completed Behavior Analysis Form (BAF) based on the case vignette.

(Continued)

		R.N.
Date: 6/25/06 Time: 1:30 p.m. Location: Hallway outside Mrs. Jackson's room Persons in Vicinity: No one in the hallway. Specifics of Interaction: Said he was bored. Walked hallways trying doorknobs to several doors. Other Events: Others were napping.	Observed Behavior: Opened the door to Ms. Jackson's room and went into the room. Asked Mrs. Jackson what she was doing in his room. Duration of Behavior: 4 minutes	Interpersonal Interaction: Mrs. Jackson screamed for help. Mr. Green fell while trying to leave. Other Environmental Interactions: Three Staff ran to the room picked him up and escorted him back to his room Recorder: Wilma Smith, R.N.

FIGURE 11.1 (Continued)

2. *Behavioral Goals*

Once we specify the target behavior to be modified, it is necessary to determine what the outcome of the behavior modification will be for the short-term as well as the long-term. Progress toward achieving the short-term goals is often measured in small, reasonably achievable steps. Progress should be reviewed at case reviews, resident rounds, or treatment team meetings. Short-term goals should be evaluated based on progress made and based on the treatment team's judgment that these goals may be modified to target greater or lesser changes than previously targeted.

Note that in this example, short-term goals describe behaviors to be decreased as well as behaviors to be increased. It is our experience that NH and ALF staff members often find it is easier to identify behaviors to suppress and even gravitate, unfortunately, to "punitive" techniques, that is, scolding, restricting movement, and so forth. In contrast they typically find it more difficult to identify socially relevant goals for the replacement behavior, that is, the positive and adaptive behaviors that should take the place of the unwanted behavior. In the case vignette,

Case Vignette (continued): Short-Term Goals

1. Suppression Goals: At the end of the first month, average frequency of walking in the hallways will decrease by 50% from baseline. Attempts to open the doors will also decrease by 50%.
2. Adaptive Goals: Mr. Green will increase social activities such as crafts and participation in reminiscence group by 90% at the end of the first month.

staff members saw Mr. Green wandering the halls and trying to turn various doorknobs. Staff might have selected a suppression goal such as "decrease the number of times per day the client is observed in bedroom." It might be tempting for the NH staff to consider punitive methods such as reprimanding Mr. Green, locking all doors, or constraining movement about the facility. In this instance, staff should focus on questions such as: "What positive behavior should replace the maladaptive behavior?" and "What skill must the resident learn to improve functioning?" These questions require more creativity and planning. For Mr. Green, the goal might be stated as "increase group participation and activity," or it could be to "increase social interactions with other people on the unit."

Long-term goals should reflect the more broadly conceived positive impact on the person's behavior. These goals are indicative of the final behavioral goal after intervention ends. The treatment plan can be terminated or maintained on a less intensive basis, when the long-term goal is accomplished. For wandering behavior, whenever Mr. Green is seen leaving his room or the dining hall, a plan that includes prompts to walk toward a group activity room may lead to increased participation in social activities and conversation.

3. *Baseline Data*

The first two steps (identifying the problem and setting the goals) often go hand-in-hand with collection of baseline data, so these three steps may seem less sequential and more simultaneous. Baseline data not only determine the extent of the problem prior to treatment but also are used to evaluate success of the treatment plan. Baseline data are usually measured in terms of frequency, magnitude or intensity, or duration, and include other details such as time of day and length of observation period during which the behavior is observed.

Many NH and ALF staff members balk at formal data collection or graphing of baseline data, thinking that it is too lengthy and tedious given their busy care schedules. Thus, when conducting training, it is necessary to provide the rationale for collecting baseline data. The rate at which behavior problems being targeted occur must be stable prior to initiating the plan. This is especially important for a resident who has just been placed in a new facility who may exhibit wandering during a period of "adaptation" to the new environment. In such cases, as adaptation progresses, wandering may decline without intervention. Should staff implement treatment without baseline data during this adaptation period, they might falsely attribute the decline in behavior to the treatment. Determination of a "stable" baseline depends on many factors: frequency of the behavior, the conditions under which it occurs, and the projected length of treatment (or length of stay in a residential treatment program). Stability in the frequency of a behavior might be considered as a fluctuation of no more than a small percentage (e.g., 5%) from the average behavior during five consecutive observations of the behavior over a specified period of time.

4. Implementing the Behavior Modification

Behavioral techniques have proven effective for many individuals in a variety of settings. In general, there are two categories of procedures: those that lead to increases in behaviors and those that lead to decreases in behaviors. These will be discussed in greater detail in the next section.

5. Evaluation of the Plan

Traditionally, behavioral approaches also involve evaluation of the treatment plan, by comparing a sequence of baseline, treatment, return-to-baseline, and return to treatment conditions, that is, an A-B-A-B design. In such an evaluation, if the return to baseline (second "A" condition) results in a return of the behavior similar to pretreatment frequency, it is likely that the treatment plan was responsible for the improvement. The second "B" condition is often a reimplementation of the treatment, but often using a gradual, fading technique in which the reinforcers might be spaced out over progressively longer periods. As noted previously, nursing assistants and other staff members may become resistant to implementing a behavioral technique if it is perceived as burdensome. As a compromise, one can train staff members to implement a simple A-B design as long as the "B" condition is modified through a fading technique. That decision must be made by the treatment team using the observation data collected over time.

As treatment progresses and criteria are met, the plan can be altered to make the short-term goals more similar to the long-term goals. Using the earlier example, there would be an increase in group participation or other appropriate social interactions, with a simultaneous decrease in wandering observed over a certain period of time. A staff member can compare the frequency of the behavior during baseline to frequency during the treatment plan.

Using the earlier example, care providers will be able to answer the question "Did Mr. Green stop wandering as a result of this intervention?" At the same time, they should be able to answer: "Did Mr. Green acquire new, more socially acceptable behaviors that are incompatible with wandering?" Staff members responsible for the resident should graph data to demonstrate to staff and others (maybe even to the resident and the resident's family) the improvements that have occurred.

TECHNIQUES FOR INCREASING BEHAVIORS

Socially acceptable or adaptive behaviors are learned when positive reinforcement techniques are used, that is, response-contingent reinforcement that leads to an increase in behaviors. Paraphrasing Thorndike's (1913) well-known Law of Effect, behaviors that are followed by satisfaction are more likely to recur, and those followed by discomfort are less likely to occur. Examples of positive reinforcers used in NHs and ALFs are compliments or praise from key staff members, food, money, and engaging in preferred activities. A staff member should not assume that everyone finds money or food to be a motivator, or that what the staff member finds rewarding is also a motivator for the resident.

Reinforcers are identified through observations of, or interactions with, the resident. What is reinforcing for one resident is not necessarily the same for another. It is important that staff reinforce a desirable behavior, such as participating in the social activity group, and that they do not try to merely deliver reinforcement for the absence of wandering, such as telling Mr. Green: "You did a great job today by not wandering around the halls." Reinforcing the absence of a behavior does not assist in teaching more appropriate behaviors. Instead, the following are positive reinforcement techniques designed to increase adaptive behaviors:

Shaping

Shaping involves reinforcement of successive approximations to the target behavior. If we are trying to teach the resident the correct way back to his or her room, we would reinforce each effort made in the direction of the room by providing a great deal of praise. The next time, they make an attempt, we might make the criteria slightly more difficult, and we would hold off on praising the effort until the newer more difficult behavior occurs. The success of the shaping technique will be affected by the level of cognitive impairment, but if the steps remain simple and repetitious, and are reinforced appropriately, learning should take place.

Premack Principle

This technique involves using a high probability behavior as a reinforcer to increase the likelihood of a low probability behavior. It is one of the most useful techniques in that it relies on behaviors the individual already does frequently. For example, one might use the high frequency behavior of wandering to reinforce a low probability behavior, such as participating in a social activity with other residents. Using the Premack Principle, we might ask the person to join us in a particular social activity and if they do so for a small amount of time (e.g., 15 minutes), then tell the resident that you will go on a walk with them. Often, time spent with a favorite staff member (as perceived by the resident) may serve as a valuable reinforcer.

Prompting

When we prompt someone, we provide cues to direct the person toward the target behavior. To reduce wandering, visual cues such as halls painted in different colors might help the confused resident to differentiate the way to his or her bedroom, or to find the way to another location of importance such as the dining hall. If the individual exhibits the desired behavior, it must be followed by social praise. Verbal prompts might be delivered by requiring all staff members to use the exact same phrase as instructed. Simple repetitious prompts followed by reinforcement increase the likelihood of the adaptive behavior being repeated.

Modeling

Modeling involves the staff member demonstrating a skill or behavior for the individual, then asking the individual to attempt the same skill. For example, a staff might say to Mr. Green, "Let's take a walk to the dining hall. Can you please follow me?" Then the staff member would walk at a pace comfortable for Mr. Green to follow, and possibly point out certain landmarks such as a potted plant, or window overlooking the garden that is on the way to the dining hall. As Mr. Green mimics the behavior, he will be reinforced for his attempts.

Chaining

Chaining involves reinforcing the person for completion of a part of a series of a behaviors. First, a complex behavior is divided into a series of steps. The individual is prompted to begin the process by attempting the first component in the sequence. After the person completes the first step successfully, the staff member prompts the second step and then reinforces. After the resident is successful at the end of both the first and the second step, the staff member prompts the third step and reinforces at the completion of that third step. When working with individuals with memory impairment, backward chaining is particularly useful to teach spatial orientation within a facility (McEvoy & Patterson, 1986). Backward chaining begins with the final step, that is, the desired destination on the unit such as the dining hall, and gradually working backward to a more distant location such as the resident's bedroom. A staff member might teach such a person how to find the dining hall in a NH by walking with the resident to within sight of the dining hall. The staff member might say: "Mr. Green can you find your way to the dining hall?" If he is successful, then the staff member will praise or compliment him for finding it. Over the next few days, the resident is reinforced for the same small step. If successful on these easy tasks, the treatment plan would dictate that the resident is ready for the next step, that is, to extend the distance a little further away, often within eyesight, of the original starting place. The staff member would reinforce Mr. Green at the end of two consecutive steps. The backward chaining steps can be increased only as far as Mr. Green is successful with the completion of prior steps.

Clinical Tips for Behavioral Interventions

- Observe the resident and define the problem in simple language.
- Identify the components of the behavior chain (A-B-Cs).
- Evaluate for degree of consensus among staff members regarding resident observations.
- Determine if the plan includes both a goal to suppress the target behavior as well as a goal to increase a socially adaptive behavior.
- Decide how staff will determine if the resident's behavior has improved.

TECHNIQUES FOR DECREASING WANDERING BEHAVIOR

Although the labels sound ominous, negative reinforcement and punishment are two techniques that have been used in long-term care to manage behavior problems. Both must be implemented with careful thought and review by all staff and especially the treatment team because of their ethical, legal, and practical implications.

Reinforcement techniques, whether positive or negative, are those that involve response-contingent application of the stimulus and must result in an increase in behavior. Negative reinforcement refers to an increase in the learning of avoidance behavior when a noxious or unpleasant stimulus is present. For example, a resident who has triggered the alarm on an exit door several times, might continue wandering elsewhere, but actually avoid going near that door in the future. Avoidance of that door might therefore be increased.

Punishment, unlike reinforcement, must result in a decrease or suppression of the target behavior. The category "Punishment Type I" refers to response-contingent application of some unpleasant stimulus that results in a decrease in the behavior.

The category "Punishment Type II" refers to response-contingent *removal* of a positive reinforcer that must result in a decrease in the behavior. Extinction is a common form of this technique and is often used when all staff members are instructed to ignore a targeted behavior problem. In such a case, the positive reinforcer to be removed would be attention of the staff, assuming that attention is, in fact, reinforcing to the resident. Whether or not extinction for wandering would be effective would depend on each resident's behavior pattern and reinforcers. In many cases, wandering occurs in the absence of attention from other people. Other forms of Punishment Type II such as "social restitution," overcorrection, or response costs (e.g., fines or removal of privileges) that have been used with psychiatric and juvenile justice populations, may be inappropriate for many residents with dementia. No matter which of these techniques is employed, the treatment plan must also involve a corollary positive reinforcement technique to increase a targeted, socially adaptive behavior.

Hussian and Davis (1985) describe management of inappropriate wandering using several of the noted techniques. Staff in an institutional setting paired a noxious stimulus with a colored symbol on the door to a hazardous area to help suppress the behavior. They also reduced sensory feedback by tightening hardware or fitting doors snugly, or even replacing knobs with handles. Using a reinforcement schedule known as differential reinforcement of other behaviors (DRO), they created opportunities for wanderers to engage in other forms of stimulation (e.g., cloth, paper, and noise producing toys) that led to reinforcement for those activities.

Modification of the Environment

Modifying the environment may reduce some stimuli reinforcing inappropriate behavior, while providing opportunity to engage in other stimulating activities incompatible with elopement or exiting the facility. For example, Hussian (1982) altered the color of hallways and elevators to help residents in one facility discriminate between hazardous areas from those areas where ambulation would be safe. Others have developed a secure, stimulating area within the NH in the form of a wanderer's lounge (McGrowder-Lin & Bhatt, 1988). Safe walking and rest areas, walking paths, and fencing may be used to provide both stimulation and rest when the resident becomes fatigued. Personalizing the resident's room and surrounding areas with family pictures and other familiar items may enhance orientation. To reduce attempts at exiting, camouflaging exits is often used.

Clinical Tips for Management of Wandering

- Identify each resident's positive reinforcement (e.g., complimenting the person for completing a task).
- Ensure that the treatment plan is implemented uniformly. Consider writing the plan on a 3 x 5 file card, and place it in the person's chart.
- Evaluate if the resident's socially adaptive behaviors increase when applying the reinforcer (e.g., will the resident increase participation in a group activity?).
- Indicate how staff members should react if they observe the resident wandering (e.g., ignore the behavior if it is not causing safety problems).
- Modify the treatment plan and goals relying on objective, observational data and consensus of the treatment team.

SUMMARY

Many of the behavior modification techniques described in this chapter have been used successfully with diverse categories of behavior problems, although few studies have focused only on wandering. When training staff members to use these techniques, there are many variables affecting successful implementation.

Implementation Issues

Several issues must be considered when evaluating the effectiveness of behavioral approaches. These are as follows:

Overestimation of Resident's Ability

Alzheimer's disease and other neurodegenerative dementias are progressive disorders. Individuals in the early stages will be able to reach more challenging goals, while those in the most severe stages of dementia are less likely to retain information or maintain skills between sessions. If the staff define goals in terms of all-or-none changes, they will become frustrated in implementing the behavioral techniques. Long-term goals for those with severe levels of dementia may focus less on complete independence and more on reducing risky behavior. Staff members must also learn the need to be patient, recognizing that a resident's abilities may fluctuate and decline over long periods of time, thereby requiring adjustments to the treatment plan.

Consistency

Regardless of the severity of memory impairment, for a plan to work effectively *all* staff at a facility must be involved and all must reinforce and extinguish behaviors exactly the same way. When inconsistency occurs, the unit no longer acts like a unit. It only takes one staff member applying the plan inconsistently for the plan to fail and the behavior to be reinforced. Inconsistency in application of the behavior modification is overcome by ongoing in-service training and treatment team meetings that permit evaluation of the treatment plan. While some staff members will try hard to implement a plan as written, others may resist because of beliefs that older adults' behavior cannot be changed for any number of reasons. A simple technique to maintain the plan is to write clear instructions on a 3 x 5 card and place it in the resident's chart. Furthermore, family members and significant others should be informed of the benefits and consequences of adhering to the plan and how to respond consistently to decrease the maladaptive behavior.

Satiation

This occurs when a reinforcer is over-used or the resident adapts to it. If food is always used as reward, the person may become full. If the person has earned several privileges that day, earning more might not be as great a motivator. For such occurrences, it is wise to consider a list of reinforcers, such that if the first one no longer motivates the person, a second or third choice on the list might. In the example of Mr. Green, if praising him for finding the correct pathway or participating in the social activity doesn't always work, the treatment team can decide if other reinforcers might work.

Generalization

Generalization is always a concern in using behavior modification. Wandering may decrease in certain locations or only when certain staff members are on duty. Uniform application of the treatment plan is the ideal remedy, and to avoid satiation, switching reinforcers may also be helpful in generalization.

GAPS IN RESEARCH

Future research needs to explore the optimal costs and benefits regarding the amount of necessary training and desired formats (e.g., video, lecture, case example, etc.) to manage wandering behavior and which staff members the training should specifically target across the variety of long-term care settings. The latter include not only NHs, but also ALFs, continuing care retirement communities (CCRCs), and medical hospitals that admit NH or ALF residents in acute need. In addition, the limited research on staff training often does not address the potential influence of family members, visitors, and other residents in those facilities and how to incorporate those individuals into treatment plans.

ALFs represent a rapidly growing segment of the housing industry. Unlike NHs, ALFs lack a common database to determine the extent of problems such as wandering. Many ALFs are privately owned and are small facilities (e.g., 16 beds or less) with a wide variety of care providers. ALF training requirements vary from state to state, with dementia-related training often depending on type of care and operating license. Some facilities have separate units or wings for individuals with dementia, while others do not. How well staff members in ALFs are trained to deal with wandering should be explored. Similarly, little is known about CCRCs and the abilities of care providers in them. CCRCs are privately owned, planned retirement communities allowing an individual to change from independent living, assisted living, and nursing home components.

Finally, there is a dearth of research about the extent to which hospitals can deal with short stay admissions of long-term care residents with dementia. Without the support of experienced long-term care staff the novel environment may disorient inpatients and place them at high risk for wandering and injury.

CONCLUSION

All forms of behavior modification take time, creativity, and monitoring. However, the payoff for the resident is an improved quality of life, independence, accomplishment, and increased self-esteem. For the staff member, the payoff may be decreased workload and reduced stress. If successful, staff will have the ability to provide greater attention to other residents who require more intensive care and assistance.

REFERENCES

Borson, S., Reichman, W. E., Coyne, A. C., Rovner, B., & Sakauye, K. (2000). Effectiveness of nursing home staff as managers of disruptive behaviors. *American Journal of Geriatric Psychiatry, 8*(3), 251–253.

Burgio, L. D., & Burgio, K. L. (1990). Institutional staff training and management: A review of the literature and a model for geriatric, long-term-care facilities. *International Journal of Aging & Human Development, 30*(4), 287–302.

Burgio, L. D., Stevens, A., Burgio, K. L., Roth, D. L., Paul, P., & Gerstle, J. (2002). Teaching and maintaining behavior management skills in the nursing home. *The Gerontologist, 42*(4), 487–496.

Cohen-Mansfield, J., Werner, P., Culpepper, W. J., & Barkley, D. (1997). Evaluation of an in-service training program on dementia and wandering. *Journal of Gerontological Nursing, 23*(10), 40–47.

Cohen-Mansfield, J., Werner, P., & Marx, M. S., & Freedman L. (1991). Two studies of pacing in the nursing home. *Journal of Gerontology: Medical Sciences, 46*(3), M77–83.

Colombo, M., Vitali, S., Cairati, M., Perelli-Cippo, R., Bessi, O., Gioia, P., et al. (2001). Wanderers: Features, findings, issues. *Archives of Gerontology and Geriatrics, Supplement 7*, 99–106.

Dawson, P., & Reid, D. (1987). Behavioral dimensions of patients at risk of wandering. *The Gerontologist, 27*(1), 104–107.

Hope, T., Keene, J., McShane, R. H., Fairburn, C. G., Gedling, K., & Jacoby, R. (2001). Wandering in dementia: A longitudinal study. *International Psychogeriatrics, 13*(12), 137–147.

Hussian, R. (1981). *Geriatric psychology: A behavioural perspective.* New York: Nostrand Reinhold Co.

Hussian, R. A. (1982). Stimulus control in the modification of problematic behavior in elderly institutionalized patients. *International Journal of Behavioral Geriatrics, 1*(1), 33–46.

Hussian, R. A. (1986). Severe behavioral problems. In L. Teri & P. Lewinsohn (Eds.), *Geropsychological assessment and treatment* (pp. 121–143). New York: Springer.

Hussian, R. (1987). Wandering and disorientation. In L. L. Carstensen & B. A. Edelstein (Eds.), *Handbook of clinical gerontology* (pp. 177–189). New York: Pergamon Press.

Hussian, R. A., & Davis, R. L. (1985). *Responsive care: Behavioral interventions with elderly persons.* Champaign, IL: Research Press.

Jackson, G. M., & Patterson, R. L. (1980). Single case behavioral treatment. In R. L. Patterson, L. W. Dupree, D. A. Eberly, G. M. Jackson, M. J. O'Sullivan, L. A. Penner, L. A., et al. (Eds.), *Overcoming deficits of aging: A behavioral approach* (pp. 89–110). New York: Plenum Press.

Kiely, D. K., Morris, J. N., & Algase, D. L. (2000). Resident characteristics associated with wandering in nursing homes. *International Journal of Geriatric Psychiatry, 15*(11), 1013–1020.

Klein, D. A., Steinberg, M., Galik, E., Steele, C., Sheppard, J. M., Warren, A., et al. (1999). Wandering behaviour in community-residing persons with dementia. *International Journal of Geriatric Psychiatry, 14*(4), 272–279.

Kramer, N. A., & Smith, M. C. (2000). Training nursing assistants to care for nursing home residents with dementia. In V. Molinari (Ed.), *Professional psychology in long term care* (pp. 227–256). New York: Hatherleigh Press.

McEvoy, C. L., & Patterson, R. (1986). Behavioral treatment of deficit skills in dementia patients. *The Gerontologist, 26*(5), 475–478.

McGrowder-Lin, R., & Bhatt, A. (1988). A wanderer's lounge program for nursing home residents with Alzheimer's disease. *The Gerontologist, 28*(5), 607–609.

Schonfeld, L. (2003). Behavior problems in assisted living facilities. *Journal of Applied Gerontology, 22*(4), 490–505.

Schonfeld, L., Cairl, R. E., Cohen, D., Kennedy-Neal, K., Watson, M. A., & Westerhof, C. (1999). The Florida Care College: A training program for long-term care staff working with memory impaired residents. *Journal of Mental Health and Aging, 5*(2), 187–199.

Schonfeld, L., King-Kallimanis, B., Brown, L. M., Davis, D. M., Kearns, W. D., Molinari, V. A., et al. (in press). Wanderers with cognitive impairment in Department of Veterans Affairs nursing home care unit. *Journal of the American Geriatrics Society.*

Snyder, L. H., Rupprecht, P., Pyrek, J., Brekhus, S., & Moss, T. (1978). Wandering. *The Gerontologist, 18*(3), 272–280.

Thorndike, E. (1913). *Educational psychology: The psychology of learning.* New York: Teachers College Press.

Wood, S., Cummings, J. L., Schnelle, B., & Stephens, M. (2002). A videotape-based training method for improving the detection of depression in residents of long-term care facilities. *The Gerontologist, 42,* 114–121.

CHAPTER TWELVE

Pharmacological Interventions Associated With Wandering

Steven Charles Castle and Michelle K. Rutledge

Medication management in persons who wander is challenging due to limited evidence of efficacy, high potential for worsening the condition, or increasing harm and mortality from commonly used medications. An effective interdisciplinary team that is aware of baseline level of functioning, establishes clear goals and targets of therapy, prospectively monitors possible adverse effects, and especially identifies any early change in condition will achieve the goal of an individualized plan of care.

The basic approach is that available therapies that address other behavioral and psychological symptoms of dementia may indirectly help with decreasing wandering. Nonetheless, when you have a team consisting of nurses, pharmacists, a primary care clinician, and a geriatric psychiatrist, they all have unique skills that are complementary in the management of the challenging and high liability issue of wandering. Effective communication among team members will improve management.

This chapter will focus on the assessment of medications in wandering (for treating wandering behaviors as well as medications that could contribute to or exacerbate wandering behaviors). Despite limited clinical evidence, the basis of recommendations is formed by

- utilizing a foundation of a careful medical assessment of the underlying dementia,

- looking for coexisting delirium or depression, and
- identifying medical conditions and medications that may make wandering a greater problem.

Once reviewed in this manner, use of medications to reduce wandering behavior will proceed with careful monitoring for efficacy and adverse events. The chapter will review the following basic principles:

- Match medication with underlying dementia type and comorbidities,
- Identify and manage medical conditions that may exacerbate wandering,
- Identify and monitor medications that may directly worsen akathisia or restlessness,
- Anticipate and proactively treat underlying medical conditions in the event of a wander event, and
- Closely monitor for efficacy for target symptoms and prospectively monitor for adverse events related to use of medications.

There is very little data to support strong recommendations, and future studies will need to specifically address novel treatment approaches beyond the use of antipsychotics, which are likely to have an increasingly diminished role, given the increased associated mortality with the use of atypical antipsychotics for behavioral management of demented patients. Medications that will need more careful study include anxiolytic agents such as buspirone, the role of different types of antidepressant/mood stabilizers, medications that improve sleep and sleep architecture, and finally the potential use of beta blockers or anti-androgen/pro-estrogen hormonal treatment. We have included a summary table (Table 12.1) to assist in developing an individualized plan of care.

SCREENING FOR WANDERING OR ELOPEMENT

Asking residents or families about wandering behavior rarely is sufficient as an assessment, as they may not be aware of the problem or may be reluctant to share the information. Some studies demonstrated that the severity of dementia correlates with wandering behavior, with a negative correlation with the Mini-Mental Status Exam (MMSE) and the Revised Algase Wandering Score, and that extroversion, distractibility, impulsivity, and executive function problems correlated with "getting lost behavior" (Chiu, 2002; Song, 2003). A comparison of dementia types with the Algase Wandering Scale-version 2 suggests that mixed dementia and

TABLE 12.1 Treatment of Behavioral and Psychological Symptoms of Dementia—Summary

Medication	Efficacy by dementia type	Potential BPSD[1] Symptom efficacy	Evidence for specific Symptom efficacy	Potential for exacerbating wandering	Key side effects to monitor
Risperidone		Insomnia, Wandering, Aggression/Agitation, Psychosis	Meguro et al., 2004 (RCT); Ballard & Waite, 2006 (R); Rabinowitz et al., 2004 (Post Hoc); Katz et al., 1999 (RCT); Brodaty et al., 2003 (RCT); De Deyn et al., 1999 (RCT); Suh et al., 2004 (RCT); Katz, Rupnow, Kozma, & Schneider, 2004 (RCT)	Agitation, Anxiety, Insomnia	Increased risk of mortality in dementia patients with *prior cardiovascular history*; sedation; caution use with Lewy body dementia; metabolic side effects—weight gain, hyperglycermia; Extra Pyramidal Symptoms, Neuroleptic Malignant Syndrome, hypotension, falls
Olanzapine		Agitation/Aggression, Hallucinations, delusion, Pyschosis	Ballard & Waite, 2006 (R); Street et al., 2000 (RCT)	Insomnia, agitation, nervousness	Increased risk of mortality in dementia patients; high sedation; caution use in Lewy body dementia; metabolic affects—weight gain, hyperglycermia, EPS, NMS, anticholingeric effects may occur, orthostatic hypotension/tachycardia, Periodic assessment of transaminases is recommended in patients with significant hepatic disease, falls

(Continued)

Donepezil	Mild to Moderate AD, Vascular dementia, Lewy body dementia, severe dementia	anxiety, apathy/indifference, irritability/lability, depression/dysphoria	Skjerve & Nygaard, 2000 (CR); Gauthier et al., 2002 (CT); Holmes et al., 2004 (CT)	Insomnia; abnormal dreams	May cause insomnia, therefore administer during the day, GI distress/loss of appetite, bradycardia
Rivastigmine	Mild to moderate AD, Lewy body dementia, severe dementia, Vascular dementia, Mild to Moderate PD	Apathy, anxiety, delusions, hallucinations	McKeith et al. 2000(RCT)		GI distress/loss of appetite, bradycardia
Galantamine	Mild to Moderate AD, Vascular dementia	Behavioral	Erkinjuntti et al., 2002 (RCT)		GI
Memantine	Moderate to Severe AD, Vascular dementia	Behavioral, agitation/aggression, eating/appetite, irritability/lability	Tariot et al., 2004 (RCT); Cummings et al., 2006 (RCT)		
Zolpidem		Insomnia; Wandering	Shelton & Hocking, 1997 (CR);		Also increase fall risk (Wang, Bohn, Glynn, Mogun, & Avorn, 2001) (CT)
Citalopram		agitation/aggression, lability/tension, depression	Pollock et al., 2002 (RCT)		Falls

[1] Behavioral and psychological symptoms of dementia.

impaired spatial discrimination were associated with higher scores on the scale. Recognizing differences in dementia types will also be important in the consideration of medications that might be more or less effective in the management of behavioral problems.

ASSESSMENT FOR MEDICAL CONDITIONS THAT CONTRIBUTE TO WANDERING

If any screening method suggests the risk of wandering, or a wandering event has occurred, then a detailed assessment is needed. The goal is to develop an individualized plan of care that can be monitored for effectiveness over time. The assessment needs to proceed along several levels, but should first evaluate for a change in condition and specifically the presence of delirium. Then assessment for dementia if not previously recognized, and a recognition of the type of dementia as best as can be determined should be addressed. Next, the assessment should focus on identifying conditions and medications that may contribute to wandering behavior. Finally, there should be an assessment of risk of injury in the wandering prone resident. Each of these steps will be briefly discussed.

Recognition of Delirium

The first level of assessment for wandering is to determine if delirium is present. Delirium is characterized by:

- A reduced awareness of the environment detected by a reduced ability to focus or shift attention
- A new impairment or abrupt worsening of existing impairment in thought processing/cognition that is noticeable over days
- Fluctuation through the day and between days
- Due to a medical condition, infection, adverse effect of a medication, or some other toxicity. (Inouye, 2006)

Surprisingly, it has been found that delirium is not well recognized by nurses in the acute care setting, and in a prospective study, nurses accurately identified the presence of delirium only 15 percent of the time when it developed (Inouye, Foreman, Mion, Katz, & Cooney, 2001). Recognition requires testing of cognition, including orientation, but more importantly attention (digit spans forward and backward, with a minimum for normal being five forward and three reverse), and changes in usual thought patterns. Part of the challenge, particularly with patients with an unknown background, is to recognize a change from usual confusion and that quiet delirium often is not recognized as a change in condition. Of note, agitation remains the highest risk for falls in the acute care setting (Oliver, Britton, Seed, Martin, & Hopper, 1997). The Confusion Assessment Method (CAM) has demonstrated good efficacy in detection of delirium by having the following conditions both a and b, with either c or d:

a. acute onset or fluctuation in decline in mental status AND,
b. inattention with an inability to focus or keep on track, with EITHER,
c. disorganized thinking OR,
d. altered level of consciousness. (Inouye et al., 1990)

Likewise, physician management of delirium is varied and lacks strong evidence for any class of medication. While use of antipsychotics is the most common method used in the United States, with two thirds of physicians surveyed (n = 270) reporting use of haloperidol alone, 20 percent reported use of lorazepam alone, 9 percent reported use of a combination, and 4 percent reported use of some other agent (Carnes et al., 2003). There are recent case series and case reports of the use of acetyl cholinesterase inhibitors in the management of acute and chronic delirium, and this will be discussed in more detail later (Lankarani-Fard & Castle, 2006).

Dementia: Is There Unrecognized Dementia, and How Is the Dementia Characterized?

To prescribe medications effectively that may reduce adverse events associated with wandering behaviors, it is important to establish an accurate diagnosis and recognition of patterns of the type of dementia. First, it must be appreciated that dementia still is often unrecognized by both family members and primary care providers, so the diagnosis should be considered in anyone who wanders. Dementia is particularly difficult to recognize in individuals that have either very high or low intelligence, patients who are affected most by executive dysfunction (cognitive processing required for problem solving and judgment) that may be sometimes difficult to resolve from long-standing personality factors, and those with severe sensory impairment, hearing or vision. The use of the Mini-Cog (Borson, Scanlan, Watanabe, Tu, & Lessig, 2005) is advocated as a quick screening test for dementia, and it or some other level of screening should be implemented in any person who has wandered and has not had a diagnosis made of dementia. The Mini-Cog entails asking a person to recall three unrelated objects, then giving them a distracter of the clock drawing test (ask the patient to draw a circle, put the numbers of a clock face in, and make the hands read 10 minutes after 11:00), and then asking them to recall the three objects. Getting all three on recall results in a pass; missing at least one item on recall and > 2 points overall (1 point for getting numbers right, 1 point for the hands on the clock drawing test) suggests more detailed testing for possible dementia is warranted. Even if screening tests are negative and there remains strong suspicion of dementia, then referral for more detailed neuropsychological testing should be done, and neuroimaging is recommended if there is an inconsistent history for dementia (particularly rapid deterioration in cognition) or focal neurological symptoms (Shekelle, MacLean, Morton, & Wenger, 2001).

It is important to recognize Lewy body dementia, because these patients usually have a very different response to antipsychotic medications. The features of Lewy body dementia include fluctuations in cognitive function (through the day and over time), persistent and well-formed visual hallucinations, with spontaneous motor features of parkinsonism, which may be hard to distinguish from motor effects of antipsychotics. What is important to realize is that many antipsychotics contribute to an increase in restlessness in some individuals, and patients with parkinsonian features are more prone to increasing stiffness, poor postural control of blood pressure, and falls due to impaired visuomotor processing.

Associated Medical Conditions That Contribute to Restlessness

Serotonin Syndrome

This syndrome is a result of excessive serotonin. Medications can release serotonin from presynaptic neurons, inhibit serotonin reuptake in the synaptic cleft, or stimulate postsynaptic serotonin receptors (Braunwald et al., 2001). Specific drugs associated with serotonin syndrome include:

- Selective Serotonin Reuptake Inhibitors (setraline, fluoxetine, fluvoxamine, paroxetine, and citalopram);
- Other antidepressant drugs (trazodone, nefazodone, buspirone, clomipramine, and venlafaxine);
- Monoamine Oxidase Inhibitors (phenelzine, moclobemide, clorgiline, and isocarboxazid);
- Anticonvulsants (valproate);
- Analgesics (meperidine, fentanyl, tramadol, and pentazocine);
- Antiemetics (ondanesetron, granisetron, and metoclopramide);
- Antimigraine agents (sumatriptan);
- Antibiotics (linezolide and ritonovir);

- Over-the-counter medications (dextromethorphan);
- Drugs of abuse (methylenedioxymethamphetamine, also known as MDMA, or ecstasy; lysergic acid diethylamide, or LSD; 5-methoxydiisopropyltryptamine, or foxy methoxy; and Syrian rue, which contains harmine and harmaline, both monoamine oxidase inhibitors);
- Dietary supplements and herbal products (tryptophan, Hypericum perforatum or St. John's wort, and Ginseng); and
- Other (Lithium). (Boyer & Shannon, 2005)

Drug combinations reported to cause SEVERE Serotonin Syndrome include:

- Phenelzine and meperidine;
- Tranylcypromine and dimipramine;
- Phenelzine and selective serotonin—reuptake inhibitors;
- Paroxetine and buspirone;
- Linezolide and citalopram;
- Moclobemide and selective serotonin-reuptake inhibitors; and
- Tramadol, venlafaxine, and mirtazapine. (Boyer & Shannon, 2005)

The symptoms of serotonin syndrome can consist of neuromuscular (myoclonus, hyperreflexia), autonomic (loose bowel movements, diaphoresis, shivering, hypertension, fluctuation of hot–cold sensation), and altered mental status symptoms including hypomania that could lead to wandering behavior. The potential triggers of the serotonin syndrome include more commonly drug overdose, and drug interactions such as concomitant use of SSRI antidepressants with MAO inhibitors.

However serotonin syndrome has been reported with a single drug use that affects serotonin activity. A waiting period of 2 to 5 weeks is necessary when changing a patient from an SSRI to an MAO inhibitor, and 2 weeks are necessary when changing from an MAO inhibitor to an SSRI (Salzman, 2005). Serotonin syndrome is diagnosed by presentation of clinical symptoms, physical examination, and drug history. Serotonin syndrome can be misinterpreted for neuroleptic malignant syndrome, anticholingergic poisoning, or malignant hyperthermia, however, it is most often misdiagnosed as neuroleptic malignant syndrome (Boyer and Shannon, 2005). Serotonin syndrome can be distinguished from neuroleptic malignant syndrome by time of onset and presence or absence of certain clinical symptoms, such as developing and resolving rapidly (onset over a period of hours from administration or addition of causative agent and then resolution over a period of hours after removal of causative agent(s)), and the presence of myclonus, hyperreflexia which is present only in serotonin syndrome (Braunwald et al., 2001).

Sleep Disorders

If wandering occurs in the evening or nighttime in particular, then evaluation for sleep disorders is warranted. This may be difficult to evaluate in persons with dementia, because self-report is not reliable and others may not be fully aware of the person's sleep habits. The key sleep disorders include restless leg syndrome (RLS), obstructive sleep apnea (OSA), and sundowning (rest–activity disorders in dementia).

Restless Legs Syndrome (RLS) is a common sleep disorder but often goes undiagnosed and is estimated to occur in 15–20 percent of the population (Jan, Erokwu, Ebose, & Strohl, 2005; Mata et al., 2006). The primary symptoms are a desire to move the extremities with paresthesias or dyesthesias, often described as crawling or jumpy sensations in the legs. The symptoms often come on in late afternoon or evening, are worsened by rest, and are temporarily relieved by movement. This is sometimes also associated with periodic leg movements, cyclical course movements of the legs at 1–3 minute intervals that may occur at rest but more commonly during sleep. There is often a family history, but physical exam usually shows no abnormalities, though there may be some overlap with parkinsonism. Treatment is unclear, and there is insufficient evidence to recommend any specific approach. The types of treatment that have been tried with varying degrees of efficacy include iron supplements (only in the presence of iron deficiency), dopaminergic agents, opioid agents, benzodiazepines, and anti-convulsants (Gabapentin, valproic acid, and others). In any event, recognition of the syndrome and attempts at management are warranted, especially if symptoms contribute to wandering behavior. No data is available on the potential impact of antipsychotic medications worsening restless legs syndrome, but this seems likely, especially in view of the apparent overlap between parkinsonism and restless legs syndrome.

Obstructive sleep apnea usually does not result in wandering as one of the key symptoms is daytime sleepiness, but it is included briefly here for completeness in discussing sleep disorders, especially because front line workers or aides in long-term care settings may witness this syndrome. Key screening questions and observations include loud snoring (heard outside the room), awaking with choking or severe shortness of breath, breathing pauses during sleep, and daytime sleepiness with difficulty concentrating (Merritt & Berger, 2004).

Sundowning has been widely discussed in the literature, but there is no consensus as to whether it really is a syndrome (Dewing, 2000).

Others have categorized it as a rest–activity disorder seen in patients with dementia, described as a syndrome that occurs when the brain attempts to process arousal when other parts of the brain, the neo-cortex in particular, are turned off, as in rapid eye movement sleep (Staedt & Stoppe, 2005). Late afternoon or early evening sleep may contribute to the shift in the diurnal cycles, resulting in generalized brain activation upon awakening following an afternoon or evening nap, but a turned off neo-cortex that results in a delirious-like state with delusions, agitation, and altered perception that may continue through the normal sleep period at night. Therefore, the foundation of management should not rely on medications but should include a careful maintenance of a normal diurnal cycle, including wake–sleep times, sleep hygiene, routine meals, and in particular careful attention should be paid to maintaining activity and awakeness in the afternoon and early evening. The use of medications should be initiated as a last option after these methods are ineffective.

If medications are used to try and correct abnormal wake–sleep diurnal cycles, it is thought that benzodiazepines and antipsychotic agents may worsen this rest–activity disturbance, while acetyl cholinesterase inhibitors may restore a more normal diurnal cycle. In the elderly, use of sedatives or hypnotics with long half-lives and other potentially harmful side effects is in general not appropriate. Particularly agents with sedating or anticholingeric effects, due to risk of fall and increase in confusion (Fick et al., 2003; Markovitz, 1993). Other agents such as buspirone or trazodone have been used with reduced falls compared to benzodiazepines in a case series, but there is very little data to determine efficacy of buspirone in particular (Cooper, 2003). The only two randomized controlled blinded studies with trazodone did not show efficacy in overall behavioral measures, though sundowning per se was not specifically investigated (Martinon-Torres, Fioravanti, & Grimley, 2006). However, one guideline recommends trazodone as the drug of choice for sundowning and insomnia (Alexopoulos, Jeste, Carpenter, Ross, & Docherty, 2005), most likely due to its short half-life and very sedating, but little anticholinergic side effects (Lacy, Armstrong, Goldman, & Lance, 2003; Wick & Zanni, 2005). Quetiapine, zolpidem, and zaleplon are listed as second line choices (Alexopoulos et al., 2005). A few studies and case reports have examined the newer agent zolpidem in improving sleep in the elderly (Shaw, Curson, & Coquelin, 1992; Roger, Attali, & Coquelin, 1993; Kummer et al., 1993) and wandering. Shelton and Hocking (1997) found that zolpidem, a nonbenzodiazepine hypnotic, was well tolerated and improved sleep patterns in two patients with dementia and severe nighttime wandering. Note it still carries a risk for falls. Wang and colleagues found use of zolpidem by older people was associated with nearly twice the risk of hip fracture, even after controlling for possible demographic and clinical confounders than nonusers (Wang, Bohn, Glynn, Mogun, & Avorn, 2001). A 1-year-long open-label trial of long-term use of zaleplon suggests it is safe for the treatment of insomnia in older patients. The authors also conclude placebo-controlled, double-blinded trials are needed to confirm results (Ancoli-Israel et al., 2005). Allain and colleagues, in a review on postural instability, falls, and hip fractures associated with use of hypnotics in the elderly, state that Z-compounds (zopiclone, zolpidem, and zaleplon) have short half-lives and have less cognitive and residual effects than older medications (Allain, Bentue-Ferrer, Poland, Akwa, & Patat, 2005). In addition, all marketed hypnotics can alter postural stability and equilibrium, thereby increasing the risk of falls and hip fractures when treated patients stand up and move around at times when they are supposed to be in a drug-induced sleep (Allain et al., 2005). Therefore, providers should be aware these newer agents may also increase fall risk compared to older sedative-hypnotics, and educate patients. Lastly, if sedatives are used to reinstate a normal diurnal cycle, then it should be periodically removed as soon as a more normal sleep–wake cycle is reinstated.

There have been a few studies linking antipsychotics and sleep behavioral problems (Ruth, Straand, Nygaard, Bjorvatn, & Pallesen, 2004; Meguro et al., 2004; Falsetti, 2000) that have shown small improvements with sundowning symptoms. One small study in persons with Alzheimer's dementia found that after the use of risperdone, aggressiveness and wandering were reduced and the nighttime sleeping hours were increased (Meguro et al., 2004). In another small study, exploring the effect of sleep–wake activity and on behavioral and psychological symptoms of dementia of the withdrawal of antipsychotic withdrawal, behavioral scores remained stable or improved in 11 of 15 patients; however actigraphy revealed decreased sleep efficiency after drug discontinuation and increased 24-hours and night activity in both groups (Ruth et al., 2004). Atypical antipsychotics are considered safer over the older agents (Bachman & Rabins, 2006), however warnings from the Food and Drug Administration (FDA) caution against use of these drugs for behavior management in dementia patients due to increased mortality associated with their use (FDA, 2005). In general, antipsychotic medications need an identified target symptom that warrants the increased associated mortality, such as severe delusions, paranoia, or hallucinations. Efficacy and potential side effects, especially anticholinergic cardiovascular effects of tachycardia and postural hypotension, should be reviewed regularly. Of note, sudden withdrawal of antipsychotic medications can affect sleep (Ruth et al., 2004).

More data on acetyl cholinesterase inhibitors and memantine in treating sundowning is needed. One case report of treatment with donepezil in sundowning in dementia with Lewy body dementia stated ratings of behavioral symptoms improved. In addition, there was a marked reduction in evening activity and an increase in daytime activity. Cognition and parkinsonism also improved (Skjerve & Nygaard, 2000). Further study is needed to determine the exact risk versus benefit of, and efficacy of treatment for sundowning. The limited support for these agents makes it a challenge in choosing the best approach for behavioral problems, and suggestions to assist in individualizing an approach will be discussed in more detail in the last section of this chapter. Suffice it to say, that these agents may in particular have use if they are helpful in restoring a normal wake–sleep cycle and are monitored for possible adverse effects.

Medications That Cause Akathisia (Restlessness) or May Contribute to Wandering

Use of medications to reduce wandering directly will be reviewed in detail later in this chapter. The focus of this section is to review medications that in particular may contribute to an increase in akathisia, otherwise known as restlessness. Akathisia is a very common side effect of neuroleptics and pyschotropics. Other medications that have been associated with akathisia are antipsychotics, antidepressants (both SSRIs and Tricyclic), benzodiazepines, memantine, bladder relaxants (anticholinergic), diltiazem, metoclopromide or prochlorperazine, some calcium channel blockers, dopamine agonists, amphetamine, buspirone, Parkinson's medications, and possibly tobacco (Nelson, 2001). While antipsychotics remain the most prescribed medication for behavioral problems in dementia patients, they provide significant challenges in dosing as response to treatment may take 6 to 8 weeks, while plasma concentrations are two to three times greater in patients over 60 years old, which is the rationale behind the go-low, go-slow approach. This is often difficult to adhere to, however, when attempting to treat a high-risk condition such as wandering. To complicate matters, akathisia, or behavior that manifests as pacing and total inability to sit still, is reported as an adverse event of antipsychotics, so wandering behavior could be due to the medication prescribed or due to an inadequate dose of the medication. That is why clear identification of target symptoms for use of an antipsychotic is so important, and why adverse effects must be prospectively monitored. This requires careful communication of the plan between the physician, nurse, and therapist as well as family members, who may best observe subtle changes in motor function.

Medication Case Reports Related to Wandering

Review of the literature will not yield much as to adverse events of medication specifically for wandering, as they will not for other geriatric syndromes, such as falls or postural hypotension. Hence, it is necessary to look for "footprints" in the literature that may lead to more awareness of medications that may exacerbate underlying tendencies for such geriatric syndromes, and in this case wandering. There are case reports of akathisia from a large number of medications including buspirone (Sathananthan, Sanghvi, Phillips, & Gershon, 1975); from diltiazem where a 62-year-old man suffered severe symptoms that resolved after discontinuing the medication and returned 2 weeks later on a re-challenge (Jacobs, 1983); and lorazepam (Roila et al., 1990). Akathisia has been reported at a 30 milligrams (mg) dose of mirtazapine, that was resolved at a lower dose but recurred when a 30 mg dose was repeated in a 73-year-old woman with chronic depression (Girishchandra, Johnson, Cresp, & Orr, 2002). While fluoxetine is a more activating SSRI and more likely to cause akathisia, akathisia was reported to occur at an incidence of 4 percent in a retrospective review of a series of patients treated with paroxetine (Baldassano, Truman, Nierenberg, Ghaemi, & Sachs, 1996). In two of the reported cases, akathisia occurred within a week of initiation of paroxetine therapy (20 milligrams per day) in which the patients described feelings of inner restlessness, insomnia, and the inability to stay still. Akathisia resolved in both cases following the addition of propranolol (40 to 80 milligrams per day) (Adler & Angrist, 1995; Baldassano et al., 1996). In addition, it is likely that restless leg syndrome will be exacerbated by SSRIs. Another case report of akathisia was reported while a patient was receiving imipramine therapy, and four others developed the same while receiving desipramine, trazodone, or tranylcypromine. The imipramine patient was a 54-year-old female who was treated for depression with alprazolam and imipramine. Once the dose of imipramine was increased to 150 mg per day, the patient complained of an uncomfortable feeling in her legs and the inability to remain still. Of note, a low dose of propranolol 10 mg three times daily resolved the symptoms completely within several hours of the first dose, and discontinuation of the propranolol resulted in a recurrence of the akathisia within 24 hours (Zubenko, Cohen, & Lipinski, 1987).

Antipsychotics

Akathisia is more frequently reported in some of the antipyschotics. A study compared akathisia induced by haloperidol or thiothixene. The haloperidol group (5 mg as test dose followed by 10 mg per day) experienced akathisia in 75 percent of cases (Van Putten, May, & Marder, 1984). Motor disturbances are reported to be less with quetiapine (Micromedex, 2006), but akathisia was reported in a 62-year-old male patient with Parkinson's disease following the administration of quetiapine at a dose of 12.5 to 25 mg daily for five days, while on levodopa at a dose of 400 mg. The patient developed severe motor restlessness and an inability to stop pacing. Quetiapine was withdrawn and symptoms of akathisia completely resolved within two days (Prueter, Habermeyer, Norra, & Kosinski, 2003). Others have reported akathisia in 15–21.5 percent of haloperidol treated schizophrenics with lower rates reported for atypical antipsychotics including risperidone (1.7%), olanzapine (7%), and quetiapine (1.1%) (Pierre, 2005).

Memantine

One other agent commonly used in dementia is memantine. Of note, depression, insomnia, increased or decreased motor activity, akathisia, and agitation were the most frequent adverse reactions reported with the use of memantine (Forest Pharmaceuticals, 2003; Goertelmeyer & Erbler, 1992). There are case reports that donepezil may actually reduce the extrapyramidal symptoms from other agents, which warrants to be tested in a randomized controlled trial (Bergman, Dwolatzky, Brettholz, & Lerner, 2005).

Anti-Emetics

The medications that may have the highest reported incidence of akathisia include metoclopramide and prochlorperazine, and it appears this is primarily from rapid and higher dose infusions of these medications in the emergency room. The impact of chronic oral use, however, particularly in individuals with dementia, is unknown. Metoclopramide-induced movement disorders such as tardive dyskinesia, acute dystonia, akathisia, and parkinsonism have occurred with both oral or intravenous metoclopramide. The neurologic complications of metoclopramide may be prevented by prolonging the rate of administration. One recommendation to prevent such occurrences is to dilute 10 mg metoclopramide in 50 ml physiologic saline and infusing the solution at 60 drops per minute or infusing the 10 mg dose as undiluted metoclopramide over 1 to 2 minutes (Corey, 1994). Another study of 300 randomized patients to the emergency room for nausea and or headache were given either a 10 mg bolus rapid infusion (minutes) of metoclopramide compared with a controlled infusion rate of 15 minutes. While control of symptoms was over 90 percent in both groups, the rate of severe akathisia reported with the bolus infusion was 30 percent versus 22.2 percent in the slow infusion group (Parlak et al., 2005).

Reports of akathisia from prochlorperazine have been reported, primarily from emergency departments where intravenous infusions of the medication are given for complaints of severe nausea. In one convenience sample of 100 subjects treated for nausea, subjects were randomized to receive 10 mg of intravenous prochlorperazine with or without the addition of 50 mg of diphenhydramine. The rates of akathisia were 36 percent in the control group and only 14 percent in the diphenydramine group (Vinson & Drotts, 2001).

Another study from a convenience sample of 100 patients with nausea seen in the emergency department were randomized to receive intravenous infusion of droperidol 1.25 mg, prochlorperazine 10 mg, or metoclopramide 10 mg, or saline. Droperidol was more effective than metoclopramide or prochlorperazine but caused more extrapyramidal symptoms in 71.4 percent. Metoclopramide and prochlorperazine were not more effective than saline placebo (Braude et al., 2006). So, if these pronounced symptoms of restlessness are commonly reported in a younger population, we must anticipate that they could have more of an impact on a frail older population with degenerative neurological conditions. The reason this discussion is included here is that anti-emetics are medications that may be added during hospitalization or over time in long-term care patients, may not have strong or clear indications for continued use, and may contribute to exacerbation of wandering behavior.

Hence, monitoring for types of movement disorders called extrapyramidal symptoms (EPS) (tremor, rigidity, akathisia, akinesia or bradykinesia, and tardive dyskinesia) must be part of the monitoring in any patient prescribed an antipsychotic, and any medication that may contribute to akathisia should be used with caution and close monitoring in any patient with a wander event. If a patient is on a medication that can cause akathisia, it should be a factor considered in the risk or presence of wandering behavior, and unless strongly indicated, a medication with less risk of akathisia should be considered. If a medication that can cause akathisia is needed, for instance an antipsychotic, and there is a risk or presence of wandering behavior, then no strong recommendations can be provided on what may lower that adverse effect, but the literature does suggest that diphenhydramine may reduce this adverse effect. Whether this should be advocated or not due to its high anticholingeric properties requires study, as whether other agents should be considered such as a beta blocker, an anxiolytic such as buspirone, or other agents. In managing patients, an agent should be chosen with specific target symptoms to monitor, potential adverse effects should be monitored, and the plan should be subsequently adjusted.

Testosterone

Given the fact that males with dementia wander more and have a higher mortality, one question in the assessment may be as to whether testosterone replacement may contribute to the risk and danger from wandering events. In one study of 50 males with dementia, there was a linear correlation with free testosterone levels and aggression and a negative correlation with estrogen levels and aggression (Orengo, Kunik, Molinari, Wristers, & Yudofsky, 2002). However, one randomized controlled study on the effect of testosterone replacement in 15 men with Alzheimer's disease and 17 men with mild cognitive impairment (aged 63 to 85 years) demonstrated significant improvement in spatial memory and constructional abilities as well as verbal memory in the testosterone treatment group (Cherrier et al., 2005).

One case report was found on the possible effects of gonadotrophin-releasing hormone agonist treatment, which reduces testosterone activity, on aggression in Alzheimer's disease. This report described apparent sustained elimination of previously treatment-resistant aggression and agitation with goserelin treatment in a 78-year-old male Alzheimer's disease nursing home resident, so the effect of anti-androgen treatment on reduction of aggression or wandering warrants further study (Rosin & Raskind, 2005). At least a retrospective review of demented patients with or without ablation of testosterone by hormonal treatment for prostate cancer and the rates of various behavioral disturbances such as wandering should be pursued.

Tobacco

Given that many patients who wander, or are prone to wander, smoke cigarettes, one question that may arise is could the nicotine be contributing or preventing wandering behavior? Current therapies for dementia that work on nicotine receptors may be of interest. We found only one randomized controlled trial, a study in college-aged students that found that a 2 mg dose of nicotine via inhaler had no effect on attention or memory, but in males it increased ratings of anxiety, discontent, and aggression, while in females, it blocked these same attributes (File, Fluck, & Leahy, 2001). However, theoretically there is much reason to consider how nicotine may affect behavior at different stages and types of dementia because of the importance of nicotine receptors in the pathogenesis of dementia. Nicotine is a cholinergic agonist that also has a presynaptic effect on releasing acetylcholine and has been shown to reverse surgically induced memory deficits in rats. Observational studies have suggested a potential effect of smoking on preventing Alzheimer's disease. In particular, a lower dose of nicotine than seen in light smokers, demonstrated improved working and reference memory in aged rats (French, Granholm, Moore, Nelson, & Bimonte-Nelson, 2006). However, a systematic review was not able to provide evidence that nicotine was an effective or useful treatment for Alzheimer's disease (Lopez-Arrieta & Sanz, 2006). One study did look at acute nicotine administration (2 mg of nicotine polacrilex) on EEG changes in Alzheimer's disease, and post nicotine EEG indices remained abnormal, but significantly shifted EEG toward normal values compared to placebo. Six of the 13 subjects were on an acetyl cholinesterase inhibitor, all were nonsmokers, and all abstained from alcohol or caffeine overnight (Knott, Engeland, Mohr, Mahoney, & Ilivitsky, 2000). However, the effect of nicotine on different types of dementia needs to be considered, given possible differences in nicotine binding in the thalamus of schizophrenics and patients with dementia with Lewy bodies (Court et al., 1999).

INDIVIDUALIZE TREATMENT TO SUBTYPES OF DEMENTIA

Importance of Individualizing Therapy, Monitoring for Adverse Events, and Efficacy

Selecting medication to treat behavioral symptoms of dementia in the elderly is challenging. The American Association of Geriatric Psychiatry (AAGP) position statement on Principles of Care for patients with dementia from Alzheimer's disease states, there is no clear standard regarding which medications to use for which types of symptoms (Lyketsos et al., 2006). And as stated previously, no pharmacologic therapy is indicated specifically for wandering. Therefore therapy should be individualized and monitored regularly for adverse events and efficacy. Data from the MDS from five states shows that antipsychotics are used 32–49 percent of the time for specifically wandering behavior (Ott, Lapane, & Gambassi, 2000), while antidepressants are reported to be used in 8–10 percent of the cases for control of wandering. However, since this recommendation was published, the FDA has issued a warning about use of atypical antipsychotics for behavior management in dementia, with an increased mortality of 60–70 percent identified in multiple studies. The cause of death is most commonly due to cardiovascular events (heart failure, sudden death) or infections (primarily pneumonia) (Kuehn, 2005). In addition, both antipsychotics and antidepressants have an increased epidemiological association with risk of falls around 50 percent higher in older adult users versus nonusers of these medications. Part of the mechanism of psychotropic medications associated with falls is speculated to be related to altered central processing, cardiovascular effects, and movement disorder that can lead to frank parkinsonism, specifically for antipsychotics. Hence, it is important to make decisions of types and classes of these medications to best match underlying types of dementia and associated abnormalities in mobility. For example, dementia of Lewy body patients are especially vulnerable to the antidopaminergic and anticholinergic actions of most conventional antipsychotics, which makes treatment of the psychotic symptoms of Dementia of Lewy body extremely difficult (Baskys, 2004).

Typical Antipsychotics: Haloperidol

Haloperidol has demonstrated decreased aggression (but not agitation), but is associated with higher adverse effects, and there is a lack of evidence to support the routine use for other behavioral and psychological symptoms or manifestations of agitation in dementia (Lonergan, Luxenberg, Colford, & Birks, 2006). In 2 trials reporting drop-out rates, there were 23/135 in haloperidol treatment compared with 10/139 for placebo, suggesting poorly controlled symptoms or other factors may cause treatment discontinuation.

Atypical Antipsychotics

Of the antispychotics, risperidone and olanzapine have strongest evidence for reduction of aggression, but with significant cardiovascular and motor side effects (Ballard & Waite, 2006). Post hoc analysis of three randomized controlled trials of risperodone vs. placebo, n = 1150, showed significant improvement with risperidone on the Cohen-Mansfield Agitation Inventory, specifically with:

- Hitting, hurting, cursing, repetitiveness, grabbing, scratching, need for constant attention;
- Pacing and aimless wandering (measured by the BEHAVE-AD scale); and
- Physical threats, violence, anxieties, agitation, tearfulness, non-paranoid delusions. (Rabinowitz et al., 2004)

Another randomized, double-blind trial comparison of risperidone and placebo for psychosis and behavioral disturbances associated with dementia, with n = 625, primarily demonstrated improvement on a variety of behavior scales versus placebo, including the Behavioral Pathology in Alzheimer's Disease rating scale (BEHAVE-AD). Each patient was randomly assigned to receive placebo, or 0.5 mg per day, 1 mg per day, or 2 mg per day of risperidone for 12 weeks. At endpoint, significantly greater reductions in BEHAVE-AD total scores and psychosis and aggressiveness subscale scores were seen in patients receiving 1 and 2 mg per day of risperidone than in placebo patients. More adverse effects were reported by patients receiving 2 mg per day of risperidone than 1 mg per day, including the most commonly reported symptoms: extrapyramidal symptoms, somnolence, and mild peripheral edema. The conclusion of the trial was that risperidone significantly improved symptoms of psychosis and aggressive behavior in patients with dementia. Results show that 1 mg per day of risperidone is an appropriate dose for most elderly patients with dementia (Katz et al., 1999). Another randomized placebo-controlled trial of risperidone for the treatment of aggression, agitation, and psychosis of dementia, with *n* = 345, concluded that treatment with low-dose (mean = 0.95 mg per day) risperidone resulted in significant improvement in aggression, agitation, and psychosis associated with dementia (Brodaty et al., 2003).

Olanzapine was examined in 206 patients with Alzheimer's disease who exhibited psychotic or behavioral symptoms. Patients were randomly assigned to placebo or a fixed dose of 5, 10, or 15 mg per day of olanzapine. Primary outcome was the core total (agitation or aggression, hallucinations, and delusions) of the NPI-NH test. Somnolence was more common among patients receiving olanzapine, and gait disturbances occurred in those receiving 5 or 15 mg per day. There was no significant increase in extrapyramidal symptoms. Authors concluded low dose olanzapine (5 and 10 mg per day) was significantly superior to placebo and well tolerated (Street et al., 2000).

Antidepressants

Citalopram has been discussed as having a possible clinical effect in agitation and emotional lability in dementia cases. The change in the Neurobehavior Rating Scale (NRS) total score was significantly greater for citalopram than placebo (10 versus 2.3 points; $P < .001$). Of 7 subscales, scales for agitation and lability significantly improved with citalopram versus placebo, but less than 1 point on a 7-point scale (Pollock et al., 2002; Sink, Holden, & Yaffe, 2005).

One study with sertraline augmented with donepezil showed no statistically significant differences at endpoint on any of the three primary outcomes. However, of the 24 patients who were treated with donepezil + sertraline, a linear mixed model analysis found modest but statistically significantly greater improvements in the CGI-I score. And in a subgroup of patients with moderate-to-severe behavioral and psychological symptoms of dementia, 60 percent of patients on sertraline versus 40 percent on placebo ($p = 0.006$) achieved a response (defined as > or = 50% reduction in a four-item NPI-behavioral subscale) (Finkel et al., 2004; Sink et al., 2005). Twelve percent dropped out in both groups due to adverse events; diarrhea was significantly more common with sertraline (27.4% vs. 11.7%, $P < .05$), and this was a Pfizer-funded study (Sink et al., 2005).

Mirtazapine is an antidepressant with some characteristics that may make it a particularly useful consideration for agitated behavior that may lead to wandering, if the agitation is thought to be due to depression. Mirtazapine tends to have a sedating effect at lower doses, but does become more activating at doses of 30 mg or higher. One study comparing total medication use in long-term care residents found that there was significantly less use of sedatives, especially lorazepam, in residents using mirtazapine. In addition, mirtazapine causes weight gain, so it would be a particularly good choice in an agitated, depressed, demented individual when you wanted to avoid using a sedative, or if weight gain would be desired (Gardner, Malone, Sey, & Babington, 2004).

Larger studies with antidepressants to treat behavioral and psychological symptoms of dementia are needed.

Trazodone

Two studies, involving 104 subjects with Alzheimer's disease (Teri et al., 2000) and frontotemporal dementia (Lebert, Stekke, Hasenbroekx, & Pasquier, 2004), were identified, with a dose of trazodone from 50 to 300 mg daily. There was no statistically significant benefit for behavioral manifestations as measured by various rating scales (Agitated Behavior Inventory for Dementia, ABID; Alzheimer's Disease Behavioral Rating Scale for Dementia, CERAD-BRSD; Cohen-Mansfield Agitation Inventory, CMAI; and Neuropsychiatric Inventory, NPI), no clinical impression of change in cognitive function, and no difference in adverse effects when compared with a placebo (Martinon-Torres et al., 2006). However, it may be that certain behavioral problems are better managed with trazodone, and more selective use may show different results, such as agitation is associated with sundowning. One study comparing trazodone (50 to 250 mg daily) in a double-blind comparison to haloperidol (1 to 5 mg per day) demonstrated that mild depressive symptoms in patients with dementia and agitated behavior are associated with greater behavioral improvement by trazodone-treated patients (Sultzer, Gray, Gunay, Wheatley, & Mahler, 2001).

Buspirone

Buspirone is an anxiolytic agent with reported lower potential for dependence and adverse effects in comparison to benzodiazepines, but no randomized controlled trials have been completed. Of note, buspirone is a serotonin agonist (partial) so care must include monitoring for serotonin syndrome, especially if other agents with serotonin activity are used. One double-blind comparison ($n = 26$) of haloperidol 1.5 mg versus buspirone 15 mg per day demonstrated a reduction in anxiety and tension with buspirone (Cantillon, Brunswick, Molina, & Bahro, 1996).

Benzodiazepines

Benzodiazepines are commonly used agents; 7–15 percent community living elderly use benzodiazepines, as do 4–15 percent long-term care facility residents (Centers for Medicaid & Medicare Services [CMS], 2001). They have both peripheral and central effects that contribute to an increased risk of falls, with an association with falls of a 1.54 Odds Ratio (Leipzig, Cumming, & Tinetti, 1999) as well as increased risk of injury from falls. The Odds Ratio of hip fracture is 2.4 in subjects that have an impaired gait and balance and use a benzodiazepine. Newer agents have not demonstrated a safer falls risk profile, including zolpidem (Wang et al., 2001). Hence, if a patient has wandering behavior and clearly has abnormalities in gait and balance, then benzodiazepines would be a poor choice of agents to treat anxiety, agitation, or sleep abnormalities.

Valproic Acid

The trials for behavior problems in dementia are regarded as preliminary. However, low-dose valproate was ineffective in treating agitation among demented patients, and high-dose therapy was associated with an unacceptable rate of adverse effects. Therefore, on the basis of current evidence, valproate therapy cannot be recommended for management of agitation in dementia (Lonergan, Cameron, & Luxenberg, 2006).

Cholinesterase Inhibitors

Cholinesterase inhibitors (CIs) are likely to take on an increasing role in the management of behavioral problems in dementia, given the increase in mortality associated with use of atypical antipsychotic medications and case reports of efficacy of cholinesterase inhibitors in delirium (acute and chronic), which is thought to represent a cholinergic deficiency. Neuroimaging and neuropsychiatric testing suggest that the "final common pathway" to delirium is lateralized to the right hemisphere in areas susceptible to changes in cholinergic activity. The reason behind the increased anticholinergic activity is unclear, but older adults with dementia have an existing cholinergic deficiency and hence are more prone to delirium. There are case reports of cholinesterase inhibitors being used to treat drug-induced delirium secondary to "nonanticholinergic medications," such as opiates and lithium, and there is evidence that cholinesterase inhibitors may be beneficial in treating agitated patients with baseline dementias or postconfusional state following traumatic brain injury. Collectively, these studies suggest that delirium may be mediated by a deficiency in cholinergic activity and therefore responsive to treatment with a cholinesterase inhibitor (Lankarani-Fard & Castle, 2006). There are currently four CIs available. Of these, Tacrine is not used due to the risk of hepatic injury and its complicated dosing schedule. The remaining three are discussed in the following paragraphs.

Donepezil

Donepezil in moderate to severe Alzheimer's disease was evaluated in 290 patients in a 24-week, double-blind, placebo-controlled study. Behavioral scales were secondary measures, which showed significant differences between the groups in favor of donepezil at week 24 (8% of donepezil and 6% of placebo-treated patients discontinued because of adverse events). Authors concluded donepezil's benefits extend into more advanced states of Alzheimer's disease with good tolerability (Feldman et al., 2001). In another study, donepezil was examined in 134 patients with mild to moderate Alzheimer's disease with marked neuropsychiatric symptoms. Patients were treated openly with donepezil 5 mg daily for 6 weeks followed by 10 mg daily for a further 6 weeks. Patients were then randomized (60:40) to either placebo or 10 mg donepezil daily. Authors concluded donepezil has significant efficacy in the treatment of neuropsychiatric symptoms in patients with mild to moderate Alzheimer's disease (Holmes et al., 2004).

Rivastigmine

Efficacy of rivastigmine in dementia with Lewy bodies was tested in a randomized, double-blind, placebo-controlled international study. Conclusion of the study was that rivastigmine at 6–12 mg daily produces statistically and clinically significant behavioral effects in patients with Lewy-body dementia and seems safe and well tolerated if titrated individually (McKeith et al., 2000).

Galantamine

Behavioral symptoms were secondary endpoints. One report suggests efficacy of galantamine in probable vascular dementia and Alzheimer's disease combined with cerebrovascular disease in a randomized trial.

Authors concluded galantamine showed a therapeutic effect on all key areas of cognitive and noncognitive abilities in this group of dementia patients (Erkinjuntti et al., 2002).

NMDA Receptor Blocker

Memantine

One randomized controlled trial of memantine treatment in patients with moderate to severe Alzheimer's disease receiving donepezil was reported with improved cognition, activities of daily living, global outcome, and behavior (Tariot et al., 2004). Another study investigated the behavioral effects of memantine in moderate to severe Alzheimer's disease in a 24-week, double-blind, placebo-controlled study. Patients stable on donepezil were treated with 20 mg per day of memantine. Measured by the NPI, patients treated with memantine had reduced agitation or aggression, appetite, and irritability or lability. Authors concluded memantine reduced agitation and aggression in patients who were agitated at baseline and delayed its emergence in those who were free of agitation at baseline (Cummings, Schneider, Tariot, Graham, & Memantine MEM-MD-02 study group, 2006).

Beta Receptor Antagonists (Beta blockers)

There are anecdotal and case reports that discuss the role of beta adrenergic antagonists (beta blockers) in the management of aggression or agitated behavior in general, and specifically in dementia. An extensive search using the general term beta blocker or beta adrenergic anatagonist, as well as individual commonly used generic beta blockade agents, together with key words of dementia, agitation, aggression, and behavior led to few articles with little evidence that evaluated the efficacy of this class of medications for behavioral and psychological symptoms of dementia. There is physiologic rationale behind the use of beta blocking agents for behavioral problems associated with dementia as enhanced behavioral responsiveness to central nervous system norepinepherine in dementia, especially Alzheimer's disease may contribute to disruptive behaviors, including pacing and wandering. One randomized, placebo-controlled study on 31 patients with probable Alzheimer's disease with persistent disruptive behavior, with a mean age of 85 years, found that a propranolol dose titration over a mean of 9 days (mean dose 106 + 38 mg per day) was significantly more effective than placebo for improving overall behavioral status, as measured by the neuropsychiatric inventory and clinical global impression of change scales. However, pressure pacing and irritability did not appear responsive to propranolol, and improvement in overall behavioral status diminished substantially after a 6-month open label propranolol treatment. Of note, 25 of the subjects were women, and only 11 propranolol and only 3 placebo subjects completed the full double-blind phase, and no propranolol subjects developed hypotension or bradycardia. These data are limited by the small sample size (Peskind et al., 2005).

There is discussion of the use of beta blockers in other areas for behavioral management, but limited objective evidence of efficacy. A Cochrane systematic review on pharmacological management of agitation and aggression in people with acquired brain injury found four randomized controlled trials using beta blockers, with beta blockers having the best evidence of others drugs, and the recommendation was that beta blockers deserve broader study (Fleminger, Greenwood, & Oliver, 2006). There are case reports of support for the use of beta blockers for the treatment of akathisia induced by various medications (Zubenko et al., 1987). However, a Cochrane database of systematic reviews of using central acting beta blockers versus placebo on antipsychotic-induced acute akathisia demonstrated insufficient data to recommend the use of beta blockers, but did not suggest adverse effects (Lima, Bacalcthuk, Barnes, & Soares-Weiser, 2006). There are also reports or guidelines that suggest the use of beta blockers for other behavioral treatment of aggression in psychiatric inpatients, intermittent explosive disorder, dementia, and panic disorders but do not include references to clinical trials (Corrigan & Storzbach, 1993; Olvera, 2002; Zamorski & Albucher, 2002).

Several issues need to be considered if a beta blocker is to be tried in the management of wandering or agitated behavior in dementia patients, and of course the first is the potential adverse effect on blood pressure, pulse, and possible exacerbation of asthma. The other issue is, what possible impact could a beta blocker have on memory and dementia itself? Usually this is not a consideration when a beta blocker is chosen to treat hypertensive or cardiac disease, but it is included here for discussion of off-label use of a medication. There is evidence of adverse effects of chronic propranolol use on memory in mice, and in particular impaired retention of spatial learning, which may have some relevance to risk of getting lost while wandering (Czech, Nielson, & Laubmeier, 2000). However, in a study the looked at effect of propranolol on cognitive function in 312 adults less than 60 years of age found only a limited adverse effect on cognitive function that was felt to not be of clinical significance, but testing in older, more impaired individuals might show a different result (Perez-Stable et al., 2000). Other approaches that may identify the impact on cognition by treatment with beta blockers was the Systolic Hypertension in the Elderly Program (SHEP) trial, which did not show a reduction in dementia as compared to placebo, and included a secondary treatment arm of the addition of atenolol. Other reviews are inconclusive about the potential effect of beta blockers on memory, but it is a definite potential adverse effect (Fogari & Zoppi, 2004).

SUMMARY TABLES

Assessment of Wandering

1. Detail what led up to the wander event and review the situation associated with the wander event.
2. Rule out component of delirium.
3. Evaluate for unrecognized dementia and type of dementia.
4. Look for associated medical conditions that contribute to restlessness:
   a. Serotonin Syndrome
   b. Sleep disorders: Restless leg syndrome, rest-activity disorder in dementia (sundowning)
   c. Medications that cause akathisia (restlessness)
   d. Restlessness associated with depression
5. Assess safety risks in the event of a wandering episode—cardiovascular disease; fall risk; chance of dehydration, hypoglycemia, or malnutrition.
6. Individualize treatment based upon the results from the previous assessment steps, monitor efficacy, and prospectively monitor for known adverse effects.
7. Limited evidence for efficacy of medications in reduction of wandering behavior—use specific criteria/improved behavior for efficacy, stop medications that are not effective.
8. Postwandering assessment: injury, dehydration or malnutrition, consider ischemic heart disease, rule out delirium, and assess for unrecognized dementia.

How to Review Medications in a Wandering Patient

1. Time of day of wander event versus medications, changes in usual dosing.
2. Determine if wandering is clearly medication related: behavior is reduced when medication is held, returns if re-initiated.
3. Indication for medications that may exacerbate restlessness, agitation, wandering.
4. Scrutinize medications that may be inappropriate for use in elderly (assess: risk vs. benefit, medication fall risk, if appropriate

dose for elderly due to renal or hepatic clearance, polypharmacy, anticholinergic or other undesirable side effects, such as, orthostatic hypotension).

5. Review pertinent lab values (drug levels, renal or hepatic function).
6. Review possible adverse effects of over the counter medications and supplements (caffeine, sleep aids—Benadryl, Tylenol PM, etc.).
7. Determine if there is a need to add medication (i.e., pain).
8. Is behavior a harm to patient or others?
9. Individualize treatment to include both nonpharmaceutical and, if needed, pharmaceutical treatment.

CONCLUSION

Review of medications in persons who wander should be performed similarly as in any older adult patient. Is there a clear indication? Is the dose and timing of regimens appropriate? Have any medications been recently discontinued or added, and why is this appropriate? Are there issues of polypharmacy, meaning identifying medications that do not take into account changes in pharmacodynamics, medications that are redundant or duplicative, are taken inconsistently or are not monitored appropriately, and are the patient and caregiver educated as to the use and possible adverse effects that need to be monitored? For instance, asking the patient and caregiver if they are aware of medications that can increase fall risk specifically should be part of a thorough medication review. For wandering patients, specific questions about impact on mood, cognition, sleep, anxiety and restlessness, appetite, and postural hypotension should be directly asked. Due to age and age-related disease-associated changes, older adults, especially those with comorbidities, are especially sensitive to drug effects and side effects, and the saying, "Start low and go slow" applies.

Behavioral and psychological symptoms of dementia such as wandering, socially inappropriate activity such as undressing in public, or hoarding frequently accompany dementia. Many of these types of behavioral activities can be helped with nonpharmacological approaches and do not respond well to pharmacologic treatment. In fact the guidelines for the code of Federal Regulations from the Nursing Home Reform Act (1987 Omnibus Reconciliation Act or OBRA) on the appropriate use of antipsychotics in the long-term care setting lists wandering as an inappropriate behavioral symptom that does not justify the use of antipsychotic medications (Buhr & White, 2006). When nonpharmacologic treatments fail, pharmacologic treatments may be considered. Although there are several pharmaceutical options that are commonly used to treat certain features or aspects of behavioral and psychological symptoms of dementia (aggression, psychosis, agitation), there is limited evidence-based data available specifically on efficacy of these agents on controlling wandering.

This is a brief summary of the current evidence-based recommendations for the treatment of behavioral and psychological symptoms of dementia. There is little evidence to support that benefits from the use of typical antipsychotics outweigh the risk of their side effects, especially in the elderly (De Deyn et al., 1999; Dolder & Jeste, 2003; Kindermann, Dolder, Bailey, Katz, & Jeste, 2002; Suh et al., 2004). The recommended approach is to match a medication to the type of dementia and co-existing chronic illnesses, monitor for efficacy in controlling the target symptom, prospectively monitor for adverse effects, and consider dosage reduction once behavior is improved.

In Summary

- Atypical antipsychotics are often used in treating behavioral and psychological symptoms of dementia, particularly risperidone and olanzapine, and there is evidence to show benefits. Atypicals are considered a safer option than conventional antipyschotics, however studies have shown an increased risk of mortality in dementia patients, possibly due to anticholinergic cardiovascular or metabolic side effects, sedation, and falls (Katz, Rupnow, Kozma, & Schneider, 2004).
- Treating dementia patients with antidepressants when depression is present may improve behavioral and psychological symptoms of dementia. Citalopram in one study did show some benefit in reducing agitation. One study with sertraline augmented with donepezil showed some benefit. Mirtazapine, because of its sedating effect and promotion of weight gain, has some features that warrant further study specifically on wandering or agitated dementia patients, and those with weight loss.
- Trazodone has not been shown to have an overall impact on behavioral and psychological symptoms of dementia, but it has low anticholingergic effect, and studies that target specific symptoms such as sundowning or sleep disturbance are needed.
- There are no randomized controlled trials for behavioral and psychological symptoms of dementia for buspirone, but case series show an historical reduction in falls. No data has been found on adverse effects on an older population, let alone in dementia.

- For insomnia, long-term use of benzodiazepine is generally not recommended in the elderly due to increase of fall risk and possible increase in confusion and disorientation due to drowsiness or sedation. Although, the newer nonbenzodiazepine agents such as zolpidem and zaleplon are considered a better option due to short half-lives and less cognitive and residual effects, these still carry an increase risk of falls.
- Valproic acid does not seem to be effective in treating behavioral and psychological symptoms of dementia and has high side effects.
- Cholinesterase inhibitors are helpful in maintaining cognition in dementia, and studies are ongoing to determine their effects on behavioral and psychological symptoms of dementia, which seem favorable.
- Limited and mixed data are available for memantine in treating behavioral and psychological symptoms of dementia, limiting support for recommending its use.
- Other off-label use of medications such as beta blockers, testosterone lowering agents, or nicotine need further study, and again efficacy may differ greatly depending on type of dementia.

In the future, randomized, double-blinded clinical trials for behavioral and psychological symptoms of dementia with acetyl cholinesterase inhibitors, memantine, beta blockers, LHRH agonists that lower testosterone levels, antidepressants (SSRIs), and possibly nicotine need to be performed as they relate to wandering behavior and other behavioral problems with dementia. Targeting of other symptoms that may contribute to wandering should also be tested. These options may be better tolerated and have less side effects than the reliance on antipsychotics. In the meantime, algorithms for behavioral management such as one developed by Sink et al. (2005) may be useful.

GAPS IN RESEARCH

a. Potential agents to reduce wandering behavior
    i. Role of antitestosterone or pro-estrogen
    ii. Role of tobacco, tobacco cessation, use of patch
    iii. Use of beta blockers in reduction of wandering
    iv. Depression detection and use of antidepressants
    v. Use of agents for akathisia when medication that causes akathisia is needed, diphenhydramine vs. anxiolytic vs. other classes such as beta blockers

Case Presentation

A 75-year-old white male with mild dementia of mixed origin, a 2-year history of Parkinson's disease, congestive heart failure controlled with medications (ejection fraction of 25%), atrial fibrillation, and a prior carotid endarterectomy (date not known) is brought into the emergency room by his daughter/caregiver for the fourth time in 3 weeks. Despite parkinsonian features, he has never had hallucinations and until now has been without significant fluctuation in cognition.

His first emergency room visit was for increasing chronic low back pain. He also needed his hydrocodone/acetaminophen renewed (it had run out due to increased usage), and he was given instructions to maintain hydration and avoid constipation. The second emergency room visit was for increasing shortness of breath, and he had vascular congestion and worsening of underlying chronic obstructive pulmonary disease. He was sent home with an increase in diuretic, potassium supplementation, and instruction to use his Atrovent® inhaler on a regular basis and his albuterol inhaler as needed. The third visit was due to a change in behavior where the patient, alone in the house, yelled out for help while seated on the couch. A neighbor came by to assist, and the patient was complaining that he was uncomfortable, but unable to express what it was. Emergency room work up was negative including head computed tomography, complete blood count, chemistries, urinalysis, chest radiography (x-ray), and urine toxicology. Because of the frequent complaints of shortness of breath, the family had decided to stop the patient from smoking. The patient became more agitated and started searching for cigarettes. He became more unstable ambulating and fell in the house, with lacerations on his knees. Finally, he started wandering out of the house, apparently in search of cigarettes, and wound up holding on to a railing near the sidewalk, unable to move and calling out for help where he was found by a neighbor. The daughter brought the patient back to the emergency room because of her fear of him wandering off and falling, and he was admitted.

The differential diagnosis was delirium versus progression of multi-infarct dementia with possible repeat stroke due to atrial fibrillation and not being anticoagulated due to fall risk. The Mini-Mental Status Exam (MMSE) was 22/30 (baseline), and he was felt to be exhibiting sundowning, wanting to leave the hospital to look for his daughter or cigarettes, and a sitter was required. No causes of delirium were identified, including possible infection, hepatic dysfunction, metabolic abnormalities, inflammatory process, or an intracranial process. Chest x-ray and blood cultures were negative;

B12, folate, thyroid stimulating hormone/thyroxine test (T4) were normal. Urine electrolytes suggested dehydration as a cause of mild prerenal azotemia above baseline. A magnetic resonance imaging was negative. Initially, haloperidol was tried to control behavior issues, and later he was given quetiapine 12.5 mg twice a day and as needed. The conclusion was the altered mental status was due to initiation of opiates for back pain, constipation, and dehydration, with possible pancreatitis that resolved. Patient was discharged home where agitation continued, and daughter was reluctant to give quetiapine. Patient was seen in a geriatric clinic where rivastigmine was restarted (it had been stopped in the hospital), the importance of quetiapine (25 mg twice daily [BID] and additional evening dose as needed) was emphasized, trazodone 50 mg was given to try and reinduce sleep at night with instruction to avoid afternoon and evening naps, and the daughter was told to allow the patient to smoke for now. The patient had improved behavior, multiple somatic complaints stopped, and he no longer wandered. The daughter was informed about the increased mortality associated with quetiapine for behavioral management of older adults, and she was willing to try a decreased dosage in the future.

REFERENCES

Adler, L. A. & Angrist B. M. (1995). Paroxetine and akathisia. *Biological Psychiatry, 37*(1), 336–337.

Alexopoulos, G. S., Jeste, D. V., Carpenter, D., Ross, R., & Docherty, J. P. (2005, January). The expert consensus guidelines series: treatment of dementia and its behavioral disturbances. *Postgraduate Medicine Special Report,* 1–111.

Allain, H., Bentue-Ferrer, D., Poland, E., Akwa, Y., & Patat. A. (2005) Postural instability and consequent falls and hip fractures associated with use of hypnotics in the elderly. *Drugs & Aging, 22*(9), 749–765.

Ancoli-Israel, S., Richardson, G. S., Mangano, R. M., Jenkins, L., Hall, P., & Jones, W. S. (2005). Long-term use of sedative hypnotics in older people with insomnia. *Sleep Medicine, 6*(2), 107–113.

Bachman, D., & Rabins, P. (2006). "Sundowning" and other temporally associated agitation states in dementia patients. *Annual Review of Medicine, 57*(1), 499–511.

Baldassano, C. F., Truman, C. J, Nierenberg, A, Ghaemi, S. N., & Sachs, G. S. (1996). Akathisia: a review and case report following paroxetine treatment. *Comprehensive Psychiatry, 37*(1), 122–124.

Ballard, C., Waite, J., & Birks, J. (2006). Atypical antipsychotics for aggression and psychosis in Alzheimer's disease. *Cochrane Database of Systematic Reviews: Reviews, 1,* CDC003476.

Baskys, A. (2004). Lewy body dementia: The litmus test for neuroleptic sensitivity and extrapyramidal symptoms. *Journal of Clinical Psychiatry, 65*(Suppl 11), 16–22.

Bergman, J., Dwolatzky, T., Brettholz, I., & Lerner, V. (2005). Beneficial effect of donepezil in the treatment of elderly patients with tardive movement disorders. *Journal of Clinical Psychiatry, 66*(1), 107–110.

Borson, S., Scanlan, J. M., Watanabe J., Tu, S., & Lessig M. (2005). Simplifying detection of cognitive impairment: Comparison of the Mini-Cog and Mini-Mental State Examination in a multiethnic sample. *Journal of the American Geriatrics Society, 53*(5), 871–874.

Boyer, E. W., & Shannon, M. (2005). The Serotonin Syndrome. *The New England Journal of Medicine. 352*(11), 1112–1120.

Braude, D., Soliz, T., Crandall, C., Hendey, G., Andrews, J., Weichenthal, L. (2006). Antiemetics in the ED: a randomized controlled trial comparing 3 common agents. *American Journal of Emergency* Medicine, *24*(2), 177–182.

Braunwald, E., Fauci, A., Kasper, D., Hauser, S., Longo, D., & Jameson, J. (2001). Poisoning and drug overdosage. In C. Linden & M. Burns (Eds.), *Harrison's Principles of Internal* Medicine (pp.2615). New York: McGraw-Hill-Medical Publishing Division.

Brodaty, H., Ames, D., Snowdon, J., Woodward, M., Kirwan, J., Clarnette, R., et al. (2003). A randomized placebo-controlled trial of risperidone for the treatment of aggression, agitation, and psychosis of dementia. *Journal of Clinical Psychiatry, 64*(2), 134–43.

Buhr G. T., & White, H. K. (2006). Difficult behaviors in long-term care patients with dementia. *Journal of the American Medical Directors Association, 7*(1), 180–192.

Cantillon, M., Brunswick, R., Molina, D., & Bahro M. (1996). Buspirone vs. haloperidol: A double-blind trial for agitation in a nursing home population with Alzheimer's disease *American Journal of Geriatric Psychiatry, 4*(3), 263–267.

Carnes, M., Howell, T., Rosenberg, M., Francis, J., Hildebrand, C., & Knuppel, J. (2003). Physicians vary in approaches to the clinical management of delirium. *Journal of the American Geriatrics Society, 51*(2), 234–239.

Centers for Medicaid & Medicare Services (CMS). (2001). *Online Survey Certification & Reporting (OSCAR) Data 2001*. Retrieved September 13, 2006, from http://www.ascp.com/resources/clinical/oscardata.cfm.

Cherrier, M. M., Matsumoto, A. M., Amory, J. K., Asthana, S., Bremner, W., Peskind, E. R., et al. (2005). Testosterone improves spatial memory in men with Alzheimer's disease and mild cognitive impairment. *Neurology, 64*(12), 2063–2068.

Chiu, Y. (2002). Getting lost behavior and directed attention impairments in Taiwanese patients with early Alzheimer's disease. Unpublished doctoral dissertation, University of Michigan.

Cooper, J. P. (2003). Buspirone for anxiety and agitation in dementia. *Journal of Psychiatry & Neuroscience, 28*(6), 469.

Corey, D. A. (1994). Adverse reaction to metoclopramide during enteroclysis (letter). *American Journal of Roentgenology, 163*(1), 480.

Corrigan, P. W. & Storzbach, D. M. (1993). Behavioral interventions for alleviating psychotic symptoms. *H&CP: Hospital & Community Psychiatry, 44*(4), 341–347.

Court, J., Spurden, D., Lloyd, S., McKeith, I., Ballard, C., Cairns, N., et al. (1999). Neuronal nicotinic receptors in dementia with Lewy bodies and schizophrenia: Alpha-bungarotoxin and nicotine binding in the thalamus. *Journal of Neurochemistry, 73*(4), 1590–1597.

Cummings, J. L., Schneider, E., Tariot, P. N., Graham, S. M., & Memantine MEM-MD-02 study group. (2006). Behavioral effects of memantine in Alzheimer disease patients receiving donepezil treatment. *Neurology, 67*(1), 57–63.

Czech, D. A., Nielson, K. A., & Laubmeier, K. K. (2000). Chronic propranolol induces deficits in retention but not acquisition performance in the water maze in mice. *Neurobiology of Learning & Memory, 74*(1), 17–26.

De Deyn, P. P., Rabheru, K., Rasmussen, A., Bocksberger, J. P., Dautzenberg, P. L., Eriksson, S., et al. & Lawlor, B. A. (1999). A randomized trial of risperidone, placebo, and haloperidol for behavioral symptoms of dementia. *Neurology, 53*(5), 946–955.

Dewing, J. (2000). Sundowning: is it a syndrome? *Journal of Dementia Care, 8*(6), 33–36.

Dolder, C. R., & Jeste, D. V. (2003). Incidence of tardive dyskinesia with typical versus atypical antipsychotics in very high risk patients. *Biological Psychiatry, 53*(12), 1142–1145.

Erkinjuntti, T., Kurz, A., Gauthier, S., Bullock, R., Lilienfeld, S., & Damaraju, C. V. (2002). Efficacy of galantamine in probable vascular dementia and Alzheimer's disease combined with cerebrovascular disease: a randomized trial. *Lancet, 359*(9314), 1283–1290.

Falsetti, A. E. (2000). Risperidone for control of agitation in dementia patients. *American Journal of Health-System Pharmacy, 57*(8), 862–870.

Feldman, H., Gautheir, S., Hecker, J., Vellas, B., Subbiah, P., Whalen, E., et al. (2001). A 24-week, randomized, double-blind study of donepezil in moderate to severe Alzheimer's disease. *Neurology, 57*(4), 613–620.

Fick, D. M., Cooper, J. W., Wade, W. E., Waller, J. L., Maclean, J. R., & Beers, M. H. (2003). Updating the Beers criteria for potentially inappropriate medication use in older adults: results of a US consensus panel of experts. *Archives of Internal Medicine, 163*(22), 2716–2724.

File, S. E., Fluck, E., & Leahy, A. (2001). Nicotine has calming effects on stress-induced mood changes in females, but enhances aggressive mood in males. *International Journal of Neuropsychopharmacology, 4*(4), 371–376.

Finkel, S. I., Mintzer, J. E., Dysken, M., Krishman, K. R., Burt, T., & McRae, T. (2004). A randomized, placebo-controlled study of the efficacy and safety of sertraline in the treatment of the behavioral manifestations of Alzheimer's disease in outpatients treated with donepezil. *International Journal of Geriatric Psychiatry, 19*(1), 9–18.

Fleminger, S., Greenwood, R. J., & Oliver, D. L. (2006). Pharmacological management for agitation and aggression in people with acquired brain injury. *The Cochrane Library,* CD003299.

Fogari, R. & Zoppi, A. (2004). Effect of antihypertensive agents on quality of life in the elderly. *Drugs & Aging, 21*(6), 377–393.

Food and Drug Administration (FDA). (2005, April 15). *Deaths with Antipsychotics in Elderly Patients with Behavioral Disturbances.* FDA Public Health Advisory. Retrieved August 24, 2006, from http://www.fda.gov.

Forest Pharmaceuticals. (2003). *Product Information: Namenda (TM).* (2003). *Memantine.* St. Louis, MO: Author.

French, K. L., Granholm, A. C., Moore, A. B., Nelson, M. E., & Bimonte-Nelson, H. A. (2006). Chronic nicotine improves working and reference memory performance and reduces hippocampal NGF in aged female rats. *Behavioural Brain Research, 169*(2), 256–262.

Gardner, M. E., Malone, D. C., Sey, M., Babington, M. A. (2004). Mirtazapine is associated with less anxiolytic use among elderly depressed patients in long-term care facilities. *Journal of the American Medical Directors Association, 5*(2), 101–106.

Gauthier, S., Feldman, H., Hecker, J., Vellas, B., Ames, D., Subbiah, P., et al. (2002). Efficacy of donepezil on behavioral symptoms in patients with moderate to severe Alheimer's disease. *International Psychogeriatrics, 14*(4), 389–404.

Girishchandra, B. G., Johnson, L., Cresp, R. M, & Orr, K. G. (2002). Mirtazapine-induced akathisia (letter). *Medical Journal of Australia, 176*(5), 242.

Goertelmeyer, R., & Erbler, H. (1992). Memantine in the treatment of mild to moderate dementia syndrome. *Arzneimittelforschung, 42,* 904–913.

Holmes, C., Wilkinson, D., Dean, C., Vethanayagam, S., Olivieri, S., Langley, A., et al. (2004). The efficacy of donepezil in the treatment of neuropsychiatric symptoms in Alzheimer disease. *Neurology, 63*(2), 214–219.

Inouye, S. K. (2006). Delirium in older persons. *New England Journal of Medicine, 354*(11), 1157–1165.

Inouye, S. K., Foreman, M. D., Mion, L. C., Katz, K. H., Cooney, L. M. Jr. (2001). Nurses' recognition of delirium and its symptoms: Comparison of nurse and researcher ratings. *Archives of Internal Medicine. 161*(20), 2467–2473

Inouye, S. K, van Dyck, C. H., Alessi, C. A., Balkin, S., Siegal, A. P., & Horwitz, R. I. (1990). Clarifying confusion: The confusion assessment method. A new method for detection of delirium. *Annals of Internal Medicine, 113*(12), 941–948.

Jacobs, M. B. (1983). Diltiazem and akathisia. *Annals of Internal Medicine, 99*(6), 794–795.

Jan, M., Erokwu, N., Ebose, I., Strohl, K. (2005). Sleep problems and the risk for sleep disorders in an outpatient veteran population. *Sleep & Breathing, 9*(2), 57–63.

Katz, I. R., Jeste, D. V., Mintzer, J. E., Clyde, C., Napolitano, J., & Brecher, M. (1999). Comparision of risperidone and placebo for psychosis and behavioral disturbances associated with dementia: a randomized, double-blind trial. *Journal of Clinical Psychiatry, 60*(2), 107–115.

Katz, I. R., Rupnow, M., Kozma, C., & Schneider, L. (2004). Risperidone and falls in ambulatory nursing home residents with dementia and psychosis or agitation: Secondary analysis of a double-blind, placebo-controlled trial. *American Journal of Geriatric Psychiatry, 12*(5), 499–508.

Kindermann, S. S., Dolder, C. R., Bailey, A., Katz, I. R., & Jeste, D. V. (2002). Pharmacological treatment of psychosis and agitation in elderly patients with dementia: four decades of experience. *Drugs & Aging, 19*(4), 257–276.

Knott, V., Engeland, C., Mohr, E., Mahoney, C., & Ilivitsky, V. (2000). Acute nicotine administration in Alzheimer's disease: an exploratory EEG study. *Neuropsychobiology. 41*(4), 210–220.

Kuehn, B.M. (2005). FDA warns antipsychotic drugs may be risky for elderly. *JAMA, 293*(20), 2462.

Kummer, J., Guendel, L., Linden, J., Eich F. X., Attalki, P., Coquelin, J. P., et al. (1993). Long-term polysomnographic study of the efficacy and safety of zolpidem in elderly psychiatric in-patients with insomnia. *The Journal of International Medical Research, 21*(4), 171–184.

Lacy, C. F., Armstrong, L. L., Goldman, M. P., & Lance, L. L. (2003). *Drug Information Handbook*. Hudson, OH: Lexi-Comp.

Lankarani-Fard, A., & Castle, S. C. (2006). Postoperative delirium and Ogilvie's syndrome resolving with neostigmine. *Journal of the American Geriatrics Society, 54*(6), 1016–1017.

Lebert, F., Stekke, W., Hasenbroekx, C., & Pasquier F. (2004). Frontotemporal dementia: A randomized, controlled trial with trazodone. *Dementia and Geriatric Cognitive Disorders, 17*(4), 355–359.

Leipzig, R. M., Cumming, R. G., & Tinetti, M. E. (1999). Drugs and falls in older people: A systematic review and meta-analysis: I. Psychotropic drugs. *Journal of the American Geriatrics Society, 47*(1), 30–39.

Lima, A. R., Bacalcthuk, J., Barners, T. R. E., & Soares-Weiser, K. (2006). Central action beta-blockers versus placebo for neuroleptic-induced acute akathisia. *Cochrane Database of Systematic Reviews, 3*, CD001946.

Lonergan, E., Luxenberg, J., Colford, J., & Birks, J. (2006). Haloperidol for agitation in dementia. Cochrane Dementia and Cognitive Improvement Group *Cochrane Database of Systematic Reviews, 3*, CD002852.

Longergan, E. T., Cameron, M., & Luxenberg, J. (2004). Valporic acid for agitation in dementia. *Cochrane Database of Systematic Reviews, 2*, CD003945.

Lopez-Arrieta J. L. A., & Sanz, F. J. (2006). Nicotine for Alzheimer's disease. *The Cochrane Library, 1.*

Lyketsos, C. G., Colenda, C. C., Beck, C., Blank, K., Doraiswamy, M. P., Kalunian, D. A., et al. (2006). *American Journal of Geriatric Psychiatry, 14*(7), 561–572.

Markovitz, P. J. (1993). Treatment of anxiety in the elderly. *Journal of Clinical Psychiatry, 54*(Suppl), 64–88.

Martinon-Torres, G., Fioravanti, M., & Grimley E. J. (2006). Trazodone for agitation in dementia. Cochrane *Dementia and Cognitive Improvement Group Cochrane Database of Systematic Reviews.*

Mata, I. F., Bodkin, C. L., Adler, C. H., Lin, S. C., Uitti, R. J., Farrer, M. J., et al. (2006). Genetics of restless legs syndrome. *Parkinsonism & Related Disorders, 12*(1), 1–7.

McKeith, I., Del Ser, T., Spano, P., Emre, M., Wesnes, K., Anand, R., et al. (2000). Efficacy of rivastigmine in dementia with Lewy bodies: a randomized, double-blind, placebo-controlled international study. *Lancet, 356*(9247), 2031–2036.

Meguro, K., Meguro, M., Tanaka, Y., Akanuma, K., Yamaguchi, K., & Itoh, M. (2004). Risperidone is effective for wandering and disturbed sleep-wake patterns in Alzheimer's disease. *Journal of Geriatric Psychiatry and Neurology, 17*(2), 61–67.

Merritt, S. L., & Berger, B. E. (2004). Obstructive sleep apnea-hypopnea syndrome: Nurses may detect a problem often overlooked by other providers. *American Journal of Nursing, 104*(7), 49–52.

Micromedex® Health Care Series USP DI®, © 1974-2006. (2006). Thomson MICROMEDEX. Retrieved September 14, 2006, from http://www.thomsonhc.com/hcs/librarian/PFPUI/kV1v3Cu1usPx12 Quetiapine.

Nelson, D. E. (2001). Akathisia–A brief review. *Southern Medical Journal, 46*(5), 133–134.

Oliver, D., Britton, M., Seed, P., Martin, F. C., & Hopper, A. H. (1997). Development and evaluation of evidence based risk assessment tool (STRATIFY) to predict which elderly inpatients will fall: case-control and cohort studies. *British Medical Journal, 315*(7115), 1049–1053.

Olvera, R. L. (2002). Intermittent explosive disorder: epidemiology, diagnosis and management. CNS *Drugs, 16*(8), 517–526.

Orengo, C., Kunik, M. E., Molinari, V., Wristers, K., & Yudofsky, S. C. (2002). Do testosterone levels relate to aggression in elderly men with dementia? *Journal of Neuropsychiatry & Clinical Neurosciences, 14*(2), 161–166.

Ott, B. R., Lapane, K. L., & Gambassi, G. (2000). Gender differences in the treatment of behavioral problems in Alzheimer's disease. SAGE Study Group. Systemic Assessment of Geriatric drug use via Epidemiology. *Neurology, 54*(2), 427–432.

Parlak, I., Atilla, R., Cicek, M., Parlak, M., Erdur, B., Guryay, M., et al. (2005). Rate of metoclopramide infusion affects the severity and incidence of akathisia. *Emergency Medicine Journal, 22*(9), 621–624.

Perez-Stable, E. J., Halliday, R., Gardiner, P. S., Baron, R. B., Hauck, W. W., Acree, M., et al. (2000). The effects of propranolol on cognitive function and quality of life: A randomized trial among patients with diastolic hypertension. *American Journal of Medicine, 108*(5), 359–365.

Peskind, E. R., Tsuang, D. W., Bonner, L. T., Pascualy, M., Rieske, R. G., Snowden, M. B., et al. (2005). Propranolol for disruptive behaviors in nursing home residents with probable or possible Alzheimer disease: a placebo-controlled study. *Alzheimer Disease & Associated Disorders, 19*(1), 23–28.

Pierre, J. M. (2005). Extrapyramidal symptoms with atypical antipsychotics: Incidence, prevention and management. *Drug Safety, 28*(3), 191–208.

Pollock, B. G., Mulsant, B. H., Rosen, J., Sweet, R.A., Mazumdar, S., Bharucha, A., et al. (2002). Comparison of citalopram, perphenazine, and placebo for the acute treatment of psychosis and behavioral disturbances in hospitalized, demented patients. *American Journal of Psychiatry, 159*(3), 460–465.

Prueter, C., Habermeyer, B., Norra, C., & Kosinski, C. M. (2003). Akathisia as a side effect of antipsychotic treatment with quetiapine in a patient with Parkinson's disease. *Movement Disorders, 18*(6), 712–713.

Rabinowitz, J., Katz, I. R., De Deyn, P. P., Brodaty, H., Greenspan, A., & Davidson, M. (2004). Behavioral and psychological symptoms in patients with dementia as a target for pharmacotherapy with risperidone. *Journal of Clinical Psychiatry, 65*(10), 1329–1334.

Roger, M., Attali, P., & Coquelin, J. P. (1993). Multicenter, double-blind, controlled comparision of zolpidem and triazolam in elderly patients with insomnia. *Clinical Therapeutics, 15*(1), 127–136.

Roila, F., Basurto, C., Baracarda, M., Picciafuco, M., Ballatori, E., Del Favero, A., et al. (1990). A pilot study of metoclopramide, dexamethasone, diphenhydramine, and lorazepam in prevention of nausea and vomiting in cisplatin-treated male patients. *Oncology, 47*(5), 415–417.

Rosin, R. A., & Raskind, M.A. (2005). Gonadotrophin-releasing hormone agonist treatment of aggression in Alzheimer's disease: a case report. *International Psychogeriatrics, 17*(2), 313–318.

Ruth, S., Straand, J., Nygaard, H. A., Bjorvatn, B., Pallesen, S. (2004). Effect of antipsychotic withdrawal on behavior and sleep/wake activity in nursing home residents with dementia: A randomized, placebo-controlled, double-blinded study. The Bergen District Nursing Home Study. *Journal of the American Geriatric Society, 52*(10), 1737–1743.

Salzman, C. (2005). Treatment of depression with new and atypical antidepressants. In C. Salzman, & G. Small (Eds.), *Clinical Geriatric Psychopharmacology* (pp. 316). Philadelphia: Lippincott Williams & Wilkins.

Sathananthan, G. L., Sanghvi, I., Phillips, N., & Gershon, S. (1975). MJ 9022: Correlation between neuroleptic potential and stereotypy. *Current Therapeutic Research, Clinical and Experimental, 18*(5), 701–705.

Shaw, S. H., Curson, H., & Coquelin, J. P. (1992). A double-blind, comparative study of zolpidem and placebo in the treatment of insomnia in elderly psychiatric inpatients. *The Journal of International Medical Research, 20*(2), 150–161; erratum, *The Journal of International Medical Research, 20*(6) following 494.

Shekelle, P. G., MacLean, C. H., Morton, S. C., & Wenger, N. S. (2001). ACOVE quality indicators. *Annals of Internal Medicine, 135*(8 part 2), 653–667.

Shelton, P. S., & Hocking, L. B., (1997). Zolpidem for dementia-related insomnia and nighttime wandering. *The Annals of Pharmacotherapy, 31*(3), 319–322.

Sink, K. M., Holden, K. F., & Yaffe, K. (2005). Pharmacological treatment of neuropsychiatric symptoms of dementia: A review of the evidence. *Journal of the American Medical Association, 293*(5), 596–608.

Skjerve, A. & Nygaard, H. A. (2000). Improvement in sundowning in dementia with Lewy bodies after treatment with donepezil. *International Journal of Geriatric Psychiatry, 15*(12), 1147–1151.

Song, J. (2003) Relationship of premorbid personality and behavioral responses to stress to wandering behavior of residents with dementia in long term care facilities. Unpublished doctoral dissertation, University of Michigan.

Staedt, J., & Stoppe, G. (2005). Treatment of rest-activity disorders in dementia and special focus on sundowning. *International Journal of Geriatric Psychiatry, 20*(6), 507–511.

Street, J. S., Clark, W. S., Gannn, K. S., Cumming, J. L., Bymaster, F. P. Tamura, R. N., et al. (2000). Olanzapine treatment of psychotic and behavioral symptoms in patients with Alzheimer disease in nursing care facilities: a double-blind randomized, placebo-controlled trial. The HGEU Study Group. *Archives of General Psychiatry, 57*(10), 968–976.

Suh, G. H., Son, H. G., Ju, Y. S., Jcho, K. H., Yeon, B. K., Shin, Y. M., et al. (2004). A randomized, double blind, crossover comparison of risperidone and haloperidol in Korean dementia patients with behavioral disturbances. *American Journal of Geriatric Psychiatry, 12*(5), 509–516.

Sultzer, D. L., Gray, K .F, Gunay, I., Wheatley, M. V., & Mahler, M. E. (2001). Does behavioral improvement with haloperidol or trazodone treatment depend on psychosis or mood symptoms in patients with dementia? *Journal of the American Geriatrics Society, 49*(10), 294–300.

Tariot, P. N., Farlow, M. R., Grossberg, G. T., Graham, S. M., McDonald, S., & Gergel, I. (2004). Memantine treatment in patients with moderate to severe Alzheimer disease already receiving donepezil: A randomized controlled trial. *Journal of the American Medical Association, 291*(3), 317–324.

Teri, L., Logsdon, R. G., Peskind, E., Weiner, M. F., Tractenberg, R. E., Foster, N. L., et al. (2000). Treatment of agitation in AD: a randomized, placebo-controlled clinical trial. *Neurology, 55*(9), 1271–1278.

Van Putten, T., May, P. R., & Marder, S. R. (1984). Akathisia with haloperidol and thiothixene. *Archives of General Psychiatry, 41*(11), 1036–1039.

Vinson, D. R., & Drotts, D. L. (2001) Diphenhydramine for the prevention of akathisia induced by prochlorperazine: a randomized, controlled trial. *Annals of Emergency Medicine, 37*(2), 125–131.

Wang, P. S., Bohn, R. L., Glynn, R. J., Mogun, H., & Avorn, J. (2001). Zolpidem use and hip fractures in older people. *Journal of the American Geriatrics Society, 49*(12), 1685–1690.

Wick J. Y., & Zanni G. R. (2005). Sundowning: disruptive behavior with many causes. The Consultant Pharmacist: *The Journal of the American Society of Consultant Pharmacists, 20*(11), 947–950, 957–961.

Zamorski, M. A., & Albucher, R. C. (2002). What to do when SSRIs fail: eight strategies for optimizing treatment of panic disorder. *American Family Physician, 66*(8), 1477–1484, 1395–1397, 1566.

Zubenko, G. S., Cohen, B. M., & Lipinski, J. F. (1987). Antidepressant-related akathisia. *Journal of Clinical Psychopharmacology, 7*(4), 254–257.

CHAPTER THIRTEEN

The Alzheimer's Association's Safe Return® Program for Persons Who Wander

Elizabeth Bass, Meredeth A. Rowe, and Monica Moreno

INTRODUCTION

In 1993, the Alzheimer's Association, a global leader in providing support and research for Alzheimer's disease, instituted Safe Return®, a national identification and support program helping adults with Alzheimer's or related dementias who wander and become lost. Since the program's initiation, more than 11,000 individuals have been reunited with their families and caregivers. Every adult with a diagnosis of progressive dementia is at risk for wandering and becoming lost, without regard to stage of disease, past behavior, age or any other characteristics (Rowe, Feinglass, & Wiss, 2004; Rowe & Glover, 2001). Of those with Alzheimer's, up to 67 percent will wander and become lost (Sink, Covinsky, Newcomer, & Yaffe, 2004). Wandering incidents are unpredictable and therefore difficult to prevent. Because a person with dementia may not have the capacity to remember his or her name and address or recognize an unsafe situation, enrollment with Safe Return® is vital. Clinicians have an important roll in familiarizing persons with dementia and their caregivers with Safe Return® and promoting enrollment in the program, because many people, particularly those unfamiliar with the condition, are unaware of Safe Return's® existence.

OVERVIEW OF THE SAFE RETURN® PROGRAM

Safe Return® facilitates the engagement of systems (i.e., local law enforcement) that speed the recovery of a demented person who has wandered and become separated from the caregiver. The return to the family is often swift since the stored data allow rapid dissemination of information. There are two general instances in which Safe Return® operates. In the first case, the caregiver realizes a person with dementia has become lost. When Safe Return® is contacted, the missing person's information and photograph is faxed to local law enforcement, prompting activation of the community support network. In the interim, clinicians at Safe Return® provide counseling and psychological support to families and friends. When the person is found, the finder (official or civilian) calls Safe Return® via a toll-free number. Safe Return® acts as a facilitator by linking the finder with the family via a conference call. During this call, plans are established for the return of the person with dementia, ensured by Safe Return®. In the second case, the caregiver may not be aware that an adverse wandering incident has occurred. A person with dementia leaves a safe environment, unbeknownst to the caregiver, and may then be identified by local police or civilians who encounter the person. When these individuals see the Safe Return® identification (described presently) and then phone the Alzheimer's Association, the individual with dementia is promptly returned to safety. This assistance is available 24 hours a day, year round. Safe Return® also provides general caregiver support in the form of literature and clinical suggestions on how to care for adults with progressive dementia. Local chapters provide assistance as well, including support groups, resource referrals, and respite care for families affected by Alzheimer's.

SIDEBAR 1

Included benefits of Safe Return® enrollment are:

- Toll-free enrollment line
- Enrollment forms in seven languages
- Access to language line with over 140 languages
- National information and photo database
- 24-hour, toll-free crisis line
- Fax alert notification system
- Links to media outlets, if permitted by family
- Local chapter support
- Wandering behavior and other safety information
- Access to Master's level clinicians (24 hours a day, 365 days a year)

- Engraved identification bracelet or necklace and iron-on clothing labels (indicating person has a memory problem)
- 5 Steps to a Safe Return® refrigerator magnet, key chain, lapel pin, stickers, and wallet cards
- For an additional $15, the caregiver is provided with jewelry that alerts others in an emergency that the wearer provides care for a person enrolled in Safe Return®

Enrolling

- All persons with dementia should be enrolled in Safe Return® regardless of whether they live in the community or a professional care setting
- Local Alzheimer's Association chapters can assist in the enrollment process
- Visit http://alz.org/Services/SafeReturn.asp for more information or to enroll

---

As of 2006, the enrollment fee was $40. For an additional $15, the caregiver is provided identification that alerts emergency personnel that the wearer cares for a person enrolled in Safe Return®. Though the actual cost of the program is much higher, the Alzheimer's Association has a grant from the Department of Justice, which covers a portion of the costs. For enrollment, accomplished by phone, fax, mail, or online, detailed information is requested; including all the enrollee's identifying characteristics, contact persons, and local law enforcement information.

PRACTICE IMPLICATIONS

The Alzheimer's Association compiles statistics on enrollees to help educate the public about trends related to wandering, for instance:

- More than twice as many Safe Return® enrollees are found than are reported missing.
- Safe Return® has enrolled approximately 145,000 individuals since 1993.
- In a given year, over 1,600 wandering incidents are reported to Safe Return® (the program receives over 6,000 calls to the Safe Return® Incident Line annually).
- The program has facilitated the recovery of 11,200 individuals with 99% success in safely returning those enrolled.

- Half of Safe Return® enrollees are found within the first four hours of reported disappearance, with 88.4% recovered within 24 hours, a critical time span for rescue efforts (based on information obtained during incidents). (Rowe & Bennett, 2003)

In addition to this notable record, enrollment in Safe Return® provides some comfort to caregivers who now have an emergency plan in place in the event of a wandering incident. The 15–30 minutes spent filling out the enrollment form and $40 fee is minimal compared to the benefits Safe Return® offers, which extend for the lifetime of the enrollee. This lifetime coverage is significant: findings from one study found that some enrollees became lost multiple times, and other enrollees eloped for the first time more than 5 years after registration (Rowe et al., 2004).

Participation in Safe Return® is not limited to community dwellers, because wandering occurs in acute, long-term care and community-based settings as well. Nursing homes and assisted living facilities can enhance their patient safety efforts by enrolling residents with dementia in Safe Return®. Enrollment ensures that residents have identification on them, which can reduce confusion when the resident leaves the facility for any reason, including physician visits, hospital stays, or outings in the community. Some larger organizations assist with or provide for enrollment into Safe Return® for members of their facility or local residents, though several have had minimal response from the community. One enrollment program done at the facility level has been underway since spring 2006 at the James A. Haley Veterans Hospital in Tampa, Florida (Tampa VA), through a partnership between the VISN 8 Patient Safety Center of Inquiry and the Alzheimer's Association. Veterans with a diagnosis of Alzheimer's or related dementias are contacted by a letter from the Tampa VA explaining the Safe Return® program and the waiver of the enrollment fee, which is paid by the hospital. Included is an enrollment brochure with a Veterans Administration stamp on the form, verifying for Safe Return® that the veteran is a veteran eligible for care at the Tampa VA. Letters are also available in the Geriatric and Memory Clinics for clinicians to give to newly diagnosed patients. The veteran or caregiver is responsible for submitting the enrollment form to Safe Return®. (In the case of nursing home residents, the assigned social worker does this paperwork.) Quarterly, the Alzheimer's Association sends an invoice to the hospital at which point the Tampa VA submits payment. By using a "scholarship" method rather than automatically enrolling patients, the responsibility of enrollment for ambulatory patients lies with the veterans and their families. In the first 6 months, enrollment was 20 percent of those eligible. The Tampa VA plans eventually to expand enrollment, collaborating with the National Center for Patient Safety to explore options to export this program nationally.

Similar registry programs have been developed by local and state governments, and several have supplementary applications. Some programs provide an ongoing, updated database for the local law enforcement agency that can be used to identify vulnerable residents. This could be important to ensure adequate services during weather disasters or other emergencies. One such example is a program in Alabama called AlaSafe (https://www.alasafe.gov/). In addition, these databases may be used to identify residents who could benefit from regular health and welfare checks by local law enforcement, such as the SARA Program with the Marion County Sheriff's Office in Ocala, FL. If these registries exist in a community, it is beneficial to enroll in both the local program and Safe Return®.

Case Study #1

In the summer of 2006, Safe Return® received a call concerning a 59-year-old woman who was last seen four days prior. She had retired from her job a year ago after being diagnosed with dementia. One morning, she woke up as usual and prepared for her day as her husband went off to work. She was planning to pick her daughter up from the airport since she was arriving from out of town for a visit. Around 9:00 A.M. the daughter called and informed her mother that the plane had arrived earlier than expected. The woman placed her dog in the basement as she routinely would when leaving home and left. A trip to the airport was routine so the family did not have any concerns. When the woman arrived at the airport, she asked a security guard for directions because she could not locate the appropriate terminal. She was provided directions, and the security guard watched her return to her car, leaving in the proper direction. She never arrived at the terminal to pick up her daughter. Later that day, the family alerted police and the National Center for Missing Adults. Although not enrolled in the program, the family contacted Safe Return® to see if the Alzheimer's Association could help them find the missing woman. The same day the woman disappeared, one of the credit card companies reported that she bought gas at a BP gas station in a western part of her home state. Later that same day she made four attempts to purchase gas again, by then two states away from her place of origin in an area where she had never lived, had no family, and had never visited. Four and a half days after the woman was last seen at home, her vehicle was found stuck in a berm along the highway in a different state. The area was very remote, approximately 70 miles from the gas station where she last tried to pay for gas. Search and rescue personnel began their search at the location where the vehicle was found and located her body in that same isolated area.

Case Study #2

A woman called her local Alzheimer's Association chapter for some guidance and support in caring for her father with dementia. During this conversation she was informed of the Safe Return® program. A friend of her father's who was dying of cancer offered to pay the $40 enrollment fee. According to the daughter, the friend wanted to do something for her father as he knew he would not be around to help in the future. A month after being enrolled in Safe Return®, the woman's father got in his car and drove away from his hometown. He was missing for two days, traveling over 75 miles, and filling up his car several times with gas using his bank card. At one point, two women noticed him getting out of his car in their neighborhood. They introduced themselves and invited him inside, offering him something to eat and drink. Noticing his Safe Return® bracelet, they immediately called the Safe Return® Incident Line. With information from the Safe Return® National database, the daughter was contacted. When she arrived to pick up her Father, he was sitting at the kitchen table of his new-found friends with a plate of freshly made cookies to take home with him.

FUTURE RESEARCH

Further research is needed to identify facilitators and barriers for enrollment to the Safe Return® program, identifying effective strategies to inform caregivers about the program, and community education to ensure Good Samaritans know how to identify and provide assistance to a lost individual. Various communities have enacted programs to improve enrollment and utilization, and it would be helpful to have an easily accessible report of those programs. More communities and states are developing their own programs, and it will be important to have materials to assist caregivers to choose the best program for their situation.

CONCLUSION

An estimated 6 out of 10 people with dementia will wander and become lost. Enrolling in Safe Return® is an additional measure to help ensure the safety of vulnerable individuals. Comprehensive, updated information on Safe Return® is available at no cost at the Alzheimer's Association's Web site, www.alz.org, or by calling 1-800-272-3900.

Web-Based Resources

For information on Safe Return®: http://alz.org/Services/SafeReturn.asp
For local chapters of the Alzheimer's Association: http://alz.org/findchapter.asp

REFERENCES

Rowe, M. A., & Bennett, V. (2003). A look at deaths occurring in persons with dementia lost in the community. *American Journal of Alzheimer's Disease and Other Dementias, 18,* 343–348.

Rowe, M. A., Feinglass, N. G., & Wiss, M. E. (2004). Persons with dementia who become lost in the community: A case study, current research, and recommendations. *Mayo Clinic Proceedings, 79,* 1417–1422.

Rowe, M. A., & Glover, J. C. (2001). Antecedents, descriptions and consequences of wandering in cognitively-impaired adults and the Safe Return (SR) program. *American Journal of Alzheimer's Disease and Other Dementias, 16,* 344–352.

Sink, K. M., Covinsky, K. E., Newcomer, R., & Yaffe, K. (2004). Ethnic differences in the prevalence and pattern of dementia-related behaviors. *Journal of the American Geriatrics Society, 52,* 1277–1283.

CHAPTER FOURTEEN

A Home Safety Program for Community-Based Wanderers: Outcomes From the Veterans Home Safety Project

Kathy J. Horvath, Rose M. Harvey, and Scott A. Trudeau

Case Illustration

A call came into the 911 operator at 6:45 A.M. reporting that an elderly woman was found lying on the sidewalk. She was dazed and confused, but responsive. When the ambulance arrived, the woman reported that she was going shopping but was unable to recall any of the events leading up to her being found. The Emergency Medical Technician noted that she was wearing a Medic Alert bracelet, as well as a Safe Return® bracelet from the Alzheimer's Association. Both systems were activated revealing that she had a cardiac history as well as dementia, and family members were notified by the staff at the emergency room.

INTRODUCTION AND BACKGROUND

For persons with dementia living in the community, the risk for wandering and becoming lost, and the potential for tragic consequences, is high. Up to 60 percent of patients with dementia will wander outside the home alone (Alzheimer's Association, 2006). Of the people who become lost, those who are missing for more than 24 hours have a 46 percent mortality rate (Koester & Stooksbury, 1995). Considering that the majority of persons with dementia of the Alzheimer's type live in the community where more than two-thirds of their care is provided by family members, wandering or the potential for wandering presents a significant problem for family caregivers.

The scenario described at the beginning of this chapter is common for families managing the care of a loved one with dementia. Fortunately for this woman, the family had registered her in the Safe Return® program (Chapter 13), but their anxiety about how this could have happened and their guilt about not being able to prevent this near tragic event were significant. What are the factors that support or oppose the capacity of informal caregivers to minimize the chances of community dwelling elders with dementia becoming lost or injured? In this chapter we will report research findings that help to answer this question.

REVIEW OF LITERATURE

Since the early 1990s, researchers have reported the importance of home safety concerns to family caregivers of persons with dementia. These initial studies described the scope of the problem of wandering outside of the home, which was the most frequent behavior problem encountered by family caregivers (Calkins & Namazi, 1991; Lach, Reed, Smith, & Carr, 1995). Family caregivers used their own ingenuity to enhance safety by controlling access to the outdoors. Various types of locks were added to doors including double-keyed locks and locks that required two steps to disengage; or locks were positioned out of the line of sight at the top or bottom of a door (Olsen, Ehrenkrantz, & Hutchings, 1993). Other strategies included using gates to block entry to an area, covering the doorknobs so they could not be opened easily and disguising the front door. Participants reported that these spontaneous strategies were often successful, but the responses also indicated that many families were unaware of all the safety options that were available such as obtaining an identification bracelet (Lach et al., 1995).

Gitlin and colleagues developed a program of research on home modifications for persons with dementia, however the focus of their interventions is on promoting patient independence and well-being rather than safety per se (Gitlin & Corcoran, 1996; Gitlin, Corcoran, Winter, Boyce, & Marcus, 1999; Gitlin, Corcoran, Winter, Boyce, & Hauck, 2001; Gitlin, Winter, et al., 2002; Gitlin, Schinfeld, et al., 2002; Gitlin, Hauck, Dennis, & Winter, 2005). The intervention consisted of an in-home skills training program to modify the environment and teach caregivers how to make adaptations to decrease the functional difficulties that the patient encounters as the illness progresses. The strategies that were implemented consisted of actions that were agreed upon by the family and the professional providers, which led to highly acceptable strategies and an overall adherence of 75 percent. Underlying their approach to home safety modifications was a collaborative approach that strived to create a partnership with the patient and family (Gitlin & Corcoran, 2000).

Implementation of recommended environmental changes by family caregivers is difficult to predict. Messecar (2000) interviewed and observed family caregivers of elders with various ailments to learn what factors were related to the use of environmental modifications. Messecar concluded that attributes of the elderly individual, attributes of the home modification, quality of the caregiver–elderly relationship, the caregiver's skills, personal resources, and available informal and formal supports all affected the caregiver's use of environmental modifications. Among these factors, the attributes of home modifications appeared to have some consistency across families, in contrast to the highly variable personal factors. Modifications that were low cost, easy to locate, and easy to use and install were more likely to be implemented.

An extensive literature review found few Alzheimer's disease education materials for adults with low literacy (Rudd, Moeykens, & Colton, 1995; Rudd, Colton, & Schacht, 2000). Health literacy involves not only the ability to read health information, but to be able to understand and act upon it (U.S. Department of Health and Human Services, 2000). Nearly half of all American adults have difficulty understanding and using health information (Institute of Medicine of the National Academies, 2004). Most health education materials are written at or above a tenth grade level, making them of limited value for a large number of Americans, especially elderly and minorities (Doak, Doak, & Root, 1996). The exception is two recent publications by the Alzheimer's Disease Education and Referral (ADEAR) Center, which developed two easy-to-read publications that meet health literacy requirements (U.S. Department of Health and Human Services, 2006a, 2006b; see also "Resources" at end of chapter).

THE VETERANS HOME SAFETY PROJECT

The Veterans Home Safety Project was begun in 1997 at EN Rogers Memorial Veterans Hospital, Bedford, MA, and supported by a grant from the

Veterans Administration Health Services Research and Development Program. Both clinicians and researchers wished to build on the preliminary studies of home safety reported in the literature and develop evidence-based recommendations that would be effective for the majority of families and would serve as a starting point for home safety education. Families were overwhelmed by the suggestions they read in the general consumer literature, which often were vague in nature, such as "secure the exits." They needed more practical information such as what and where to purchase low-cost home safety devices. Both professional care providers and family caregivers needed a better understanding of how to manage the care recipient with dementia in a home environment for as long as possible without increased risk of accident, injury, morbidity, and mortality for either the caregiver or care recipient. We began a series of research studies with the overall goal to intervene before an injury by providing an environmentally safe home living situation for the care recipient and providing the caregiver with the know-how and self confidence to prevent risky behaviors that lead to injuries. The Veterans Home Safety Project utilized the Home Safety/Injury Model as the conceptual framework to address these issues.

Home Safety/Injury Model

The Home Safety/Injury Model (Figure 14.1) was developed to guide clinical practice and research to prevent accidents and injury to persons with dementia living at home in the community (Hurley et al., 2004). The model uses the concept of a safety platform to protect the person with dementia of the Alzheimer's type (DAT) from risky behaviors that lead to accidents and injury. The safety platform can be extended to protect persons with DAT from injury due to risky behaviors such as wandering within the home or exiting the home alone and becoming lost. The safety platform is extended by creating a protective physical environment and increasing caregiver competence.

The first study of the Veterans Home Safety Project utilized a qualitative design to explore the concept of caregiver competence. Caregiver competence was defined as the effective performance of caregiving actions that are associated with the care recipient's safety and the related knowledge and skills (Horvath et al., 2005). Key informants consisting of 17 professional interdisciplinary care providers of persons with dementia described clinical incidents with a range of caregiver competency represented. The following factors were found to influence family caregiver competence to prevent home injury: educational attainment of the caregiver, self-confidence to make modifications (i.e., perceived self-efficacy), family support and resilience to make role changes, alliance with professional care providers, and use of community resources.

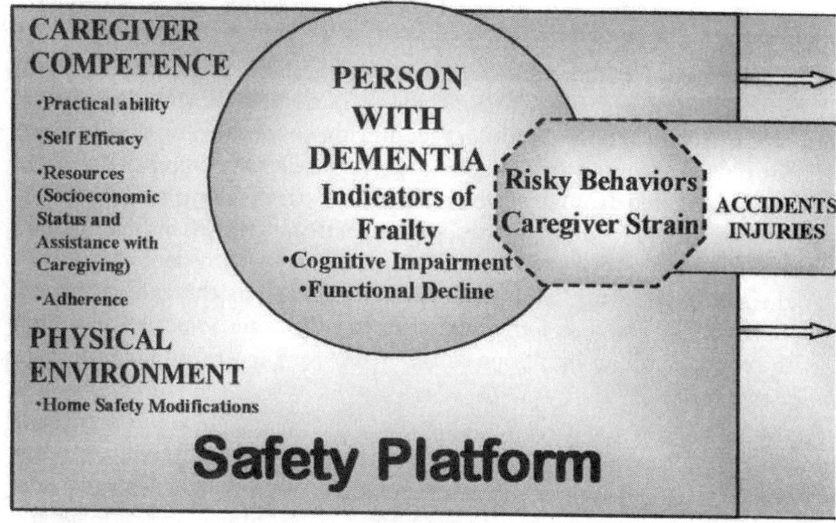

FIGURE 14.1 Home safety/injury model.

The Home Safety/Injury Model incorporates a collaborative decision-making process with the informal caregiver in order to increase the likelihood of adherence to home safety recommendations (Hurley et al., 2004). The decision-making process includes six steps: (1) assessment of the environment's protectiveness; (2) an initial plan for safety modifications initiated by the professional provider; (3) negotiation of recommendations for change with the family caregiver(s); (4) logistics and resources to evaluate practical considerations; (5) a proposed plan that includes negotiated changes and resources for an action plan; and (6) application or implementation of the plan by the caregiver.

Engaging the caregiver in a plan that they perceive to be beneficial is an important element of adherence and reflects a change in basic assumptions underlying patient/family implementation of treatment recommendations. Adherence, versus compliance, connotes a participative rather than a subservient role for the patient and family that is essential in an environment where treatment recommendations increasingly require elements of self-care responsibility (Bosworth, Weinberger, & Oddone, 2006). The collaborative decision-making process of the Home Safety/Injury Model became the central communication strategy with families in order to provide a safer physical environment and improve caregiver competence through increased knowledge and self-efficacy.

METHODS

The study reported here aimed to identify the high frequency and high severity environmental risks for accidents in homes, the home modifications to which families would agree, and those modifications that were effective in preventing risky behaviors. A consecutive, convenience sample was recruited from the Dementia Out-Patient Clinic at a Veterans Administration Hospital in the Boston metropolitan area. The sample consisted of primary family caregivers of a person with dementia of the Alzheimer's type who lived in the same residence as the care recipient. Data collection included two home visits to each family, six months apart, with monthly follow-up phone calls.

Assessment

A home safety assessment was conducted by a nurse researcher and occupational therapist at the first home visit in order to negotiate a plan for modifications needed in the home. Each room was assessed using a tool called The Home Safety Checklist, which was developed for this study and incorporated the most frequently, cited safety recommendations in the literature and the experience of expert clinicians (VA New England Geriatric Research Education and Clinical Center, 2004). The home visit was an opportunity to demonstrate the application of home safety recommendations in the caregiver's own home.

Initial Plan: Protective Physical Environment

The initial recommendations for making exits and entrances safer used suggestions found in the research and general consumer literature and included the following: Place an extra lock high or low on exit doors; Disguise the door with a print or picture; Register the person with dementia in the Safe Return® program; and Give a picture ID to the local police station (U.S. Department of Health and Human Services, 2005).

Negotiation

In many ways, the most challenging part of the home safety visit was the negotiation process with the family caregiver to implement the safety recommendations. Throughout the home safety assessment, we tried to maintain the integrity of the care recipient, the caregiver and the home environment. We identified specific problems in the negotiation process and developed some approaches that were helpful for solving them.

Problem: Lack of Understanding of AD and Its Progression

Some caregivers were reticent to accept the need to implement change without first-hand experience of wandering or other risky behaviors. They took a "it will never happen" perspective with regard to the potential of the care recipient to become lost. Putting locks on doors or removing stove knob covers was perceived to be demeaning to an adult and revealed a tension between concerns for personal dignity and autonomy and the need to restrict access to risky areas.

Approach. A useful approach to this problem was to frame the importance of safety measures from a preventative standpoint. An "it only takes once" approach is useful. It also helped to share real life examples of caregivers who were surprised by risky behaviors (without revealing personally identifiable information). In this sample of primarily older men who were socialized into traditional male roles of breadwinner rather than homemaker, both researchers and caregivers were surprised by care recipients who took a sudden interest in the stove. It is important to express understanding of the caregiver's reluctance and how some of the safety measures could be perceived to be demeaning to an adult who did not have Alzheimer's disease and the brain changes that interfered with a person's previously good judgment. Without infantilizing the care recipient, we reminded the caregiver that they needed to take preventative approaches similar to what was done for small children who could not distinguish between safe and risky behaviors. Assuming this protective role for the care recipient was often a significant role change for the caregiver, whether they were a spouse or an adult child.

Problem: Lack of Understanding of the Safety Recommendations

Caregivers may agree to make changes and assure you that "yes" they understand the recommendations. They may state their willingness to make any and all modifications but not really understand the rationale or purpose.

Approach. It became important for the researchers to remain aware that many caregivers would perceive a hierarchical relationship rather than a collaborative one. Caregivers would often manifest this perception with apologies, "Oh, you're right, I'm sorry, I should have taken care of that." We would first need to assure the caregiver that we were not the "safety police" and that it was not our purpose to criticize or punish but rather to support and assist. We began by capitalizing on the apparent interest and enthusiasm of the caregiver. In order to avoid overwhelming the caregiver, we focused on preventing unsupervised exits as one of the most critical issues. We asked the caregiver to summarize their plan and the reasons for making changes. In order to avoid a paternalistic role, we would instead encourage the caregiver to prioritize the recommendations in order to avoid becoming overwhelmed. Indeed, some homes had such extensive home safety issues that the researchers had to be even more selective than usual during the safety assessment to help the caregiver prioritize the implementations. Caregivers of the veterans in our study were very appreciative of the telephone follow-up calls to reinforce key issues and provide support for the progress made.

Problem: Reluctance to Make Changes

Some caregivers stated that they did not see the need to make changes. Often, they anticipated the concerns that were raised and were ready with reasons why they did not have to be addressed. Occasionally, the caregiver assumed a somewhat confrontational or defensive posture during the home safety assessment. These caregivers might list things they are unwilling to change before entering an area of the home. This was especially poignant in one caregiver who tearfully explained, "I have waited all my life to have my beautiful bathroom. We just finished it before he was diagnosed—it may not be perfect, but I am not changing anything in here."

Approach. A change that seems logical to the professional caregiver may evoke feelings of loss in the family caregiver and care recipient. It is important for the professional to be aware of all the emotions related to the disease of a loved one. Changes in the arrangement of rooms or routines should be minimal unless there is a real potential for wandering or other injury. Caregivers frequently told us that they wanted to preserve a sense of "normality" for as long as possible and maintain the appearance of the home as they remembered it. We tried to align ourselves with the part of the caregiver that recognized the hazards. As suggested by Gitlin and Corcoran (2000), we guided the caregiver to implement changes incrementally, beginning with the high frequency/high severity risks for injury. The caregiver was reminded that many of the safety modifications were appropriate for themselves, not just the care recipient with dementia, and that the caregiver's safety was essential to the continued well-being of their loved one.

Logistics and Resources

Family caregivers selected from a "toolkit" the safety items that they were willing to use to make the exits safer such as slide bolt locks, padlocks, and deadbolt locks. A database of items and their cost and distribution was maintained to monitor the total expense of home safety devices and provide a reference list should an item be recalled and the family needed to be notified. The primary family caregiver was encouraged to enlist the assistance of other family members to implement the home safety recommendations, or to use a local business that specialized in small household tasks, such as installing grab bars.

Proposed Plan

Following the initial home visit, we sent the caregiver a written summary of the agreed upon plan along with illustrations provided by digital photos of the areas for change. The nurse researcher telephoned the caregiver monthly to answer further questions or concerns about home safety to reinforce the teaching. A follow-up home visit was conducted in 6 months to evaluate the application or implementation of the negotiated plan.

RESULTS

Sixty-two caregiver/care recipient dyads were enrolled in the study. Ten families did not complete the study at 6 months because of caregiver illness, institutionalization, or death of the care recipient. One family was lost to follow-up. Of the 52 caregiver/care recipient dyads that completed the study, all were Caucasian except for one family, reflecting the population of veterans in this suburban community. The caregivers in the sample were primarily female spouses of the care recipients (83%) and adult children (12%) with an average age of 69. Care recipients were male veterans with an average age of 77 and cognitive impairment as measured by the Mini Mental State Exam (X = 16; S.D. = 7.7; Folstein, 1975). Participants lived in the following types of residences: 67 percent in a single family home; 19 percent in a multiple family home; 12 percent in a condominium; and 2 percent (one family) lived in an apartment house.

Providing a Protective Physical Environment

Leaving the home unsupervised was one of the two most frequent risks for injury in the home of a person with dementia of the Alzheimer's type (Table 14.1). The first 17 home visits provided initial evidence of what the family caregivers would find acceptable to secure exits and entrances and decrease the likelihood of the person with dementia getting lost or wandering into a room with risky items. The remaining 35 home visits confirmed that the interventions were acceptable and effective for all care recipients in the sample.

Despite the frequent recommendation in the literature to consider using double-keyed locks, we learned during the conduct of the study that such locks do not conform to the Massachusetts state fire safety code. There is a prohibition against any lock that requires a key or tool to unlock. Using the database of distributed items, we contacted the families that had chosen a double-keyed lock and recommended that a slide bolt lock be used instead. One caregiver decided to continue with the double-keyed lock because of the repeated and persistent attempts by the care recipient to leave the home.

Slide bolt locks that were placed on the door above or below the line of vision, that is high for shorter patients or low for taller patients, became the standard. More importantly, we learned that locks, regardless of type or number, were not sufficient to make exits safer without a motion sensor. Even very advanced patients who were passive and withdrawn had moments of lucidity when they attempted to leave the home. Family caregivers are often spouses who have hearing impairment, and without a warning that the patient was at an exit door, an elopement could happen before the caregiver realized where the patient was.

The standard recommendation for safer exits and entrances became an extra slide bolt lock *with* a motion sensor placed at the door. The motion sensor that was preferred by families was one that was developed originally for travelers and thus was relatively small and could be hidden behind a plant or lamp. The motion sensor had both a chime and a continuous alarm. The chime sound was surprisingly loud and caregivers appreciated the volume, with a pleasing, familiar sound that did not scare the patient. Hearing-impaired caregivers used the alarm option at

TABLE 14.1 Summary of Risky Behaviors in Veterans Home Safety Study

Behavior	# incidents reported
Falls/Tripping	>10
Exiting Alone	10
Stove incidents	6
Firearm incidents	1
Knife incidents	2
Driving incidents	1
Toxic substances	2
Fires (1 smoker; 1 clothes dryer)	2

night when they feared they would not hear the patient leave the sleeping area for an exit door. Surprisingly, this sample of family caregivers did not choose to use a mural or poster to disguise exit doors. However, in contrast to locks and motion sensors, we did not have a door disguise to give to families immediately and would have had to order one. Because the locks and motion sensors were readily available and effective, the caregivers did not try using the door disguise, which might have worked just as well.

Even a safer exit area cannot be absolutely elopement safe, and thus we included recommendations to obtain an identification bracelet and register the patient in the Safe Return® Program. Caregivers often needed advice about how to convince the care recipient to wear the Safe Return® identification bracelet. Five strategies proved effective: (1) tell the care recipient that "all veterans are wearing these now"; (2) obtain a second identification bracelet for the caregiver that notifies others that there is a dependent person at risk if something happens to the caregiver; (3) tell the care recipient that the doctor ordered it for him, or tell the caregiver to bring the bracelet to the clinic and have the physician place the bracelet on the patient; (4) obtain a necklace instead of a bracelet, which for this population of veterans, was perceived as new "dog tags"; or (5) have a beloved child or grandchild give the bracelet as a special gift. Caregivers were also advised and agreed to provide a recent photo to local police. However, most of the care recipients in the sample who exited the home unsupervised were returned by a neighbor; thus family caregivers were encouraged to inform neighbors that their loved one had "memory loss" and to call the caregiver if they saw the person with dementia in the community alone. Making this recommendation, however, required the family caregiver to have an understanding of the illness and enough comfort with the diagnosis to discuss it with others in the community.

Wandering Within the Home

Even with close supervision, a caregiver can be distracted at times, or will need to attend to personal needs and will not be in the same room as the person with dementia. Caregivers also were concerned that the care recipient would wander into the kitchen at night instead of returning to the bedroom after using the toilet. Many families used the motion sensor in a hallway that would warn them if the care recipient was headed in the direction of the kitchen instead of the bedroom or bathroom during the night. The caregivers preferred not to lock the bedroom door or use a door alarm, because their own sleep would be interrupted frequently, thus they placed the motion sensor in a hallway or on a wall outside the bedroom. In a spontaneous effort to promote safety, many caregivers would leave lights or nightlights on around the home, in case the care recipient wandered about. We advised these caregivers to limit nightlights to the route of the bathroom. Placing one nightlight in the bathroom to focus the care recipient's attention from the bedroom and one in the bedroom to light the way back—leaving other areas of the home dark. Darkness sensor lights that turn on automatically were most effective for this.

The primary concern of caregivers for nighttime safety and safe wandering in the home was making the kitchen safer. Indeed, as shown in Table 14.1, the kitchen stove and knives were both a frequent and serious source of risky behaviors. The standard recommendations for making the kitchen safer that were effective in preventing accidents were: Remove stove knob covers and put one in a nearby drawer for the caregiver to use as needed, or alternatively, use "child proof" covers for stove knobs; limit the number of knives to one or two; hide knives in the back of a drawer where they would be concealed from sight by other items such as foil and plastic wrap; and hide medication in a cabinet that is accessible to the caregiver but not used by the care recipient. The principle, "Out of sight, Out of mind" worked surprisingly well and provided a safer environment for the care recipient without burdening the caregiver with additional locks or devices. The findings were incorporated into a clinical teaching tool called *Worksheet for Making the Home Safer for a Person With Memory Loss* (VA New England Geriatric Research Education and Clinical Center, 2002). The *Worksheet* addresses the basic safety measures for all families with a care recipient with dementia of the Alzheimer's type.

Cost of Home Safety Items

The most popular safety items and their typical costs are listed in Table 14.2. Items such as locks and motion sensors, used to prevent the care recipient from leaving the home alone, were the first concerns of the caregivers. The total cost of home safety items for this sample of 52 care recipient/caregiver dyads was $4,576. The average cost per family was $88 with a range of $10 to $249.

Increasing Caregiver Competence

All families except two stated that the home safety assessment and information was very helpful because they now knew what risks to be concerned about. Previously, they did not know where to begin or how to make home safety modifications. The two families who were upset initially by the home visit found it anxiety-provoking, because they had not considered the many safety hazards in their home. The recommendation to

TABLE 14.2 Popular Safety Items and Average Prices

Item	Average Price
Motion Sensor	$24.99
Slide Bolt Lock	$6.99
Smoke Alarm	$16.99
Grab bars	$24.00
Colored Duct Tape (4 rolls)	$3.99
Stove knob covers	$7.99
Tub Chair	$57.45
Portable Bathtub Rail	$49.99
Nightlights	$3.99

hide knives and other sharp objects was particularly disturbing, because these two caregivers could not conceive of their care recipient as being a danger to anyone.

The primary caregivers in this sample relied mostly on the monthly follow-up phone calls by the nurse researcher to review the recommendations and discuss any problems they were having with implementation. The written materials were used more often to share information with other members in the family, usually adult children, and enlist their assistance with implementation. All caregivers found the home safety toolkit very helpful, because going to a store and not knowing what to buy, where an item could be found, or whether it would be effective was so time-consuming.

Factors That Enhanced or Inhibited Implementation

At the second home visit, 42 family caregivers in the sample agreed to an interview by the nurse researcher to learn what factors enhanced or inhibited implementation of the safety recommendations (Harvey, Horvath, Foley, Hurley, & Trudeau, 2005). We concluded that modifications were most likely to be implemented when:

1. The caregiver perceived positive outcomes for the function and safety of the veteran.
2. The modification was easy and did not disrupt routines.
3. The modification led to benefits for the caregiver such as making care giving easier, safer, or less worrisome.

Conditions that decreased the likelihood of implementation were:

1. The task was difficult and the caregiver lacked the resources (e.g., time, money or carpenter) to implement it, such as grab bars or an extra railing.
2. The caregiver perceived the modification to be unnecessary at this time based on the veteran's condition.
3. The veteran (care recipient) objected to the modification.

Cultural and Literacy Appropriate Booklet

We developed an illustrated, learner-verified home safety booklet that presents the standard, basic home safety recommendations in a format that meets health literacy guidelines (Figure 14.2). Guidelines for health education materials include specific techniques, such as showing the reader what action should be taken, presenting information in bite-size steps, and using a clear background with simple line drawings (Doak et al., 1996). The new booklet *Keeping the Person With Memory Loss Safe at Home* was developed with a home safety "toolkit" that enhances

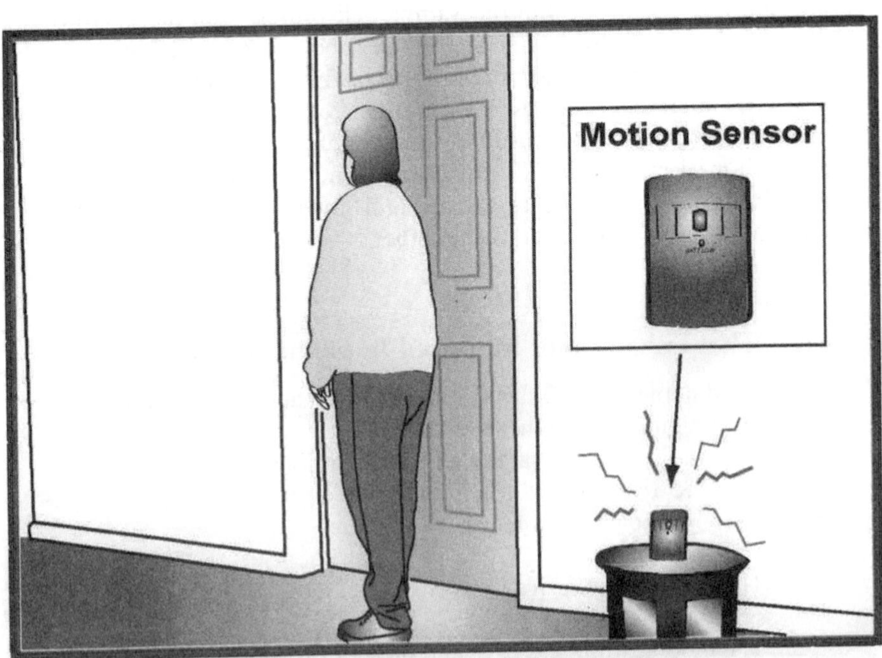

FIGURE 14.2 Exit safety.

caregiver competence through practical knowledge and skills about simple, affordable devices to enhance home safety.

IMPLICATIONS FOR PRACTICE

Environmental modifications to prevent wandering and the potential for accidents and injuries and increased caregiver competence are essential components of an effective plan for home safety. Yet, few clinical providers have the opportunity to make a home visit and environmental assessment for the person with dementia of the Alzheimer's type. However, the *Worksheet for Making the Home Safer for a Person With Memory Loss* addresses the basic safety measures for all families caring for a person with dementia and can be used as a starting point for discussing home safety. The *Worksheet* includes a practical list of home safety items with average prices that can be purchased in a hardware store and medical distributors who will deliver specialty items, such as a bath bench, to a residential address. The *Worksheet* is a text-based document that is most effective when given to families within the context of a clinical encounter where the professional provider can discuss issues for a particular patient and home circumstances. The new cultural and literacy appropriate booklet, *Keeping the Person With Memory Loss Safe at Home,* has illustrations and simplified directions that can be used for the general public, when it is ready for distribution.

The influence of the home setting on the implementation of safety interventions cannot be overstated. When structural changes to a home are recommended, other issues such as privacy, dignity, and autonomy become salient in addition to the issue of safety. Clinicians must respect the fact that they are practicing in someone else's domain. A change that may make perfect sense to the clinician may be thwarted by the caregiver if it challenges their sense of personal space or their understanding of the care recipient's preferences. The home setting also has to incorporate the competing demands on family caregivers who may have other dependents and who have to live themselves in this new dementia-safe environment. Providers need to negotiate a plan for home safety modifications with the family caregiver in order to anticipate potential barriers to implementation.

IMPLICATIONS FOR RESEARCH

The primary outcome of this study was an empirically derived home safety intervention that includes a cultural and literacy appropriate booklet and a home safety toolkit, which warrants further testing. A comparison group with random assignment to different treatment conditions is needed to know what factors were most influential in caregivers' adherence to home safety modifications. There could have been a treatment effect because the families knew that they were in a research study and wanted the results to be successful. It is possible that adherence would have been successful for any family that had the benefit of two home visits and monthly follow-up calls with unlimited time to discuss their concerns about home safety. A double-blind clinical trial is not possible in a study of home safety, because the treatment conditions cannot be hidden from the investigators like a placebo-controlled drug trial. Nevertheless, there are techniques that can provide some protection against threats to validity in a single-blinded study, including generation of a random allocation sequence, concealment of the treatment allocation prior to enrollment, explanation of any exclusion of subjects after randomization, and blinding of group identity (Chow & Liu, 2004; Schulz, Chalmers, Hayes, & Altman, 1995).

Home telehealth is a growing part of clinical care and can be incorporated into a home safety strategy. Technologies to monitor medication adherence can be adapted to enable the professional provider to follow-up with caregivers regarding implementation of safety modifications. The reminders might not have the same impact as the negotiation of a plan within the context of a home visit, but testing this possibility would provide further evidence of the most effective clinical processes that are necessary to achieve desirable outcomes.

CONCLUSION

A descriptive, exploratory study enabled the authors to develop an empirically derived list of essential home safety modifications that caregivers found acceptable and practical. This baseline of home safety recommendations provides a starting point for families to focus on the most important changes to address the high frequency and high severity risks for accidents and injuries in homes. A list of recommendations, however, is limited if the caregiver has an inadequate understanding of the nature of dementia of the Alzheimer's type and the cognitive changes in the care recipient that require balancing values for individual autonomy with safety needs, and may necessitate role changes within the family structure. The experience of this study underscores the importance of professional caregivers to actively engage family caregivers in the negotiation of interventions to optimize in-home care of persons with Alzheimer's disease.

RESOURCES

Administration on Aging, Alzheimer's Resource Room. http://www.aoa.gov/alz, or 1-202-619-0724.

Alzheimer's Disease Education and Referral (ADEAR) Center. Understanding Memory Loss; Understanding Alzheimer's Disease; Home Safety for People with Alzheimer's Disease. http://www.alzheimers.nia.nih.gov, or 1-800-438-4380.

Family Caregiver Alliance. http://www.caregiver.org, or 1-800-445-8106.

National Eldercare Locator (Eldercare services). 1-800-677-1116.

Worksheet for Making the Home Safer for a Person With Memory Loss. http://www.bu.edu/alzresearch/documents/HomeSafetyWorksheet.pdf

REFERENCES

Alzheimer's Association (2006). *Wandering*. Retrieved September 5, 2006, from http://www.alz.org/Care/SafetyIssues/wandering.asp

Alzheimer's Disease Education and Referral (ADEAR) Center (2002). Understanding Memory Loss; Understanding Alzheimer's Disease; Home Safety for People with Alzheimer's Disease. Retrieved from http://www.alzheimers.nia.nih.gov.

Bosworth, H. B., Weinberger, M., & Oddone, E. Z. (2006). Introduction. In H. B. Bosworth, E. Z. Oddone, & M. Weinberger (Eds.), *Patient treatment adherence: Concepts, interventions, and measurement* (pp. 3–11). Mahwah, NJ: Lawrence Erlbaum Associates.

Calkins, M. P., & Namazi, K. H. (1991). Caregivers perceptions of the effectiveness of home modifications for community living adults with dementia. *Journal of Alzheimer's Care & Related Disorder Research, 6,* 25–29.

Chow, S. C., & Liu, J. P. (2004). *Design and analysis of clinical trials: Concepts and methodologies* (Second ed.) Hoboken, NJ: John Wiley & Sons, Inc.

Doak, C. C., Doak, L. G., & Root, J. H. (1996). *Teaching patients with low literacy skills.* Philadelphia: J. B. Lippincott Company.

Folstein, M. F. (1975). Mini-mental state. A practical method of grading the cognitive state of patients for the clinician. *Journal of Psychiatric Research, 12,* 189–198.

Gitlin, L. N., & Corcoran, M. A. (1996). Managing dementia at home: The role of home environmental modifications. *Topics in Geriatric Rehabilitation,* 28–39.

Gitlin, L. N., & Corcoran, M. (2000). Making homes safer: Environmental adaptations for people with dementia. *Alzheimer's Care Quarterly, 1,* 50–58.

Gitlin, L. N., Corcoran, M. A., Winter, L., Boyce, A., & Hauck, W. W. (2001). A randomized, controlled trial of a home environmental intervention: Effect on efficacy and upset in caregivers and on daily function of persons with dementia. *The Gerontologist, 41,* 4–14.

Gitlin, L. N., Corcoran, M., Winter, L., Boyce, A., & Marcus, S. (1999). Predicting participation and adherence to a home environmental intervention among family caregivers of persons with dementia. *Family Relations, 48,* 363–372.

Gitlin, L. N., Hauck, W. W., Dennis, M. P., & Winter, L. (2005). Maintenance of effects of the Home Environmental Skill-Building Program for family caregivers and individuals with Alzheimer's disease and related disorders. *The Journals of Gerontology. Series A., Biological Sciences and Medical Sciences, 60*(3), 368–374.

Gitlin, L. N., Schinfeld, S., Winter, L., Corcoran, M., Boyce, A., & Hauck, W. W. (2002). Evaluating home environments of persons with dementia: Interrater reliability and validity of the Home Environmental Assessment Protocol (HEAP). *Disability and Rehabilitation, 24*(1–3), 59–71.

Gitlin, L. N., Winter, L., Dennis, M. P., Corcoran, M., Schinfeld, S., & Hauck, W. W. (2002). Strategies used by families to simplify tasks for individuals with Alzheimer's disease and related disorders: Psychometric analysis of the Task Management Strategy Index (TMSI). *The Gerontologist, 42*(1), 61–69.

Harvey, R., Horvath, K., Foley, M., Hurley, A., & Trudeau, S. (2005). Implementation of home safety recommendations by dementia caregivers: The veterans home safety study (abstract). *The Gerontologist, 45*(Special Issue II), 348.

Horvath, K., Hurley, A., Duffy, M., Gauthier, M. A., Harvey, R. M., Trudeau, S. A., et al. (2005). Caregiver competency to prevent home injury to the care recipient with dementia. *Rehabilitation Nursing, 30,* 189–196.

Hurley, A., Gauthier, M. A., Horvath, K., Harvey, R., Smith, S., Trudeau, S., et al. (2004). A model to promote safer home environments for persons with Alzheimer's disease. *Journal of Gerontological Nursing, 30,* 43–51.

Institute of Medicine of the National Academies (2004). *Health literacy: A prescription to end confusion.* Washington, D.C.: The National Academies Press.

Koester, R. J., & Stooksbury, D. E. (1995). Behavioral profile of possible Alzheimer's disease patients in Virginia search and rescue incidents. *Wilderness and Environmental Medicine, 6,* 34–43.

Lach, H., Reed, T., Smith, L. J., & Carr, D. B. (1995). Alzheimer's disease: Assessing safety problems in the home. *Geriatric Nursing, 16,* 160–164.

Messecar, D. C. (2000). Factors affecting caregivers ability to make environmental modifications. *Journal of Gerontological Nursing, 26,* 32–42.

Olsen, R. V., Ehrenkrantz, E., & Hutchings, B. (1993). Creating supportive environments for people with dementia and their caregivers through home modifications. *Technology and Disability, 2,* 47–57.

Rudd, R. E., Colton, T. C., & Schacht, R. (2000). *An overview of medical and public health literature addressing literacy issues: An annotated bibliography* (NCSALL Report #14, pp. 1–61). Cambridge: Center for the Study of Adult Learning and Literacy.

Rudd, R. E., Moeykens, B. A., & Colton, T. C. (1995). Health and literacy a review of medical and public health literature. In J. Comings, B. Garners, & C. Smith, (Eds.), *Annual review of adult learning and literacy.* New York: Jossey-Bass.

Schulz, K. F., Chalmers, I., Hayes, R. J., & Altman, D. G. (1995). Empirical evidence of bias: Dimensions of methodological quality associated with estimates of treatment effects in controlled trials. *Journal of the American Medical Association, 273,* 408–412.

U.S. Department of Health and Human Services. (2000). *Healthy people 2010: Understanding and improving health.* Washington, D.C.: Author.

U.S. Department of Health and Human Services. (2005). *Home safety for people with Alzheimer's disease* (MH Publication No. 02-5179). Washington, D.C.: Author.

U.S. Department of Health and Human Services. (2006a). *Understanding memory loss* (NIH Publication No. 06–5442). Washington, D.C.: Author. Also available at http://www.alzheimers.nia.nih.gov.

U.S. Department of Health and Human Services. (2006b). *Understanding Alzheimer's disease* (NIH Publication No. 06–5441). Also available at http://www.alzheimers.nia.nih.gov.

VA New England Geriatric Research Education and Clinical Center. (2002). *Worksheet for making the home safer for a person with memory loss.* Retrieved September 5, 2006, from http://www.bu.edu/alzresearch.

VA New England Geriatric Research Education and Clinical Center. (2004). *Home Safety Checklist.* Requests to kathy.horvath@med.va.gov.

Warner, M. L. (1998). *The complete guide to Alzheimer's-proofing your home.* West Lafayette, IN: Purdue University Press.

CHAPTER FIFTEEN

Technologies to Manage Wandering

William D. Kearns and James L. Fozard

INTRODUCTION

Wandering within and around the home, becoming lost within the home, and elopement from the home are one class of problem behaviors exhibited by persons with dementia. Others include repetitive questioning, inappropriate vocalization, rejection of sustenance, and inappropriate toileting and sexual behavior (Mace & Rabins, 1999). Caregivers have the difficult task of discerning which problem behaviors of the person with dementia are amenable to behavior and environmental modification and which are not.

The present chapter reviews technologies, existing and potential, used to assist caregivers to manage wandering behavior. The technologies are categorized according to how they implement three behavioral approaches used to manage the actions of persons with dementia. The chapter is organized into the following sections: the prevalence of wandering; a description of the three approaches to managing problem behaviors of persons with dementia; existing and emergent technologies to manage wandering; and conclusions and ethical considerations.

When evaluated in formal institutional care settings (Day, Carreon, & Stump, 2000), commercial wanderer management technologies have been shown to enable residents to access safe areas of their environment while preventing or discouraging them from wandering into unsafe areas or leaving the facility (Polisher Research Institute, 2005). No published evaluations of the effectiveness of these technologies have been found for home use. Managing wandering at home will become an increasingly salient problem for caregivers and policy makers as the maturing baby boom generation strains state and federal Medicaid nursing home budgets. Persons with dementia may suffer for many years (Holtzer et al., 2003; Hope et al., 2001) and enter a nursing home (NH) early because they wander. Once transferred to formal care, the average NH cost exceeds $49,000 annually (Holahan, Wiener, & Lutzky, 2002). Delaying NH entry may produce significant cost savings; wanderer management technologies for the home will play an important role in the management of dementia for caregivers seeking to control costs.

Nonpharmacological interventions for wandering behaviors that have been empirically evaluated in institutional settings include subjective barriers, enhanced environments, behavioral interventions, music, and security devices such as alarms and more recently anti-elopement technologies. Technologies that are designed to alert caregivers to the occurrence of elopement can vary in complexity from a stand-alone device with a local alarm monitoring one door, to networked systems that monitor many doors and areas. Some systems provide complete monitoring of the facility environment, residents, and caregivers by working in conjunction with other systems and hardware. Some of these technologies, especially local alarm monitoring of exit doors, concealed door openers, and camouflaged doors and exits, are recommended for home settings, but no systematic studies of the frequency of adoption of these interventions or their effectiveness has been published. In the following discussion we briefly review the recommendations for using no-tech or low-tech interventions to manage wandering in the home and subsequently review the literature evaluating applications of technology to manage wandering in institutions that provide care for patients with dementia and discuss the implications for home care.

THREE APPROACHES TO MANAGING WANDERING

The management of problem behaviors in persons with dementia is a key theme in *The 36 Hour Day* (Mace & Rabins, 1999), a text for caregivers that describes three principal approaches to managing problem behaviors. The first approach emphasizes the importance of *reassurance and reducing stimulus overload;* agitation and confusion related to one's decreased cognitive processing capability can be particularly upsetting for the person with dementia who might be exposed to a noisy environment filled with unfamiliar persons, or those whom the person no longer recognizes. This agitation may be made worse by changes in familiar routines, disrupted sleep patterns, or changes in medication. Under these circumstances removing the person with dementia to a quiet location and providing calm reassurance is the most appropriate action.

The second and third approaches rely largely on the caregiver's ability to envision behaviors they consider optimal and desirable for the person with dementia to exhibit. We often know which undesirable behaviors we wish would disappear, but we may be less willing to prescribe behaviors we deem desirable for the person with dementia, perhaps out of concern for violating social taboos or a misplaced belief that the person with dementia "knows the right behavior to engage in and would do so if they really wanted to" but doesn't.

The second approach relies on *diverting the attention* of the person with dementia to activities that are incompatible with disruptive behaviors. One technologically mediated approach to this problem has been tried by Japanese researchers (Tamura et al., 2001) who found that the introduction of lifelike, inexpensive plastic baby dolls to persons with dementia showing agitation and wandering had the effect of increasing the rate of an incompatible behavior (nurturing) in their subjects. Recipients of the dolls held them closely during the study period, and the researchers observed declines in wandering and other problem behaviors while the recipients "nurtured" the dolls. Removing the dolls resulted in an increase in disruptive behaviors. A similar diverting tactic could use structured activities, such as well-learned games that don't require short-term memory in order to play, listening to music or watching television, taking a walk, or light exercise.

The third approach discussed in *The 36 Hour Day* consists of providing *referential cue stimuli in the person with dementia's environment* to ensure that appropriate behaviors are performed at the correct time and place. The cues may be temporal (clocks, calendars, etc.) or spatial (e.g., attaching the person's photograph to their bedroom door, putting signs pointing to the bathroom) to help ensure that the person is anchored with respect to time and place. Persons with dementia live their lives very much in the present, and events of only a few moments ago are not stored, while well-learned behavior patterns established over a lifetime remain retrievable and deteriorate more slowly. The cuing approach grew out of earlier efforts by Dr. James Folson and others to link cues with programs that help persons with dementia relearn their orientation to time and place. Dubbed "reality orientation," the in-class instruction was intended to facilitate the hoped-for relearning.

Reassurance, diversion, and cued behavior show promise for being integrated into machine mediated behavioral interventions in the elderly; a hallmark of the nascent field of gerontechnology (Fozard & Kearns, 2007). Before beginning the discussion on the integration of these approaches into gerontechnology, a caveat is essential concerning using aversive control to manage problem behaviors in persons with dementia. Coercion, berating, and abuse should never be used in the management of problem behaviors in persons with dementia, either by a human or a piece of technology. Persons with dementia cannot learn that undesirable behavior will be consequated by punishment irrespective of the number of pairings and will not remember such learning experiences even if they occurred only a few minutes before. Neither will they register a steadily escalating frustration and rising tone of voice of the caregiver as they repetitively provide the same piece of information to the person with dementia (Follette & Linnerooth, 2001).

BASIS FOR EXISTING RECOMMENDATIONS FOR MANAGING WANDERING IN THE HOME

The literature on which the existing recommendations are based comes from the revised edition of *The 36 Hour Day* (Mace & Rabins, 1999) and from the Web site of the Alzheimer's Association (2006a) and its many associated Internet links. The recommendations from the various sources overlap considerably but vary widely in the degree to which interventions are linked to the multiple causes of wandering. Two recommendations are present in all or almost all of the sources. One is to provide a means for the person at risk for wandering to be identified; an identification bracelet, identification card, or identification labels sown into the person's clothing are essential to allow the wandering person to be identified. The Safe Return® program established by the Alzheimer's Association (2006b) has done an exemplary job of accomplishing this goal in the United States. The bracelet or other means of identification should be accompanied by current photographs to help authorities or other persons identify the wandering person.

The second caveat is to avoid interventions that result in what Mace and Rabins call catastrophic events—unwanted outbursts of anger, heightened agitation, or other extreme reactions to the intervention by the person with dementia. Such reactions can occur in response to caregiver instructions to cease wandering, or encountering door locks and door openers, or discovering missing appliance controls. Collectively, the recommendations often appear self-contradictory and attest to the wide range of individual differences in patient responses to interventions. Mace and Rabins (1999) note that many of the interventions and recommendations derive from the ingenuity of particular caregivers and may not work for everyone.

TECHNOLOGIES FOR MANAGING WANDERING

In the Home

The interventions are roughly divided into two overlapping groups, those for managing wandering within the home and those addressing exiting the home. A secondary classification distinguishes purposeful and aimless wandering in both groups. It is widely believed that persons with dementia who initially wander within the home will eventually progress to exiting the home. Recommendations for managing wandering within the home include providing diversionary activities such as helping a caregiver with tasks; providing entertainment such as music, TV, or dancing; and creating a safe place for wandering within the home or yard. Familiar places in the home should be made more distinctive by including signs on the bathroom door indicating its function and one or more pictures of the person with family members on their bedroom door to remind them of the location of their sleeping quarters. Disabling stove controls and other potentially dangerous appliances is recommended if wandering into unsafe areas such as the kitchen occurs. Nightlights for safety and devices to awaken and alert a sleeping caregiver are frequently mentioned. One caregiver reported tying her and her husband's ankles together with a string that would waken her when he left the bed.

Preventing or Managing Exiting and Elopement

Interventions to prevent exiting the home are based on the principles of the diversionary principle of camouflage or concealment of exits, disabling exits, or by alarms signaling the caregiver of a successful exit. These recommendations are mostly borrowed from interventions used in institutional settings or control of prisoners under house arrest or on probation. Examples of camouflage include concealing doors with curtains or other materials, Velcro across the doorknob, painting the door the same color as the adjacent wall, and so forth. Camouflage and concealment achieve their effect by removing visible stimuli from the environment that have long-term associations with exiting the building.

Recommended interventions involving disablement of exits include placing locks at the bottom or top of the door rather than the usual location in the middle or the door, deadbolt locks requiring a key to operate, childproof locks or locked doors that require keypads to open, gates across exits, and locks on windows. The use of locks to disable doors relies upon the principle of cued behavior sequences; however the individual must first test the door to determine that it is locked, a process that will doubtless be repeated frequently. (A better strategy might involve placing a "Do not enter" or "Door is locked" sign in front of the locked door in order to minimize door testing behavior.)

Alarms for exit doors can be activated by door openings, pressure activated sensors beneath the approach to a door, or manipulation of door opening devices. Alarms are usually for the benefit of the caregiver to alert them to a potential elopement; loud alarms run counter to the principle of reassurance and calming and may precipitate catastrophic emotional events for the person with dementia. As of March 2007, dual function devices that signal the exit of the wandering person and monitor their location have not been discussed in the literature.

In Institutions

Elopement Management Systems

Warner (1999a, 1999b) has defined elopement management systems (EMS) as those that alert caregivers when wanderers leave monitored areas, may automatically lock doors, or incorporate radio frequency technologies to sound alarms. EMSs vary from stand-alone devices with local alarm coverage to sophisticated networked systems providing complete facility coverage.

Seven EMS subtypes were identified by Warner: *Pressure activated systems* respond to an external load applied to or removed from a pressure pad. These are usually floor mats laid next to the wanderer's bed, or before a doorway, and stepping on the mat triggers an alarm. External pressure removed from a pillow, bed pad, or chair cushion may also trigger an alarm indicating the wanderer has moved. They operate at point of placement and may miss movement events if inadvertently relocated.

Pull tab alarms connect a detachable tab to the wanderer's clothing and fix the monitor to a bed or chair. Movement pulls the tab from the monitor and sounds an alarm, which the person with dementia may find emotionally upsetting. Some play personally recorded messages instead of alarms to prompt the wanderer to sit down or return to bed, which may be reassuring to the person with dementia. The weakness of the technology is the connection to the person's clothing which may detach leading to missed detections.

Audible alarms sound when a door is opened or a wanderer traverses a doorway; some alert by triggering household lamps. Most cannot distinguish who passes through the doorway and give frequent false alarms. Advanced systems detect wristbands worn by the wanderer and alert caregivers only when the wanderer traverses the monitored doorway. *Optically activated alarms* alert when a wanderer approaches or traverses a monitored zone. Passive infrared technology (PIR) motion detectors detect a wanderer up to 50 feet away and may trigger audible alarms or play prerecorded messages. Others sound alerts if a wanderer interrupts a light beam when attempting to leave a bed. PIR is usually reliable but works by detecting body heat and so may miss events in warmer rooms.

Visual deterrents may be large, bright warning signs (STOP or DANGER) stretched across a doorway to deter passage and may sound an audible alarm if the barrier is crossed. They may also be camouflaged wallpaper depicting bookshelves or kitchen pantries that make the discovery of a doorway difficult for wanderers. Visual deterrents, as mentioned earlier, make use of the principle of diversion to achieve their objectives.

Eight studies, all conducted in institutional settings, investigated the effects of door visual barriers (mural, cloth or mirror door disguises) or floor visual barriers (taped grid patterns affixed to the floor in front of an exit doorway that alter the appearance of the doorway) to reduce a person with dementia who wanders (PDW) approaching or opening the door (Dickinson, McLain-Kark, & Marshall-Baker, 1995; Kincaid & Peacock, 2003; Mayer & Darby, 1991; Hussian & Brown, 1987; Hussian, 1988; Hewawasam, 1996; Namazi, Rosner, & Calkins, 1989; Feliciano, Vore, LeBlanc, & Baker, 2004). A ninth report asserted that both types of barriers were helpful in reducing exiting behavior in institutional and community settings, but no details were provided to support the assertion (Roberts, 1999). All of the eight studies had one or more methodological shortcoming in design, analysis, or sampling including small sample size, not characterizing participants with respect to degree of impairment, not accounting for the effect of co-morbidities, no use of control groups, inadequate description of the physical environment of the exit door and the style of door used in the study, and a failure to independently evaluate reasons for the results beyond speculation. Seven of the studies have been systematically reviewed and critiqued by Siders et al. (2004) and Price, Hermans, and Grimley (2001). None of the studies met the criteria for a controlled or randomized clinical trial. All used a serial design with each subject as his own control comparing exit approaching or exit seeking in one or more baseline conditions to the effects of one or more interventions. Carryover effects from multiple interventions when measured by repeated baseline conditions were inconsistent across studies. Control groups were not used as would be expected in the ward settings used in the studies.

Irrespective of the formal limitations of the studies, the interventions described provide leads for further research. With that goal in mind, the results and descriptions have been organized for presentation in Table 15.1. The first five studies listed describe door visual barriers. The two studies that disguised door opening mechanisms with cloth panels eliminated exit seeking by PDW during the designated observation periods used in the study. The continued effectiveness of door barriers over time cannot be evaluated from the studies, and the mechanism of door barrier effectiveness is unknown.

TABLE 15.1 Summary of Visual Barrier Studies to Reduce Elopement

Study	Intervention	Sample	Dependent Variable	Findings
Door Visual Barrier Studies				
Dickinson, McLain-Kark, & Marshall-Baker (1995)	Mini-blinds matched to door color, covered windows, covering the bar opener with cloth the same color as door	Five ambulatory males and two females (70-78 years in age), clinically diagnosed with dementia (type and MMSE scores unspecified)	Exiting attempts through an unlocked exit door of a 30-bed nursing home unit dedicated to dementia care	Of the 198 recorded exit attempts, 58% occurred in the three baseline conditions while 32%, 2%, and 7% occurred in the mini-blind, cloth, and combined interventions, respectively. 74% of the exit attempts were made by two participants.
Kincaid & Peacock (2003)	Mural on a locked exit door	10 females, 2 males out of 20 residents (mean age 78)	Door testing behaviors	Of the 829 door tests, 81% occurred in the baseline condition, 21% with the mural. Individual differences were striking—3 of the 12 participants accounted for 72% of events.
Namazi, Rosner, & Calkins (1989)	Two types of cloth camouflage strips spanning the door and covering the doorknob	5 female and 4 male (mean age 76) were selected from a ward with 14 ambulatory residents. Most were severely demented.	Nursing staff recorded each exit attempt whenever the alarm sounded	During 9 periods there were 242 exits. 27% occurred during two baseline conditions. In the two conditions with the cloth hiding the knob, no exit attempts occurred. The percentage of exits with the

				painted doorknob was 6% and with the restrictive cover, the percentage was 3%. The remaining 64% of the exits occurred in the paper grid conditions. No statistical analyses were reported. The second baseline condition had half as many exits as the first, indicating some carryover effects of the successive treatments.
Mayer & Darby (1991)	Free-standing, full-length mirror 30 cm in front of main unlocked exit door; for control the mirror was reversed.	Nine residents of a nursing home identified as "wanderers." Mean age = 77.8 and all MMSE below 12.	Exit approaches were defined by a PDW passing a defined point beyond entrance to a hallway to the door. Observations by six observers conducted from 10 A.M. and 4 P.M.	313 approaches to the door were recorded. During control days, 76.2% approaches occurred; the corresponding percentages for the reverse condition and the mirror condition were 51% and 35.7%, respectively, the latter reported as being a statistically significant difference from the control condition. Individual differences were large. The mirror increased the number of approaches by four participants.

(Continued)

TABLE 15.1 Summary of Visual Barrier Studies to Reduce Elopement (Continued)

Study	Intervention	Sample	Dependent Variable	Findings
Feliciano, Vore, LeBlanc, & Baker (2004)	A narrow strip of cloth that matched the door color was placed across an open doorway.	53-year-old female with moderate mental retardation, bipolar disorder and probably dementia. MMSE score = 0.	Entries into an open-door, restricted area	Entries were eliminated during the first intervention phase and were reduced to an average rate of 0.4 per hour during all days of intervention and follow-up combined, representing a 95% decrease in entry behavior.
Floor Visual Barrier Studies				
Hussian & Brown (1987)	Grid pattern variations of horizontal tape strips on the floor.	Eight males (mean age 78 years, mean MSQ scores 0–6 of a possible 11). One of the participants had a diagnosis of moderate dementia, the remainder, severe.	The ambulation of the selected patients was studied, observers noting whether or not the patient stepped to or reached to within 15.2 cm of the end of the hallway.	97% of the walks ended with the participant turning the doorknob or manipulating a light switch. During intervention, 139 walks were observed over a 2-month period. In comparison to the 98% crossings observed in the first baseline, the percentage of crossings with the combined 3, 4, or 6, strip or 8 strips conditions was 45% and 30%, respectively. In the 8-strip condition, the number of crossings in the intervention was lower than in the first baseline for

				every participant. In an 8-strip grid that ended 15.2 cm to the door as opposed to .91 m and a vertical stripe condition, the percentages of crossings were 51% and 57%, respectively.
Hussian (1988)	Alternated two baseline periods with two grid-floor barriers	Five males (mean age 71.2 years) diagnosed with dementia	Number of attempts to open an exit door	The number of attempts to open an exit door in a 1-hour period was 21, 11, 29, 2, respectively, in the first baseline, first intervention, second baseline, and fourth baseline. It was concluded that the grid was successful in reducing attempts to open the door.
Hawawasam (1996)	Eight-strip vertical and horizontal grid patterns used by Hussian and Brown	Seven females and three males (mean age 76, six with severe dementia, four with moderate) were selected by staff as being wanderers.	Observers noted the frequency of door contacts (touching, attempting to open) during quiet times.	In three baseline conditions, 22% of the monitored walks resulted in contacts with the door. The percentage of times the grid WAS NOT crossed was 42% and 59%, respectively, for the horizontal and vertical grids. The text and table were in conflict as to whether door contacts or no crossings were measured. Because the

(Continued)

TABLE 15.1 Summary of Visual Barrier Studies to Reduce Elopement (Continued)

Study	Intervention	Sample	Dependent Variable	Findings
Hawawasam *(Cont.)*				text stated that the vertical grid was less effective than the horizontal one, the figures cited previously should probably be 58% and 41%, respectively. Statistical tests comparing baseline and intervention data on a participant by participant basis cannot be interpreted as described.
Namazi et al. (1989)	Horizontal grid pattern first used by Hussian and Brown.	Nine residents of NH dementia unit, four males and five females; mean age = 76.0, with a previously successful exit.	Staff rates exits per day; study uses frequency counts and no statistics.	Compared to 27% of the total exits occurring in the two control conditions, 22%, 21%, and 21%, respectively, occurred in the brown tape, beige tape, and black tape (45-degree stripes) conditions.
Chafetz (1990)	Grids affixed to the floor in front of full-pane double-glass doors	Thirty patients with dementia, not all identified as wanderers. Mean age 81.	Staff counts patient exits and exits stopped by staff. Observations made 7 A.M. to 7 P.M.	Failed to replicate the Hussian and Brown study results.

Although not independently evaluated in the studies, it was speculated that a contributing factor is the impaired recognition of object identity common in persons with dementia. In a study that disguised the door with a mural, the "door testing behavior" was significantly reduced, but not as much as in the case of the cloth barriers. Judging from the picture of the protected door shown in the report of that study, the door opening controls were visible in the mural barrier. In the study using a free-standing mirror in front of the door, the reduction in exiting behavior was the least effective of the door barrier interventions. From these studies, we may conclude that: (a) there is a need for attention to the location, function, and external view provided by the door; (b) concealing the most distinguishing feature of a door, such as its doorknob or lever bar opener, is necessary and perhaps sufficient for a door visual barrier; and (c) a visual barrier affixed to the door itself is more effective than installing a free-standing barrier in front of the door.

The last five studies listed in Table 15.1 summarize the results of floor barriers, or grid patterns affixed to the floor in front of exit doorways. Except for the 3–6 stripe conditions used by Hussian and Brown (1987), the variations in grid configuration made little difference in exit-seeking control. The rationale for using grid patterns in front of doorways is based on empirical observations indicating that PDW are more likely to avoid high contrast edges of flooring. In some of the studies reviewed, it was speculated that visuospatial deficits in dementing illnesses may cause 2-D objects to be perceived as 3-D (Hinton, Sadun, Blanks, & Miller, 1986). The competing explanations for the modest effectiveness of floor barriers include PDW inattention to the floor, adaptation to the intervention, and inadequate brightness and color contrast between barrier and floor.

From these studies we may conclude that: (a) attention needs to be given to the color and brightness contrast between the floor and the floor barrier, and to the lighting of the floor area of the barrier; (b) floor barriers should have visual interest sufficient to capture the attention of typically distracted and disoriented persons with dementia; and (c) the floor visual barrier should be wide enough so that an individual cannot easily step over it in one stride.

As indicated previously, there are several formal problems with the studies described in Table 15.1. Although these studies were forms of interrupted time series, they provided little information about carryover and adaptation effects. Longer term evaluations would permit an assessment of carryover effects or accommodation, that is, whether the efficacy of the intervention declines as the PDW becomes more familiar with the barrier. While visual agnosia and altered depth perception in dementia were offered as explanations for the use of camouflage and grid patterns, respectively, there was no independent verification of these problems in the participants used in the studies. All studies took place in an institutional environment (nursing home or hospital). Definitions of wandering and wanderers varied across studies, and the studies were conducted in environments that included nonwandering patients. Exiting and exit seeking was defined in different ways across studies, and outcomes were described narrowly in terms of increased or decreased number of exits. No study included a broader assessment encompassing quality of life issues, psychological aspects (agitation) or caregiver-focused outcomes (time, stress, nursing home placement), or cost evaluation. Despite the limitations of the studies reviewed in Table 15.1, overall findings offer fairly convincing evidence for the value of door camouflage for reducing exiting and exit seeking in institutional settings and less convincing evidence for the effectiveness of the grid pattern interventions. Anecdotal evidence indicates that the interventions or variations of them are now being used in a variety of institutional settings. The extent that they are being used in home settings is unknown.

Tracking systems locate wanderers before or after elopement, and are either radio frequency (RF) range finding (Miskelly, 2004) or global positioning systems (GPS). RF systems use transmitters worn by the wanderer and tracked by a hand-held device, which triangulates location over a range of 1–40 miles. GPS systems combine satellites, wireless networks, and the Internet to precisely locate a wanderer and may have national coverage. GPS-based technologies provide a discreet means for a caregiver to monitor a person with dementia outside the home, enabling a caregiver to recover a person who wanders at a time and place of their choosing. The wanderer wears a transmitter shaped like a watch, pager, ankle bracelet, or a box-like device in a fanny pack or rucksack and is located by computer, mobile phone, PDA, or central monitoring station. Tracking devices may provide the position of a wanderer at any moment, report if they have fallen, or be an elopement management system if linked with alarm systems.

Some GPS systems developed as house arrest solutions or locators for lost children have been adapted to senior populations. In a novel application of GPS-enhanced cybernetic technology, Digital Angel, Inc. has developed an entire system to manage wandering in persons with moderate dementia. Digital Angel's solution uses a cellular telephone's onboard advanced computational abilities and built-in GPS to establish a perimeter (termed a "geofence") around the home (Munson & Gupta, 2002). Wanderers wearing the cellular telephone, who cross the geofence, automatically reveal their position to their caregivers through a server-based notification system of e-mail, pager, and automated telephone calls using synthesized voices. Caregivers can locate the missing wanderer to within

100 feet, and coverage is dependent upon cellular telephone service and GPS satellite availability. One intriguing variant of their approach is that a wanderer who crosses a geofence could be redirected to his home by verbal directional cues delivered by a networked system similar to the Patterson, Etzioni, Fox, and Kautz (2002) "Activity Compass." Such a system would acquire data on a wanderer's location and vector and might issue specific prompts contingent on their response to verbal instructions. For example: "Please turn around and face the house. Walk back to the house. Enter the house." Patterson et al.'s technology has the potential to perform all three principle functions of reassurance, diversion, and cued performance of well-learned behaviors in persons with dementia depending upon its programming.

Advanced systems incorporate many features into one multifunction device to monitor a predefined area and activate an audible or visual alarm or send the caregiver digital messages via e-mail or pager when a wanderer leaves. Some lock external doors, and most require transmitters be worn to differentiate wanderers. They are sophisticated technologies requiring caregiver training for successful operation and are usually found in professional care organizations.

Two new variants, location aware systems and robotically mediated diversionary technologies were not mentioned by Warner but are included in this discussion because they represent emerging technological solutions to the problem of wandering. *Location aware systems* can be used to prompt behaviors as has been shown by several demonstration projects, including the University of Florida's "Smart House," which employs tiny radio frequency identification devices (RFIDs) located in the physical environment or occupants' clothing to prompt wearer behavior contingent on their location by proximity to a scanning device (Helal et al., 2005). In practice, such devices might warn an elder with dementia that he or she was in the kitchen, that the hot stove would potentially burn them, and then cue them to withdraw from the area. When the RFID scanner device itself has been incorporated into a glove, it provides cues to the wearer with dementia as to the uses of touched objects (Philipose et al., 2004), increasing the likelihood that a user might successfully carry out an ADL. Similarly, intelligent devices incorporating computer vision can verbally prompt the resumption of complex behavioral sequences such as hand washing, which can be interrupted if the elder with dementia becomes distracted (Mihailidis, Carmichael, & Boger, 2004).

Outside of the home, location aware services may rely on GPS-enabled devices. Patterson et al.'s (2002) "Activity Compass" verbally prompts the elder with dementia or mild cognitive impairment to perform an ADL at that set of geographical coordinates. This system is sophisticated enough to recognize when a person becomes lost on the way to a commonly traveled destination and can verbally prompt him or her "Were you going to the store? If so you'll want to turn right just up ahead." Verbal prompting provides direct cuing of behaviors and can be reassuring if presented in a calming voice that is respectful of the person.

Robotically mediated diversionary technologies can also offer relief to caregivers tending to the needs of persons with dementia who wander. Robotic dolls may play a role by stimulating communications in persons with dementia, but they can also provide programmed cues and guidance to persons with memory disorders and act as a type of electronic guide dog. Sony's newest version of AIBO (Sony, Inc., 2005) includes touch sensors, cameras, wireless networking, and artificial intelligence that learn its environment, causing the robot's "personality" to change over time. It presents six unique "emotions": happiness, sadness, fear, dislike, surprise, and anger in order to stimulate contact by people. AIBO's onboard sensors and data recording capability may also allow easier gathering of longitudinal behavioral data in home and community settings where obtaining information on the progression of dementing disorders might otherwise prove difficult or unreliable. Besides their diversionary role, these robots provide tactile comfort and reassurance and can offer verbal cues to guide behavior, thus integrating all three approaches of reassurance, diversion, and cued behavioral recall.

Tamura et al. (2001) demonstrated that simple baby dolls and toy animals can reduce agitation and increase social interactions among persons with moderate to severe dementia. Tamura et al. (2004) has found that animating the dolls produced significant increases in verbal interaction by demented persons. These investigators presented an AIBO robotic dog dressed in baby clothes or an inexpensive electronic toy dog to 13 severely demented men and women. Patients increased communication with both toys, but more communication was observed with the inexpensive electronic toy dog than with the AIBO. Patients referred to the dressed AIBO dog as either a dog or baby, and the investigators concluded that the robot's ambiguous identity may have reduced patients' communications with it, because they were unsure which behaviors were appropriate in the presence of the AIBO. In contrast, the simple electronic toy dog reliably elicited behaviors characteristic of pet owners.

Wada, Shibata, Saito, and Tanie (2002) presented a robotic harp seal replica to 26 residents of a nursing facility over a period of 5 weeks; approximately 38 percent of the residents had some level of dementia. The robot was programmed to learn from its environment and increase behaviors for which it was rewarded and decrease those for which it was punished. The investigators reported statistically reliable improvements in resident affect for weeks 2–5 among the residents using the Profile of Mood States questionnaire and found that persons with prior histories of breeding animals were more likely to benefit from exposure to the robot. Unfortunately, a placebo condition was not included to evaluate the effect of additional attention paid to the residents. A subsequent study by Saito, Shibata, Wada, and Tanie (2003) measured urinary stress hormones in nursing home patients interacting with the behaviorally complex seal robot or a version having only a minimum set of programmed stereotyped behaviors and incapable of learning. Their analysis showed reduced stress hormone levels in elders who interacted with the more behaviorally complex robot compared to elders who interacted only with the simpler version, which emitted stereotyped behaviors.

Takanori (2004) has eloquently described these variants of service robots as *human interactive robots for psychological enrichment.*

> Human interactive robots for psychological enrichment are a type of service robot that provides a service by interacting with humans while stimulating their minds and we, therefore, tend to assign high subjective values to them. It is not necessary for these robots to be exclusive, but they should be as affordable as other new luxury products. In addition, accuracy or speed is not always of prime importance. Their function or purpose is not simply entertainment, but also to render assistance, to guide, to provide therapy, to educate, [and] to enable communication. (p. 1751)

Takanori's (2004) psychological enrichment robots offer the promise of direct reassurance and calming, the diversion of attention, and behavioral cuing contingent on temporal, spatial, or environmental (behavioral) triggers. In this respect, these robots represent what could be the best technological means to address wandering in persons with dementia. One can imagine a cuddly electronic "pet" or companion, capable of emitting a soothing purr and being completely captivating, thereby lessening the likelihood a person with dementia will wander away. This same "pet" might resist being taken out of the home by whimpering convincingly when taken outside, or by verbally requesting that the person with dementia please take it back home because it was frightened of the outdoors. Because the "pet" could also be a node on a larger network of services, it could also reveal its location and other information about elder agitation levels (i.e., whether there has been recent stroking of the pet's "fur" and whether the "pet" has been dropped or sustained an impact resulting from having been thrown) to the caregiver who may then take appropriate action to calm and reassure the person with dementia.

CONCLUSIONS AND ETHICAL CONSIDERATIONS

This chapter has classified a wide variety of interventions used to manage wandering in dementia according to the three principles outlined by Mace and Rabins (1999)—reassurance and reducing stimulus overload, diverting attention, and providing referential cue stimuli in the person with dementia's environment. This organizing scheme was applied to existing technologies and to future oriented technologies throughout this chapter.

The use of technology for surveillance and control of wandering and other behaviors raises significant ethical issues. Dementia is a highly destructive progressive disorder that robs a person of their memories, intelligence, dignity, and ultimately their life. It can be highly destructive to family relationships, also, and places large demands on caregivers, who may themselves be elderly and in ill health. Many excellent discussions have been presented on ethical issues and technology (for example, Fogg, 2003), and our intent is not to revisit them here.

We contend technologies employed for the management of wandering should follow the Hippocratic Oath of "First, do no harm." This means surveillance, monitoring, and behavioral management techniques should not be the first resort, but should be introduced only if a person with dementia's wandering presents a clear danger to themselves or to other family members or caretakers and then only as needed. The essential dignity and privacy of the person with dementia must be respected, and only the minimum monitoring necessary to keep them safe should be employed. Cameras in people's homes in particular are considered extremely invasive and are viewed negatively (Haigh et al., 2003). In order to make the invasion of privacy less unpalatable, monitoring devices relying on pressure transducers and switch closures and other devices have been employed instead of cameras. Unfortunately, sensors such as passive infrared devices, pressure pads, and door switches often lack the ability to accurately discern who triggered them and may lead to inaccurate information and false alarms (Haigh et al., 2003).

There appear to be several avenues emerging for robotic devices capable of reassuring, entertaining, and gently directing persons with dementia. These devices may or may not be part of larger sensor networks at the discretion of their owners and caregivers. Caregivers should carefully consider the ethical considerations of continuous monitoring of a person with dementia. As research continues into the applicability of robotics to the management of wandering in persons with dementia and the use of robots in the home becomes more mainstream, we may expect significant improvements in home care for persons with dementia. In the short term, however, it is likely that technologies such as camouflage wallpaper, pressure pads, and door alarms will constitute the bulk of the approaches used by caregivers to manage wandering in persons with dementia. Their relative ease of use, cost, and availability makes them the most attractive alternatives for caregivers with limited resources. As our understanding of dementia progresses and technology costs decline, more technologically advanced alternatives to traditional wanderer management approaches will be adopted by caregivers with a resulting improvement in quality of care.

REFERENCES

Algase, D. L., & Struble, L. (1992). Wandering: What, why & how? In K. Buckwalter (Ed.), *Geriatric mental health nursing: Current and future challenges* (pp. 61–74). Thorofare, NJ: Slack.

Alzheimer's Association (2006a). Publications, fact sheets and reports. Retrieved May 31, 2006, from http://www.alz.org/Resources/FactSheets.asp.

Alzheimer's Association (2006b). Fact sheet: Alzheimer's Association project Safe Return®. Retrieved May 31, 2006, from http://www.alz.org/Resources/FactSheets/SRfactsheet.pdf.

Cancro, T. (1968). Elopements from the C.F. Menninger Memorial Hospital. *Bulletin Menninger Clinic, 32,* 228–238.

Chafetz, P. K. (1990). Two-dimensional grid is ineffective against demented patients' exiting through glass doors. *Psychology and Aging, 5*(1), 146–147.

Day, K., Carreon, D., & Stump, C. (2000). The therapeutic design of environments for people with dementia: A review of the empirical research. *Gerontologist, 40*(4), 397–416.

Dickinson, J., McLain-Kark, J., & Marshall-Baker, A. (1995). The effects of visual barriers on exiting behavior in a dementia care unit. *Gerontologist, 35*(1), 127–130.

Feliciano, L., Vore, J., LeBlanc, L. A., & Baker, J. C. (2004). Decreasing entry into a restricted area using a visual barrier. *Journal of Applied Behavior Analysis, 37*(1), 107–110.

Fogg, B. (2003). *Persuasive technology: Using computers to change what we think and do.* Amsterdam: Morgan Kaufman.

Follette, W., & Linnerooth, P. (2001) Positive psychology: A clinical behavior analytic perspective. *Journal of Humanistic Psychology, 41*(1), 102–134.

Fompa-Loy, J. (1988). Wandering: Causes, consequences, and care. *Journal of Psychosocial Nursing & Mental Health Services, 28,* 8–11, 15–18.

Fozard, J.L., & Kearns, W. D. (2007). Impacts of technology interventions on communication in aging and aged persons. In G. Lesnoff-Caravglia (Ed.), *Gerontechnology: Growing old in a technological society* (pp. 271-291). Springfield, IL: Charles C. Thomas.

Haigh, K., Kiff, L., Myers, J., Guralnik, V., Krichbaum, K., Phelps, J., et al. (2003). The independent lifestyle assistant TM (I.L.S.A.): Lessons learned. Technical Report ACS-P03–023. Minneapolis: Honeywell Laboratories.

Hawawasam, L. (1996). The use of two-dimensional grid patterns to limit hazardous ambulation in elderly patients with Alzheimer's disease. *Nursing Times Research, 1,* 217–228.

Hebert, L., Scherr, P., Bienias, J., Bennett, D., & Evans, D. (2003). Alzheimer disease in the U.S. population: Prevalence estimates using the 2000 census. *Archives of Neurology, 60*(8), 1119–1122.

Helal, S., Mann, W., El-Zabadani, H., King, J., Kaddoura, Y., & Jansen, E. (2005). The gator tech smart house: A programmable pervasive space. *IEEE Computer Magazine, 38*(3), 64–74. Retrieved January 26, 2006, from http://ieeexplore.ieee.org/iel5/2/30617/01413118.pdf?arnumber=1413118.

Hinton, D., Sadun, A., Blanks, J., & Miller, C. (1986). Optic-nerve degeneration in Alzheimer's disease. *New England Journal of Medicine, 315*(8), 485–487.

Holahan, J., Wiener, J., & Lutzky, A. (2002). Health policy for low-income people: States' responses to new challenges. Retrieved November 8, 2005, from http://content.healthaffaiars.org/cgi/content/full/hlthaff.w2.187v1/DC1.

Holtzer, R., Tang, M. X., Devanand, D. P., Albert, S. M., Wegesin, D. J., Marker, K., et al. (2003). Psychopathological features in Alzheimer's disease: Course and relationship with cognitive status. *Journal of the American Geriatrics Society, 51*(7), 953–960.

Hope, T., Keene, J., McShane, R., Fairburn, C., Gedling, K., & Jacoby, R. (2001). Wandering in dementia: A longitudinal study. *International Psychogeriatrics, 13*(2), 137–147.

Hussian, R. (1988). Modification of behaviors in dementia via stimulus manipulation. *Clinical Gerontologist, 8*(1), 37–43.

Hussian, R., & Brown, D. (1987). Use of two-dimensional grid patterns to limit hazardous ambulation in demented patients. *Journal of Gerontology, 42*(5), 558–560.

Jost, B. C., & Grossberg, G. T. (1996). The evolution of psychiatric symptoms in Alzheimer's disease: A natural history study. *Journal of the American Geriatrics Society, 44*(9), 1078–1081.

Kincaid, C., & Peacock, J. (2003). Effect of a wall mural on decreasing four types of door-testing behaviors. *Journal of Applied Gerontology, 22*(1), 76–88.

Mace, N., & Rabins, P. (1999). *The 36 Hour Day.* Baltimore, MD: Johns Hopkins University Press.

Mayer, R., & Darby, S. (1991). Does a mirror detect wandering in demented older people? *International Journal of Geriatric Psychiatry, 6,* 607–609.

Mihailidis, A., Carmichael, B., & Boger, J. (2004). The use of computer vision in an intelligent environment to support aging-in-place: Safety, and independence in the home. *IEEE Transactions on Information Technology in Biomedicine, 8*(3), 238–247.

Miskelly, F. (2004). A novel system of electronic tagging in patients with dementia and wandering. *Age and Ageing, 33*(3), 304–305.

Munson, J., & Gupta, V. (2002). Location-based notification as a general-purpose service. Retrieved January 26, 2006, from http://delivery.acm.org/10.1145/580000/570713/p40-munson.pdf?key1=570713&key2=6728038311&coll=GUIDE&dl=ACM&CFID=63489869&CFTOKEN=97325999.

Namazi, K., Rosner, T., & Calkins, M. (1989). Visual barriers to prevent ambulatory Alzheimer's patients from exiting through an emergency door. *Gerontologist, 29*(5), 699–702.

Patterson, D., Etzioni, O., Fox, D., & Kautz, H. (2002). The activity compass. *Proceedings of UbiCog '02: First International Workshop on Ubiquitous Computing for Cognitive Aids,* Gothenberg, Sweden. Retrieved January 26, 2006, from http://www.cs.washington.edu/homes/djp3/AI/AssistedCognition/publications/compass03tr.doc.

Philipose, M., Fishkin, K., Perkowitz, M., Patterson, D., Fox, D., Kautz, H., et al. (2004). Inferring activities from interactions with objects. *IEEE Pervasive Computing Magazine, 3*(4), 50–57.

Polisher Research Institute. (2005). *Technology for long term care: Wander Management.* Retrieved November 1, 2005, from http://www.techforltc.org/ltc.cfm?pageid=154&CareIssue=9.

Price, J., Hermans, D., & Grimley, E.. (2001). Subjective barriers to prevent wandering of cognitively impaired people. *Cochrane Database of Systematic Reviews,* Issue 1. Chichester, UK: John Wiley & Sons.

Rheaume, Y., Riley, M. E., & Voliver, L. (1987). Meeting nutritional needs of Alzheimer's patients who pact constantly. *Journal of Nutrition for the Elderly,* 7(1), 43–52.

Roberts, C. (1999). The management of wandering in older people with dementia. *Journal of Clinical Nursing, 8,* 322–324.

Saito, T., Shibata, T., Wada, K., & Tanie, K. (2003). Relationship between interaction with the mental commit robot and change of stress reaction of the elderly. *Proceedings of the 2003 IEEE International Symposium on Computational Intelligence in Robotics and Automation.* July 16–20, Kobe, Japan.

Siders, C., Nelson, A., Brown, L., Joseph, I., Algase, D., Beattie, E., et al. (2004). Evidence for implementing nonpharmacological interventions for wandering. *Rehabilitative Nursing, 29*(6), 195–206.

Sony, Inc. (2005). *ERS-7M3.* Retrieved January 29, 2006, from http://www.sony.net/Products/aibo/.

Soverini, S., & Borghesi, E. (1968). On a strange case of wandering in an arteriosclerotic demented patient. *Gerontology, 16*(8), 846–851.

Stokes, G. (1986). *Wandering, common problems with the elderly confused.* Bicester, UK: Winslow Press.

Takanori, S. (2004). An overview of human interactive robots for psychological enrichment. *Proceedings of the IEEE, 92*(11), 1749–1758.

Tamura, T., Nakajima, K., Nambu, M., Nakamura, K., Yonemitsu, S., Itoh, A., et al. (2001). Baby dolls as therapeutic tools for severe dementia patients. *Gerontechnology, 1*(2), 111–118.

Tamura, T., Yonemitsu, S., Itoh, A., Oikawa, D., Kawakami, A., Higashi, Y., et al. (2004). Is an entertainment robot useful in the care of elderly people with severe dementia? *The Journals of Gerontology Series A: Biological Sciences and Medical Sciences, 59A*(1), 83–85. Retrieved January 26, 2006, from http://biomed.gerontologyjournals.org/cgi/content/abstract/59/1/M83.

Wada, K., Shibata, T., Saito, T., & Tanie, K. (2002). Analysis of factors that bring mental effects to elderly people in robot assisted activity. *Proceedings of the 2002 IEEE/RSJ International Conference on Intelligent Robots and Systems.* EPFL, Lausanne, Switzerland.

Warner, M. (1999a). *Alarms: Precautions for wandering.* ElderCare Online. Retrieved August 10, 2006, from http://www.ec-online.net/knowledge/articles/wandering2.html

Warner, M. (1999b). *Deterrents and diversions: Precautions for wandering.* ElderCare Online. Retrieved August 10, 2006, from http://www.ec-online.net/knowledge/articles/wandering3.html.

CHAPTER SIXTEEN

Environmental Design

Bettye Rose Connell and Margaret P. Calkins

INTRODUCTION

As discussed in other chapters in this book, dementia-related wandering is a broad term that encompasses a number of distinct behaviors observed in persons with dementia. According to one view, *pacing* (including aimless wandering) is characterized by unrelenting walking or wheeling, often up and down hallways or around rooms during activities such as meals. Pacing has been hypothesized to provide needed stimulation not otherwise available (Cohen-Mansfield & Werner, 1998). Others characterize *pacing* more discretely as back and forth locomotion between two endpoints (Martino-Saltzman, Blasch, Morris, & McNeal, 1991) and use Martino-Saltzman's term *random* to refer to the more erratic and often unrelenting form of wandering (Algase, Kupferschmid, Beel-Bates & Beattie, 1997), attributing it to a broader set of precipitating and contributing factors (Algase et al., 1996). *Shadowing* describes the behavior of persons with dementia who closely follow another person, often a caregiver, as they engage in daily activities. Shadowing has been explained as a means of receiving attention and providing a sense of security (Perez, Proffitt, & Calkins, 2001). *Rummaging* involves entering someone else's space and going through drawers and closets, ostensibly looking for something familiar to the individual (Perez et al., 2001). When the term wandering is used by long-term care staff to refer to a specific behavior, they often are referring to *wayfinding failures*. Wayfinding failures include difficulty finding or recognizing a desired destination, which previous research has linked to both dementia-related deficits in cognitive abilities as well as to environmental complexity (Algase, 1992; Liu, Gauthier, & Gaither, 1991; Passini, Rainville, Marchand, & Joanette,

1995). *Exiting* entails leaving an area designated by caregivers as safe, without the knowledge of caregivers. Exiting incidents are complex and have been explained as the exercise of autonomy (e.g., go outdoors when individual wants to), a means to escape stimuli that are aversive to the individual (e.g., avoid a bath), reenactment of life-long behaviors (e.g., go to work/home after work), and disorientation to time and place (e.g., go to a home that is no longer owned, seeking a deceased parent) (Connell, 1992; Perez et al., 2001). As these examples suggest, the wandering behavior of persons with dementia is closely linked to the environmental conditions they experience.

The purpose of this chapter is to review current research and best practice with regard to environmental issues impacting wandering in persons with dementia in long-term care. Research on dementia-related behavior problems, including wandering, has been accompanied by debates about whether care practices and care environments should prevent or accommodate them. Arguments for prevention emphasize the potential health and safety hazards some wandering, for example exiting, may pose for the individual. Arguments for accommodation emphasize the idea that wandering may be adaptive behavior (e.g., a means to cope with stressors) or a source of stimulation. The goals of dementia care and dementia care environments are important, because the architecture of prevention is quite different from the architecture of accommodation. Prioritizing prevention tends to increase the institutional nature of long-term care at the expense of humanizing and normalizing it for residents. Prioritizing accommodation tends to emphasize independence and autonomy of the individual, supporting long-term care residents' use of preserved abilities to the extent possible.

The approach taken here is guided by Lawton and Nahemow's Environmental Press Model (1973). In that view, observed behavior and affect reflect the interaction of individual "competence," or ability to perform an activity, and the "press" or demand placed on the individual by the environment during the conduct of that activity. The model hypothesizes that "maladaptive behavior and affect" occur when individuals experience either excessive *or* insufficient environmental press, in relation to their competence. When press exceeds competence, individuals experience "excess disability," functioning as if they are more impaired than they really are. Importantly, excess disability can be reversed. In principle, environmental demands can be modified to a level that permits full use of preserved abilities. The model also suggests that when competence exceeds press, individuals are not challenged or stimulated to use preserved abilities and may subsequently lose them at an accelerated rate.

For the purpose of this chapter, wandering is treated as a "maladaptive behavior" and indicative of "excess disability." This implies that wandering is not an intractable outcome of dementia and that under different conditions the frequency, duration, extent, and even occurrence of wandering behaviors can be lessened. Thus, whether wandering is an adaptive behavior or an expression of unmet needs, whether it leads the individual into hazardous situations, is disruptive to others or is benign in its effect, the Environmental Press Model suggests that under environmental conditions that better match individuals' preserved abilities, wandering would occur less often, because the situations that trigger these behaviors would have been modified.

Briefly, persons with dementia experience age as well as dementia-related deficits in a number of cognitive functions relevant to wandering, including spatial cognition, attention, information processing, various aspects of memory, and executive functioning. Directly related to the focus of this chapter are findings that older adults with dementia are susceptible to the effects of visual and auditory distractions on working memory (West, 1999), use less-systematic, task-oriented scanning of visual scenes than do those without dementia (Hutton, 1985; Mosimann, Felblinger, Ballinari, Hess, & Muri, 2004), experience spatial orientation and cognitive mapping deficits (Henderson, Mack, & Williams, 1989; Liu et al., 1991; Passini et al., 1995), and have difficulty planning and carrying out goal-directed travel and recognizing a destination and disengaging from wayfinding (Allen, 1999; Passini et al, 1995; Ryan et al., 1995). Also important with regard to the focus of this chapter are the effects of aging on learning new environments (Kirasic, 2000), and the finding that anxiety has a greater effect on divided attention in older, rather than younger, people (Hogan, 2003). Additionally, sensory functioning is important with regard to "competence" and wandering. Vision impairment is a significant predictor of mobility in long-term care residents with dementia (Connell, McConnell, Mancil, & Coombs, 2001) and has implications for other issues important in discussions of wandering, such as access to wayfinding cues and meaningful stimulation.

"Environmental press" associated with wandering is attributable to demands from proximate physical and social environments in relation to preserved abilities. The Professional Environmental Assessment Protocol (PEAP) (Norris-Baker, Weisman, Lawton, Sloane, & Kaup, 2000) provides a framework of eight environmental goals that can be used to describe different aspects of the environmental press side of the equation. These domains are: maximize awareness and orientation, enhance safety and security, provide privacy, regulate stimulation and coherence, support functional abilities, provide opportunities for personal control, enhance continuity of self, and facilitate social contact. Each domain is defined in terms of its particular relevance for individuals with dementia, with myriad examples of environmental features and characteristics that are supportive of the needs and preserved abilities of this population.

Persons with dementia retain the ability to do some things for themselves, if given appropriate assistance, until late in the disease process (Dawson, Wells, & Kline, 1993). However, because dementia involves a progressive loss of cognitive abilities, environmental demands as well as care practices also must be modified over time to allow the individual to continue to capitalize on preserved abilities (Connell & McConnell, 2000). In long-term care settings, abilities vary across people as well as time. However, the design of the physical environment of long-term care settings can only be partially individualized as a strategy for balancing abilities and environmental demands. Staff members play an important role in providing assistance to residents in their use of environmental supports and in managing environmental conditions for residents no longer able to do it for themselves. Activities programming also is important in providing structure and meaningful stimulation during discretionary time.

This chapter is structured by six environmental features of long-term care units (nursing homes and assisted living facilities), suggested by research and best practice literatures as associated with wandering behaviors: (1) unit layout, (2) hallways, (3) doorways (to spaces on the unit), (4) unit exits, (5) directional and destination signage, and (6) ambient conditions. For each feature, we describe environmental characteristics common in many long-term care facilities that are potentially problematic for persons with dementia who wander and discuss why they pose a problem for residents (and sometimes for staff). Then, recommendations are made for modifying problematic environmental characteristics. Many of these recommendations come from the structure of the PEAP, described previously, along with research and best practice resources. Two case studies that integrate the preceding information are presented and discussed, followed by a discussion of implications for practitioners interested in the physical environment as a tool in the management of wandering in long-term care. Finally, methodological issues of importance in evaluating existing research and gaps in research are presented.

REVIEW OF LITERATURE

Interest in the impact of the physical environment on people with dementia generally dates back to the early 1980s, although some pioneering work was done earlier. Early efforts reported on the apparent sensitivity of persons with dementia to environmental conditions, evaluated the effect of environmental changes on dementia-related behavior, and documented the effect of relocation on function, behavior, and affect in persons with dementia. (See, for example, Anthony, Proctor, Silverman, & Murphy, 1987; Hanley, 1981; Hussian, 1987; Lawton, Fulcomer, & Kleban, 1984.) Although the therapeutic role of the physical environment for persons with dementia is now widely accepted, research is surprisingly limited. For a review published in 2000, only 71 published, empirical research articles, of which two-thirds were published between 1991 and 1999, were identified (Day, Carreon, & Stump, 2000). In addition, several design guidelines were published in the 1980s and 1990s (Brawley, 1997; Calkins, 1988; Cohen & Weisman, 1991). It is not always appreciated that these design guidelines are research-based in only a limited way. Nonetheless, the experience, expert consensus, and extrapolations from research in other fields that they embody have influenced research in several ways. As noted elsewhere (Day et al., 2000), these guidelines should be viewed as testable hypotheses. The activation of new facilities that were designed in accordance with these guidelines has lead to global evaluations of the impact of these innovative care environments on the behavior, functioning, and well-being of persons with dementia (Hoglund, Dimotta, Ledewitz, & Saxton, 1994). They also continue to be an important source of evidence of the expected impact of usual and improved environmental conditions on specific outcomes, such as wandering.

Wandering has been a long-standing topic of interest among environmentally oriented geriatric researchers. In some studies, wandering was classified as one of an extensive list of agitated behaviors (Cohen-Mansfield, 1986, 1991) and in other cases, research focused on wandering as a distinct dementia-related behavior (Algase, 1992). However, different wandering behaviors have not received equivalent attention, leading, for example, to complaints about the limited attention given to pacing (Cohen-Mansfield & Werner, 1998). The bulk of the research has focused on exiting behavior and disorientation or wayfinding problems.

Unit Layout

Traditionally, long-term care units have been designed with resident rooms arrayed along one or more long hallways, with shared spaces (e.g., lounges, TV rooms) located apart from resident rooms. Some shared spaces are usually centrally located near nurses' stations with the intention of making the spaces accessible to all *and* of making it easier for staff to monitor residents and respond quickly in the event of an emergency.

Some types of shared spaces (e.g., activity rooms, dining rooms) may be located off-unit, and used by residents from several units.

One result of this typical long-term care unit layout is that spaces used by residents are out-of-sight of each other—you often cannot see a desired destination from your point of origin—and wayfinding is involved in traveling to them. In long-term care units designed for individuals with dementia, the excessive environmental demands thought to be created by out-of-sight destinations are often addressed by increasing visual access of frequent destinations. Because dementia special care units are usually planned for fewer residents than is typical of traditional long-term care, resident rooms and shared spaces can be grouped close together, often around a shared social space (Cohen & Weisman, 1991; Day & Calkins, 2002). More open layouts enable residents to see frequent destinations from different points of origin, rather than having to remember what is out-of-sight, how to get there, and remain task-oriented along the way. These types of units have been associated with higher levels of orientation (Netten, 1989).

This approach to reducing environmental demands usually is not feasible in existing facilities in the absence of extensive renovations. An alternative approach is to increase visual access, to the extent possible, of locations staff want to encourage residents with dementia to access and use independently, such as by leaving doors open that normally are closed. In a study that compared daytime use of in-room toilets under usual conditions (toilets not visible from outside resident rooms) and with toilets visible from outside rooms (doors to resident rooms and curtains surrounding in-room toilets were purposefully left open), independent toilet use increased dramatically under the experimental high visibility conditions (Namazi & Johnson, 1991a). Visual access also can be enhanced through choices about where to (re)locate new and existing functional spaces on existing units. For example, if an on-unit dining area is to be added for residents with dementia and the choice is to locate it in a quiet room at the end of a resident room hallway, or in a room used for equipment storage across the hall from a frequently used lounge, the latter is the better choice in terms of supporting residents' wayfinding to meals.

Hallways

The layout of most traditional long-term care units results in two or more resident room hallways with identically spaced doors. Two of the most noticeable characteristics of many long-term care unit hallways are how much they look alike and how little meaningful stimulation they afford.

Distinctiveness

If residents with dementia are to move around a unit independently, they must make choices about which hallway to follow to reach their room, a lounge, or other desired destination. When residents make the wrong choice, they are at risk for several adverse outcomes. They may not recognize they have made a mistake, continue to search for a space that is not there, and in the process intrude into the spaces of others. There are anecdotal reports that territorial intrusions have lead to resident-to-resident aggression. Even if residents are able to recognize they are on the wrong hallway, they may be unable to work out where they went wrong and correct the error. The feeling of being lost is frightening and exhausting, further adding to the stresses experienced by residents. It also may discourage a resident from future attempts to wayfind, encouraging more passivity and solitude as he or she stays in the bedroom unless accompanied by staff.

Facility hallways are usually differentiated in some way. However, in many facilities the means of differentiation are too abstract or otherwise lack meaning for residents with dementia, increasing the demands experienced by residents during wayfinding. For example, some facilities incorporate floor and orientation into hallway signage designations ("1-East" and "1-West"), and staff refer to hallways in this way when giving directions to residents. Other facilities use designations that have another meaning for some residents with dementia and may produce confusion. For example, calling unit hallways "Pods A, B, and C" may puzzle residents who are retired gardeners or farmers and who know pods grow on plants or trees and have seeds inside. Moreover, hallway designations are often provided to residents verbally, but visual differences among the referenced hallways are subtle (e.g., different shades of blue) or absent.

Landmarks, such as a large plant, a distinctive piece of furniture, or a wall hanging, are widely used in facilities designed for people with dementia to visually signal choice points and differentiate hallways (Baskaya, Wilson, & Ozcan, 2004; Bertram, 1989; Coons, 1988) (see Figure 16.1). Landmarks have the additional advantage of being readily incorporated into wayfinding prompts from staff. Painting hallways significantly different colors also adds to the distinctiveness of hallways, although vision changes associated with aging and dementia may reduce the effectiveness of color as a wayfinding cue, particularly if used alone (Cronin-Golumb, 1995; Gilmore & Whitehouse, 1995). These strategies can be easily adopted for the same purposes in existing facilities not planned for, but now serving, people with dementia, as in newly planned and constructed dementia special care units.

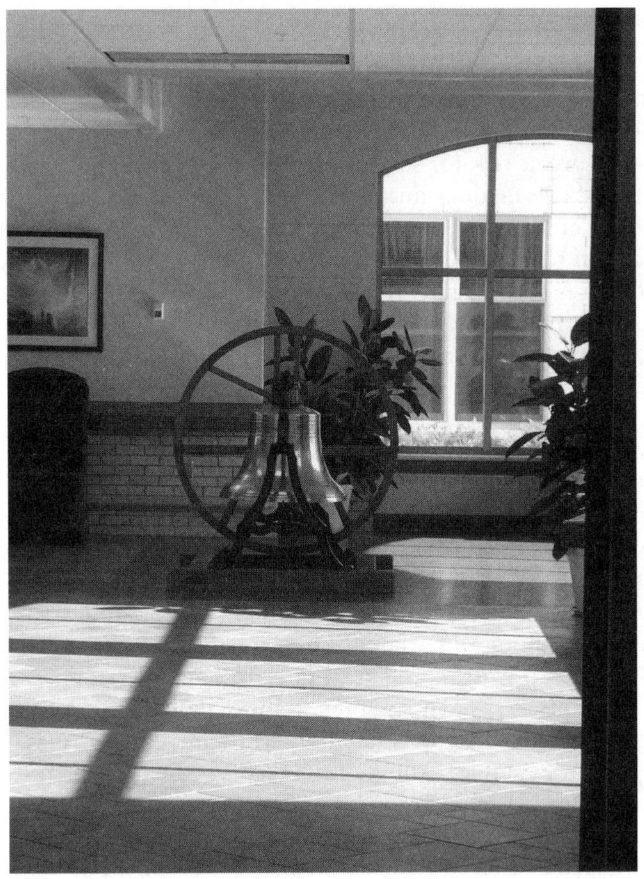

FIGURE 16.1 Landmark (series of 3).
In this facility, there are three hallways leading to three separate "neighborhoods." They used distinctly different landmarks—the old farm bell that was used to call the workers back when the facility was the county poorhouse, a fountain, and a greenhouse/front porch—to help people easily identify which direction to go. Notice even the window treatment is different in terms of design and mullion pattern.

Meaningful Stimulation

Design guidelines and environmental assessment protocols (Brawley, 1997; Calkins, 1988; Cohen & Weisman, 1991; Norris-Baker et al., 1999; Sloane et al., 2002; Zeisel, Hyde, & Levkoff, 1994) make an important distinction between the quality and quantity of stimulation for people with dementia.

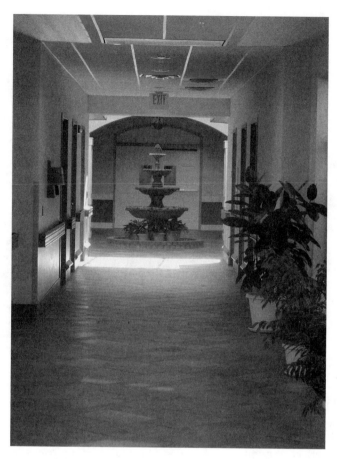

FIGURE 16.1 (Continued)

Hallways in long-term care facilities are typically painted a neutral color and have a uniform appearance for their entire length. Hallways seldom afford residents a place to sit, enjoy an attractive view, look at artwork, feel tactile wall hangings, listen to music, and so forth. When attractive, stimulating views are present in hallways, they often are seen through glass panels in or near exit doors—locations that staff discourage residents who wander from frequenting. When artwork is present, too, often it is visually inaccessible to residents as a result of small size and low contrast of images, the height it is hung, and poor lighting. Additionally, there may be medicine and supply carts, soiled linen containers, and lifts or other equipment temporarily stored in hallways, blocking access to handrails. If the facility uses an overhead pager system, these speakers are usually located in hallways as well as at other locations. In general,

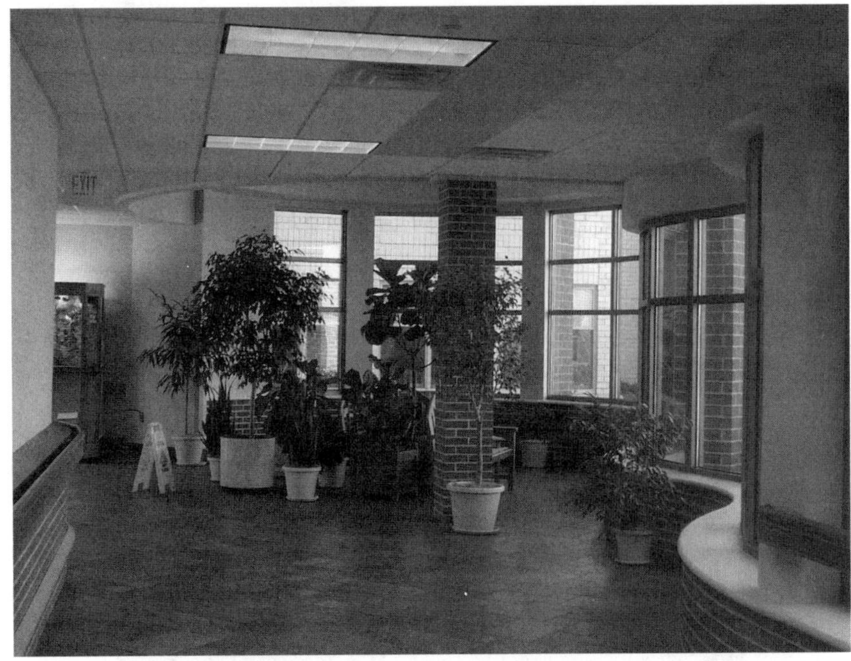

FIGURE 16.1 (Continued)

typical long-term care hallways offer residents with dementia insufficient positive stimulation and expose them to excessive meaningless stimulation, all at the same time.

The effect of two hallway simulations that used multisensory stimuli to enhance hallway environments were compared with usual institutional hallway environments to determine the effect of the enhanced environments on observed wandering behavior (Cohen-Mansfield & Werner, 1998). One enhancement simulated a nature scene and the other a scene of home and people. Both enhancements provided visual (e.g., murals, period photos), auditory (e.g., bird calls, music), and olfactory (e.g., forest and citrus aromas) stimulation, and were installed near existing seating. Residents were attracted by the simulated environments, as evidenced by the significant increase in time spent in the hallways when the simulated environments were in place, and reductions in time spent in all other locations except the dining room. Additionally, residents spent more time sitting on the benches when the simulations were in place, and the increase was significant for the home and people simulation. When the simulations were in place, less exiting and trespassing as well as other types of agitation were observed, although these differences were not significant, possibly due to sample size. No differences were observed in pacing.

In a second study relevant to positive environmental stimulation (Yao & Algase, 2006), subjective ratings of "environmental ambience," consisting of "engaging" and "soothing" subscales, were completed by trained observers at study sites (nursing homes and assisted living facilities). Controlling for mobility and cognitive status, ambience scores were used to predict walking behavior among residents. High ambience scores were associated with lower frequency and duration of walking and longer duration of sitting. Further analyses suggest that the "engaging" subscale scores were primarily responsible for the observed effects of ambience on walking. Environments perceived as "simulating, warm, embellished, welcoming, colorful and novel" rated higher on the engaging subscale than did environments that were not perceived by raters as having these qualities.

Research on reduction of meaningless stimulation associated with light, noise, and smell is discussed later under ambient conditions.

Doorways to On-Unit Spaces

In long-term care units, multiple doorways leading to private, shared, and staff spaces are often in close proximity to one another. These doorways are largely undifferentiated, except by room numbers. When residents with dementia are presented with too many similar choices that look alike, they make mistakes. Entering another resident's room while looking for one's own can lead to rummaging and confrontation. Failing to find the bathroom in a timely way can lead to incontinence episodes and embarrassment. Repeated incidents can lead to staff restrictions on independent mobility.

Resident Room Doorways

Painting proximate resident room doors different colors makes each room entry visually distinctive from a distance. Although the effect of this strategy on residents' wayfinding has not been validated empirically, it remains a recommended best practice. An alternative approach, supported by research, is to personalize or individualize the space around a resident room doorway to make it distinctive. This is most often accomplished by displaying memorabilia in cases installed beside resident room doors. Memory cases are typically filled with objects and pictures from a resident's past. The rationale for using this type of memorabilia is that it is expected to resonate with a resident's long-term memory, supporting an individual in identification of his or her room (see Figure 16.2).

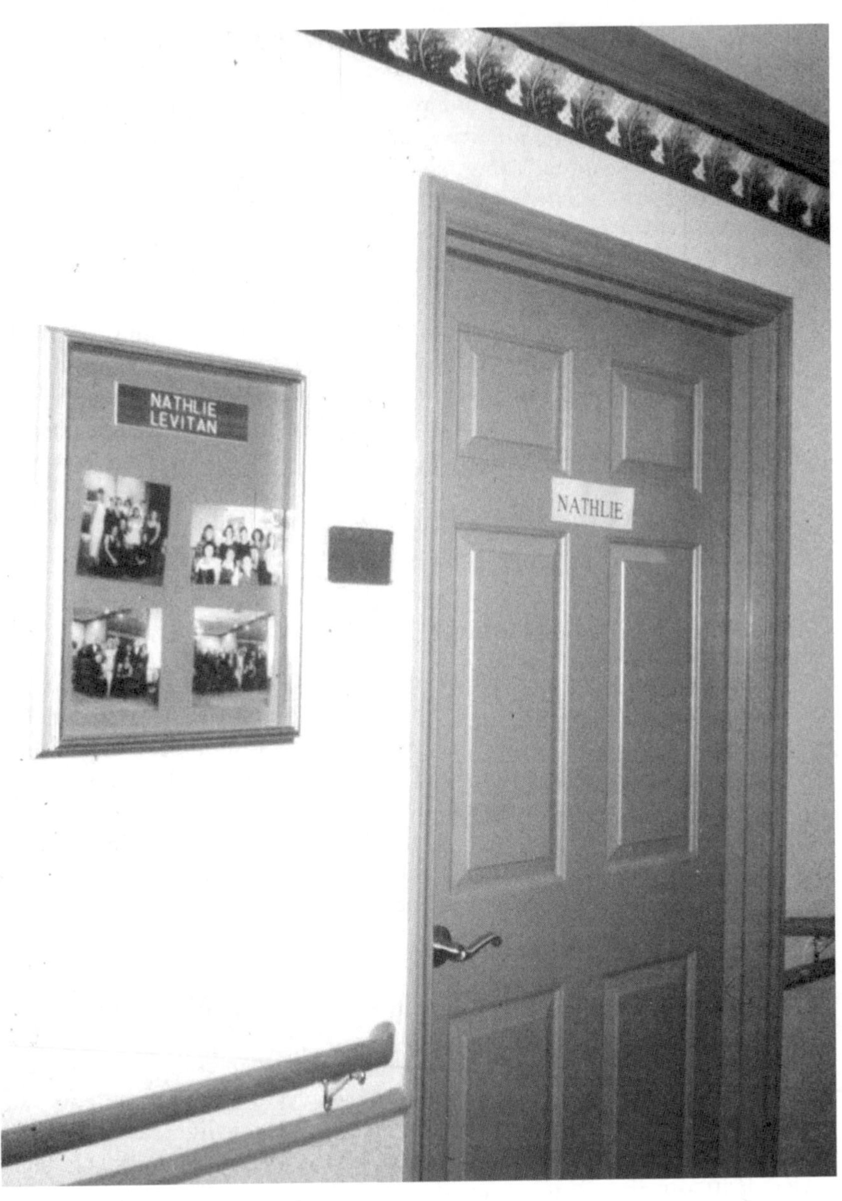

FIGURE 16.2 Bedroom orientation.
A simple frame that holds several photos is a relatively inexpensive solution. Notice the high contrast for the name in the frame and on the door. The small plaque next to the door, in gold and blue, is very low contrast, and, according to staff, meant only for the fire department to be able to identify doors in an emergency. The frame is hung too high for someone who uses a wheelchair.

Two research projects evaluating the effect of personalized cues at resident room entries were identified. In the first, the effect of two types of memorabilia, personally significant versus distinctive but not personally significant, on a resident's success in finding their room were compared over 10 trials (Namazi, Rosner, & Rechlin, 1991). Results were mixed, with some residents at each stage of dementia doing slightly better with personalized items, and some residents doing equally well under both conditions. The other study achieved an average 57 percent improvement in finding the bedroom when the display included a large (usually 8" x 10") photograph of the resident from an earlier time (50 years ago) (Nolan, Mathews, Truesdell-Todd, & VanDorp, 2002).

In practice, the contents of memory cases are often poorly lit, and the size of cases dictates the number and type of things that can be displayed. However, given the prevalence of age- and disease-based vision loss in long-term care populations, the effectiveness of memory cases is likely to be enhanced by use of easy-to-see larger objects and high contrast photographs.

Shared Space Doorways

Indistinct doorways to shared spaces, such as hallway toilets, pose problems for residents with dementia, especially when doors are routinely kept closed and several closed doors are located close together (see Figure 16.3).

One best practice approach to making doorways to shared spaces easier for residents with dementia to identify entails making doorways distinctive, such as by painting the door a distinctive color, adding a canopy over the door, or using dementia-friendly signage (see Figure 16.4 and discussion below). In some states, it is possible to have a shared social space open directly onto the hallway (i.e., without doors) as long as both areas are equipped with sprinklers. This increases visual access of the shared space from the hallways and helps residents maintain better orientation to these destinations.

All On-Unit Doorways

The identity of a room behind a closed door is often difficult to determine without opening the door and entering the room. In many cases, doors are closed out of habit and cultural convention. Keeping resident room doors closed, whether rooms are occupied or not, respects the privacy of occupants and affords them some degree of control over intrusions into their space. However, the trade-off is that it may make it harder for residents to correctly distinguish their room from the rooms of others. One best practice compromise is to use "Dutch" doors for resident room

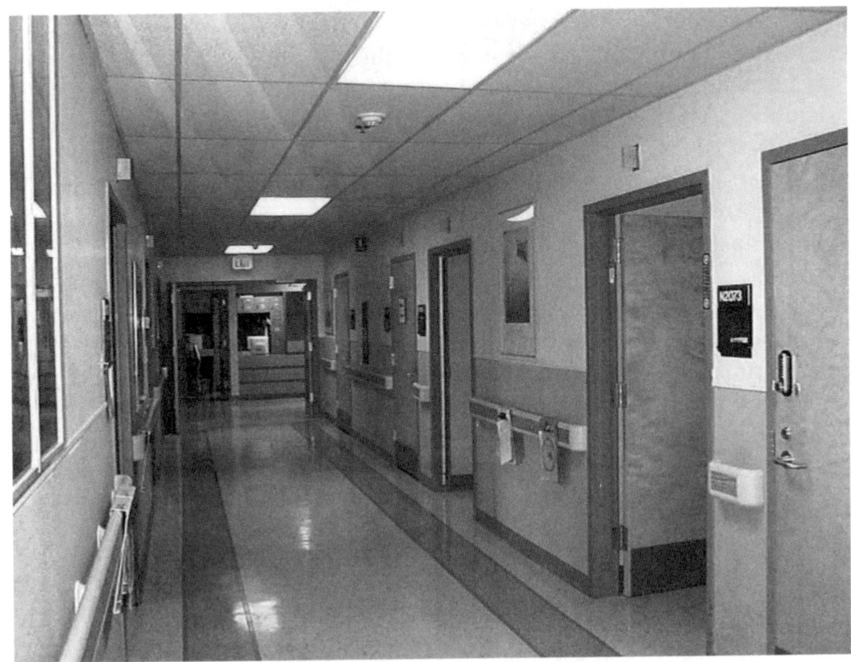

FIGURE 16.3 Poor signage in hallway.
This is a classic example of a hallway with a series of identical doorways, making it highly unlikely that someone with dementia will be able to find the bathroom, which is the last door on the right.

entries. Keeping the bottom door closed and top open during the day reduces intrusions and rummaging while affording residents a view into the room (Hoglund et al., 1994).

As mentioned earlier, when resident room doors and curtains around toilets were opened to allow in-room toilets to be seen from outside resident rooms, residents entered and used the toilets more often (Namazi & Johnson, 1991a). Leaving doors open on hallway toilets is more difficult because often these doors open outward into the hallway to prevent the door from being blocked from the inside (unless the door has double-swing hinges). Hallway toilet doors also usually have automatic closers to provide privacy and ensure they do not obstruct the hallway if left partially open. One possible concern is that leaving hallway toilet room doors open may create a potential safety hazard (life safety codes specify the width of hallways that must be free of obstructions for emergency egress). Another concern is that some staff and families may be uncomfortable with leaving toilet room doors open.

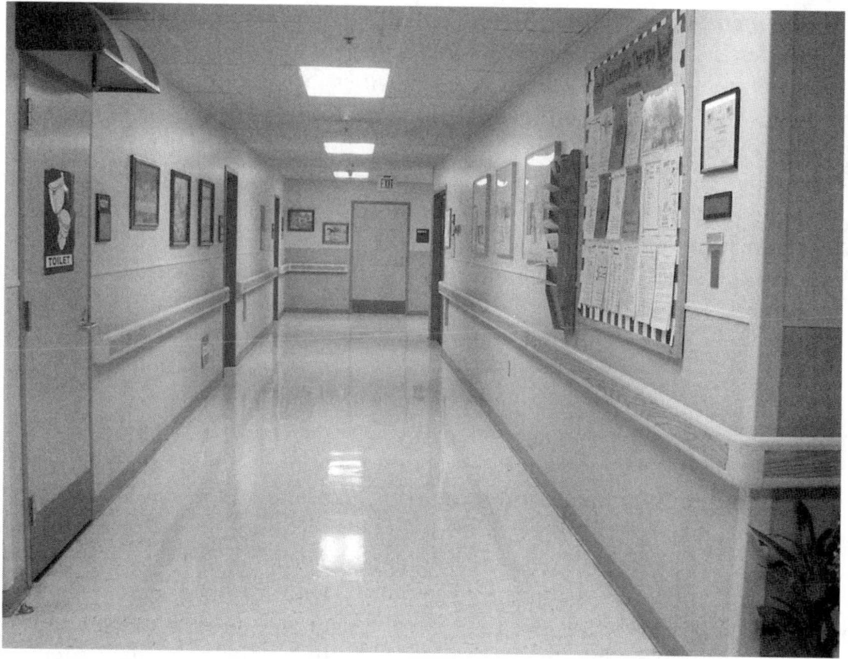

FIGURE 16.4 Toilet canopy.
The dark canopy over the door to the toilet, along with the large and high-contrast sign on the door, make it easier for people with dementia to find the toilet in this facility.

Unit Exits

Memory, executive function, and spatial orientation deficits in residents with dementia make doorways that lead outdoors or to parts of a facility where a resident might not be recognized a source of great concern for long-term care staff. Residents with dementia who exit the unit may be disoriented to time and place, have poor judgment, and lack the ability to find their way back safely. Some residents with dementia who exit care facilities have experienced adverse outcomes including medical complications from missed medications, urban violence, dehydration, hypothermia, and death (Connell, 1992).

Long-term care facilities differ in the number and location of exits leading off the unit or to the outdoors, and in the architecturally based opportunities they afford residents with dementia to use these exits without the knowledge of staff (Connell, 1992). In units with hallway-based circulation, at least one emergency exit is usually located on each hallway, often at the end and perpendicular to the route of travel. These exits are often distant from nurses' stations and care locations, and unit layout may limit architecturally based opportunities for staff to visually monitor exits as they move around the unit providing care (Connell, 1992). Units also have one or more exits connecting them to the rest of the facility. In some but certainly not all, nurses' stations are located adjacent to exits leading off the unit to other parts of the facility, or these exits can be easily seen from locations frequently used by staff. In other cases, resident rooms and even TV rooms have been located adjacent to exits leading off the unit (Connell, 1992).

Dementia Special Care Units

Although special care units differ, many limit problems with exiting in one or more ways. First, many are self-contained with on-unit dining, activity space, and programming and often have access to secure outdoor space (Judd, Marshall, & Phippen, 1998). By consolidating these functions on the unit, the number of times residents may leave for legitimate reasons is limited, thus decreasing their familiarity with how to leave. Second, exits are often secured, or egress by residents without a staff or family escort is controlled by use of cognitively complex door operating systems or wanderer alarm systems that trigger magnetic door locks if a resident approaches an exit. Third, special care units often have higher staffing levels and more activity programming than do traditional units, making it easier to monitor residents who wander and to keep them engaged. Special care unit staff also often receive training not provided to staff on traditional units that helps them to avoid unintentionally triggering exiting behavior.

Traditional Long-Term Care Units

In long-term care units with mixed populations of residents with and without dementia, there generally are greater architecturally based opportunities for exiting than is the case in special care units. Perhaps the most widely adopted strategy to manage exiting from these units is the use of wanderer alarm systems.

Wanderer alarm systems provide traditional long-term care units with residents with dementia an important tool for managing exiting, but they cannot prevent exiting unless equipped with an automatic door-locking feature. However, door-locking features, that are automatically overridden in the event of a fire or other emergency, are not fool-proof. Wanderer alarm systems also vary in the amount of information provided to staff (e.g., whether or not alarm signal is exit specific, whether or not a resident is identified), the way staff are notified (e.g., loud, burglar alarm type auditory signal vs. signal sent to staff via in-house pager system), and the ease of resetting the system after an alarm (e.g., whether or not staff have to travel to exit to turn off alarm). Loud auditory alarms, typically greater than 90 dB, were common in earlier wanderer alarm systems and introduce stimulation onto units that is meaningless and aversive to residents with dementia. High levels of meaningless stimulation are generally believed to trigger dementia-related agitation. Newer wanderer alarm systems are available that send quieter auditory or vibrating notifications to pagers worn by staff. Different features likely impact how quickly and effectively staff are able to respond, as well as the disruptiveness of alarms to other residents.

The layout of a wanderer alarm system should, but often does not, result in a secure perimeter around routinely used spaces. Layouts that result in perimeters that have to be crossed frequently to reach routinely used spaces are problematic. If residents must be routinely taken across the perimeter, for example, to reach the dining room, residents are, in effect, being repeatedly shown how to leave. Additionally, unless the wanderer alarm system can be easily turned off and reset on both sides of the perimeter, staff escorting residents may soon not bother, inviting false alarms and reduced staff vigilance (Sanford, Fazenbaker, & Connell, 1992).

A different approach to managing exiting is to minimize the detectability of exits that should not be used without an escort. One strategy is to paint the door and frame the same color as surrounding walls, and to use door hardware of a similar color, thus relying on the reduced contrast perception deficit of individuals with Alzheimer's disease to be unable to see and recognize the door (Gilmore & Whitehouse, 1995).

A second strategy entails use of visual barriers. One type of visual barrier capitalizes on dementia-related deficits in depth perception. Two-dimensional grid patterns applied to the floor at exit points are seen by some persons with dementia as three-dimensional (i.e., negative space in the grid looks like it is at a lower level). Research results have been mixed, showing reduction, increase, and no change in exiting (Chafetz, 1991; Hussian & Brown, 1987; Namazi, Rosner & Calkins, 1989). There have been repeated anecdotal reports of residents jumping or awkwardly stepping over 2-D grids, rather than not crossing it.

A second type of visual barrier obscures exit doors or exit hardware. One study compared two differently colored and patterned pieces of fabric attached with Velcro® across the center of the door, effectively covering the door handle—one the same color as the door and one in a contrasting color and pattern across the center of the door. Both were equally effective in reducing the number of times residents exited through the door (Namazi et al., 1989). Although visually obscuring doors and hardware are generally effective, life safety codes prohibit blocking access to emergency exits. Sometimes, visual barriers are not allowed in practice for this reason. Interestingly, some long-term care units unwittingly draw attention to exits by placing large stop signs on them, with the expectation that residents will turn around. However, as one resident reported, stop signs mean you stop, look both ways, then go (Calkins, 2006).

Another approach to reducing exiting is to *increase* the demands placed on cognitively impaired residents who try to operate exit doors. Keypad controls, remote door openers, and multistep door operating sequences have been used to make it difficult for cognitively impaired residents to open doors or call elevators (Calkins, 1988). Cognitively intact residents and visitors can follow posted instructions, but cognitively impaired residents are unable to do so, or the time it takes them to complete the task increases the chance a staff person will observe them and intervene.

Glass panels and large windows that are located near exit doors and provide views of the outdoors or other interesting scenes have been associated with exiting (Morgan & Stewart, 1998). If the view is more interesting than what is going on inside, residents may be attracted to what they see and seek ways to go outside. In one study, exiting was cut in half when blinds were added to windows in exit doors (Dickinson, McLain-Kark, & Marshall-Baker, 1995). Views through glass panels beside doors can be blocked by adding blinds or placing a tall plant in front of the panel, unless this blocks the exit route.

Exiting in conjunction with entry onto the unit by a visitor also has been reported as a problem, particularly for residents who pace. At one facility, the main unit entry–exit door was on axis with a hallway used by residents who paced. One resident exited when he arrived at the exit as a visitor was entering. The visitor who was entering the unit thought the resident was an elderly visitor and held the door open for him (Connell, 1992).

Access to Secure Outdoor Space

Traditional long-term care units do not typically provide direct access to a secure outdoor space. In focus groups with staff from several facilities to discuss previous exiting incidents in their facility, one of the most frequently reported scenarios involved residents wanting to go outdoors when no staff was available to escort them (Connell, 1992). This suggests that access to secure outdoor space may provide an alternate means to satisfy some residents' desire to go outdoors, thereby reducing exiting attempts through unsecured exits. However, in a study that added a wanderer alarm system and provision of secure outdoor space, wanderers were not relocated away from exits to the outdoor space (Connell, Sanford, Megrew, & Engel, 1997). Although the outdoor spaces could be accessed directly from each of the study units, it was not feasible at any of the sites to locate the outdoor space or the entrance to it so they could be easily observed by residents or staff from frequently occupied indoor locations.

The perceptions of staff about the appeal of outdoor space is somewhat countered by studies of usual bright light exposure in long-term care residents that indicate most residents, including resident with dementia, seldom go outdoors (Ancoli-Israel et al., 1997). However, seldom going outdoors actually strengthens the importance of providing secure outdoor space, perhaps not so much as an exiting deterrent, but as a means to provide bright light exposure (important for entraining circadian rhythms and Vitamin D metabolism) to long-term care residents. Secure outdoor space also is a potentially important venue for providing meaningful stimulation to residents with dementia. However, even when a secure outdoor space is available, some residents with dementia may require encouragement and assistance from staff to go outdoors (Connell & Calkins, 2004). When residents are accustomed to going outdoors, preventing them from doing so may have negative consequences. One study found that agitation and pacing increased when doors to the outside, which were normally not secured, were locked (Namazi & Johnson, 1992).

Directional and Destination Signage

The likelihood that signage will be useful to people with dementia in wayfinding is related to three factors: its legibility, its comprehensibility, and the potential that it will be seen. Signage in most long-term care facilities is selected to be code-compliant and to fit in with the facility's décor. Accessibility codes govern some aspects of the design of official signage systems, including the minimum size of letters, the inclusion of equivalent information in Braille, and the height of signs above the floor.

Legibility

Age- and disease-based impairments in visual acuity, contrast sensitivity, color discrimination, glare sensitivity, and visual fields are common in older people (Brawley, 1997). In addition, Alzheimer's disease independently worsens vision impairment (Cronin-Golumb, 1995; Gilmore &

Whitehouse, 1995). Lighting is also important to being able to clearly see signage. Facilities with lower lighting levels in public areas have been found to be associated with more wayfinding problems among long-term care residents (Netten, 1989).

There is an extensive body of research on vision in older adults and in persons with dementia, and recommendations for the design of visual information, including signage, for older populations are available (Arditi, 2005). In short, signage in long-term care settings intended to be helpful to residents needs to use high contrast color combinations and font styles and sizes that are legible to older adults (see Figure 16.5).

Comprehensibility

Cognitive impairment affects the ability to decode abstract concepts and symbols. People with dementia may have difficulty understanding icons and euphemisms that younger adults take for granted, such as use of a

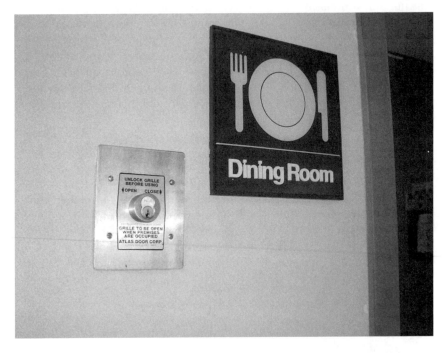

FIGURE 16.5 Dining room sign.
Very high contrast, large lettering, and exceptionally clear graphics make this an excellent sign. The lock next to the sign is somewhat distracting, although the silver color does not have much contrast with the white wall, which makes it somewhat less visible.

crossed knife and fork to indicate the dining room, and the word restroom to indicate the location of a toilet. One study compared the effect of different ways of conveying wayfinding information about a public toilet (e.g., word "restroom," word "toilet," a literal graphic showing a toilet, and directional arrows) on locating and using the toilet (Namazi & Johnson, 1991b). The sample of mildly and moderately impaired subjects were most successful in wayfinding when arrows with the word "toilet," executed in high contrast, primary colors, were placed on the floor at intervals of about three feet (see Figure 16.6). In general, signage should use literal words and actual images of objects (i.e., photographs).

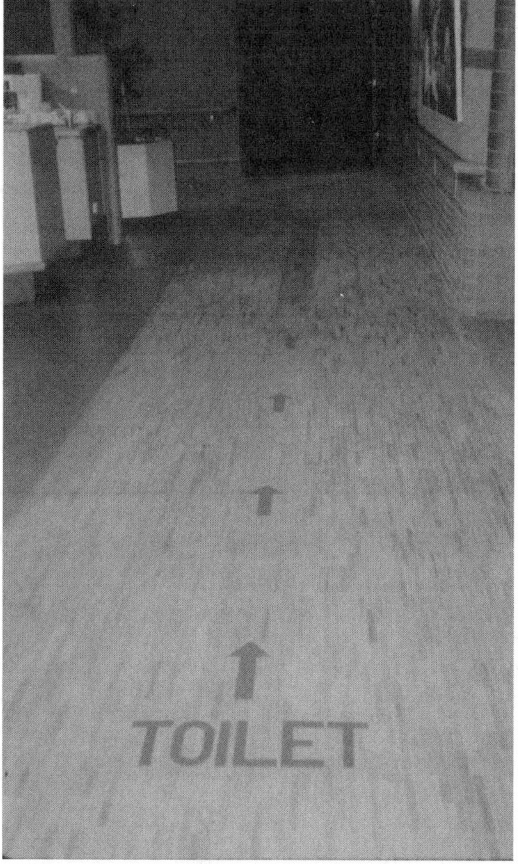

FIGURE 16.6 Toilet sign on floor.
Given the postural stance of older adults, signage on the floor may be more visible to and therefore effective than signs that are posted at typical heights.

Likelihood of Detecting Wayfinding Information

For people with dementia, wayfinding information is likely used not only to reduce errors in task performance, but also as a prompt to cue the task at hand. Individuals with dementia have been shown to use less systematic, task-oriented scanning of visual scenes than do those without dementia (Hutton, 1985; Mosimann et al., 2004). In addition, postural change and restrictions in upward gaze may influence where long-term care residents look for (or serendipitously are likely to see) wayfinding information (Hutton, 1985).

A portable, wireless eyetracker system was used to assess visual scanning patterns of nursing home residents with and without dementia during wayfinding tasks. Surprisingly, where participants looked most often was more closely related to their mode of ambulation than cognitive status. Ambulatory subjects looked most often at the lower wall and floor, and, wheelchair users looked most often at the area immediately above the handrail. The side-to-side scanning patterns of participants with cognitive impairment, while moving down a hallway searching for test signage, were less systematic than were those of participants without cognitive impairment. Some fixated on one wall, suggesting that directional signage needs to be placed on both walls. Directional signage also needs to be repeated, although an optimal interval was not examined in this study. The locations with code-compliant signage were looked at infrequently by all subjects. Additionally, test signs perpendicular to the route of travel were looked at twice as often as those parallel to the route of travel (Connell, Schuchard, & Griffiths, 2005).

Ambient Conditions

The ambient environment of long-term care facilities includes lighting conditions, noise levels, and smells encountered as one moves about a unit. Ambient conditions are important considerations in dementia care settings for two distinct reasons.

First, lighting and acoustics directly impact everyday vision and hearing functioning, which in turn influences independence in daily activities, communication, mobility, and falls risk. General and task lighting levels in long-term care settings often are lower than levels recommended for settings occupied by older adults (Brawley, 1997). There also are anecdotal reports of quieter environments improving communication and understanding between residents and staff.

Second, ambient conditions are a source of sensory stimulation. Meaningful, pleasant, and age- and culturally appropriate stimulation are believed to contribute to use of preserved communication, social, and task abilities by evoking powerful memories and cuing appropriate behaviors. In contrast, quantitatively excessive, meaningless, painful, and unpleasant stimulation may trigger agitation and behavioral disturbance in persons with dementia and should be reduced or eliminated (Hall, 1999; Hall, Kirschling, & Todd, 1986; Lawton, 1981; Perez et al., 2001). Frequently implicated sources of auditory overstimulation include alarms and auditory signals and other loud noises that have little or no meaning for residents (e.g., PA systems, call systems that use an auditory signal, housekeeping and maintenance equipment, and wanderer alarm system alarms). Staff talking loudly to each other from a distance also may fall in this category. Additional sources of overstimulation are glare and reflections that impair vision and can be painful, and unpleasant smells.

Limited research has assessed the effect of enhancing ambient conditions in persons with dementia. Cohen-Mansfield and Werner (1998) incorporated pleasant smells in their enhanced environment intervention. Although the effect of aromas could not be separated from the impact of other components, residents spent more time sitting when the enhanced environments were in place, and there was a declining trend toward reduction of some wandering behaviors.

More research has focused on quantifiable aspects of ambient conditions. Several studies of low-stimulus dementia care units that combined reductions of all types of stimulation with structured, consistent caregiving practices for residents with dementia report mixed results for reducing wandering (Cleary, Clamon, Price, & Shullaw, 1988; Swanson, Maas, & Buckwalter, 1993). Quiet long-term care environments have been associated with improved orientation (Netten, 1993).

CASE STUDIES

Case Study 1

Mrs. Barry is a 78-year-old, retired university librarian who has lived in a nursing home in her community for the last 2 years. She has a number of chronic health problems including hard-to-manage diabetes, depression, and a history of cardiovascular disease. She is frequently incontinent, has vision loss due to macular degeneration, and uses a walker. Routine testing done in the nursing home indicates she has mild–moderate cognitive impairment.

All her adult life, Mrs. Barry has walked daily "to get her exercise." When she moved into the nursing home, she incorporated walking into her daily routine, which takes her to all three floors of the nursing home, several times on most days. The dining room, patio, and one of the rooms used for planned activities are on the first floor; her room and a small lounge she uses as a living room are on the second floor; and the room of a long-time neighbor who spends most of her time in bed is on the third floor. Although staff are aware Mrs. Barry has some cognitive impairment, they have never been concerned about her walking routine. Her schedule and route are fairly predictable, and when she goes outdoors, she has never gone further than the patio.

However, Mrs. Barry recently has had some problems finding intended destinations during her daily routine, even though these are destinations she visits frequently and has done so since moving into the home. Once, while going to visit her friend on the third floor, she entered the wrong room, saw it was occupied by someone else, and became upset when she thought her friend had died and no one had told her. She had a similar problem finding her own room on returning from an evening activity on the first floor. Twice, she had incontinence episodes in the hallway on the first floor while looking for the bathroom she knew to be near the dining room. Once, she got confused traveling from her friend's room to the dining room, a departure from her usual routine, and was late arriving for dinner.

Discussion

Mrs. Barry relies on a routinized sequencing of destinations and travel routes to wayfind successfully. This reduces her need to rely extensively on vision and to some extent her memory when she is moving about the unit, and works fairly well for her except under certain circumstances. When she deviates from her usual routes, or when she needs to visually augment her wayfinding decisions, she has problems. If she gets off the elevator on the wrong resident room floor, she has difficulty readily detecting and correcting her error because both floors look alike, as do the hallways and entries to resident rooms on them. Because the elevators are placed across from each other, the direction she turns when she reaches a floor depends on the elevator she rode. She tries to avoid getting "turned around" by using only one of the elevators, but that is not always possible.

Making the elevator lobby on each floor distinctive, adding landmarks at hallway intersections, adding directional signage from the elevator and dining room to the toilet on the first floor, and personalizing resident room doors would likely be very helpful to Mrs. Barry and other residents with similar wayfinding problems. Finally, although the staff are aware of Mrs. Barry's cognitive deficits, they think of her as a dedicated exerciser, not as a person who has problems wayfinding some of the time. Consequently, they have not recognized her need for verbal cues and prompts, particularly at the times of day and under the circumstances she is tired, stressed, or breaking her routine. The danger is that when they realize she does have wayfinding problems, they will overreact, classifying her as at risk of exiting and restricting her walking range. A more appropriate response would be to identify the times of day and circumstances when Mrs. Barry has wayfinding problems and to provide verbal prompts accordingly. Because Mrs. Barry travels to all parts of the nursing home, it will be important to enlist the cooperation of all staff in providing cueing when and where it is necessary. It also is important for staff to work with Mrs. Barry to help her learn to recognize the new landmarks and room cues and to incorporate them into the verbal assistance that is provided.

Case Study 2

Mr. Allen is a retired plumbing contractor. When he retired, he and his wife relocated to a small town in another state in order to be near their only daughter and her family. Almost exactly 1 year after moving, Mr. Allen's left leg was amputated below the knee due to cardiovascular disease, and he began to use a wheelchair. They made a few home modifications to make it easier for him to get in and out and around the house in his wheelchair. Two years later, he was diagnosed with probable Alzheimer's disease. Over the next year, he became increasingly uncooperative when Mrs. Allen tried to assist him with transfers, and he began to leave the house without Mrs. Allen's knowledge. Mrs. Allen was afraid he was going to be hit by a car, or get lost and not be found. Her daughter, whose job and family prevented her from helping her mother much, was afraid the stress her mother experienced as a caregiver was detrimental to her health. After several months of escalating problems, Mrs. Allen was persuaded it was time to place her husband in long-term care. The area is fairly rural, and the closest facility that admitted persons with dementia was 20 miles away.

At any time, at least half the residents of the facility have dementia and many of them wander. After one resident left and was not found for 3 days, a wanderer alarm system was installed. Now, all new residents with a history of wandering away from home are fitted with a wanderer alarm system tag on admission. Emergency exits at the end of resident room hallways are equipped with automatic locking devices, but if a resident wearing a wanderer alarm system tag exits through a unit's main exit, only the alarm goes off, at 90 dB or louder so staff will be sure to hear it. Each unit's main exit can be observed from the unit's nurses station, but staff spend little time there except when charting. Each unit's main exit opens into a lobby area, which provides access to the central dining room and to several exits to the outside.

Several years ago, the units were painted different colors (pale blue, pale green, pale yellow) and some families decorate resident room doors, but there is little other evidence of environmental modifications for residents with dementia. Staff are warm and caring, but training in dementia caregiving techniques has been limited, although the orientation for new employees includes review of facility procedures for locating residents who exit. The activities program is staffed by a fairly new employee who used to work at an independent living facility. She has limited experience in programming for people with dementia, although she tries to include these residents into the programs she offers now and has offered a few programs specifically for residents with dementia.

Most residents, including those who are at risk of wandering, go off-unit daily for meals in the central dining room. Residents with dementia also attend scheduled activity programs in the central activities room, also located in the lobby. Staff turn off the wanderer alarm system while they transport residents to and from meals and activities.

Mr. Allen's disorientation worsened following admission. He continues to frequently ask staff "who are you" and "what is this place?" He remains highly mobile in his wheelchair, but frequently appears to have no apparent destination. He has been found in other residents' rooms on several occasions looking through their chest of drawers. When staff determined that Mr. Allen routinely woke up around 5 A.M., for a while he was one of the first residents to receive morning care. However, this resulted in his being dressed and in his wheelchair by 6 A.M., even though breakfast is not served until 7:30. Some mornings Mr. Allen followed staff from room to room; other mornings he exited the unit and triggered the wanderer alarm system while staff were completing morning care with other residents. When staff tried delaying his morning care until closer to time for breakfast, his agitation as well as incontinence increased.

Mrs. Allen is only able to visit two or three afternoons a week, but most days Mr. Allen begins asking about and looking for his wife shortly after lunch. Staff try to get him to join after-lunch activities, but he usually fidgets and never stays long. Recently, he has begun to go outside during the time residents are being transported to and from the dining room and activity room, and has been found in the parking lot, stating that he is looking for his wife.

Discussion

Outside of his wife's visits, little happens to engage Mr. Allen. He is functioning at a lower level than he was at home. Personalizing his room door with pictures from his past (e.g., of his wife when they were first married, his daughter when she was young, his old Army buddies, his employees) would help to make his room entry personal and distinctive. However, staff would need to work with him, such as by engaging in repeated conversations about the pictures and referring to the pictures when directing him to his room, for the pictures to become functional as a wayfinding aid. Adding landmarks to make choice points more distinctive would be simple to do.

Mr. Allen's greatest need is for access to resources that engage his preserved abilities and provide an alternative to going outside to look for his wife as a means to obtain meaningful stimulation. However, unlike most of the residents, Mr. Allen has no history with other residents or with the staff. They know little about him or his past. However, Mrs. Allen and her daughter, if asked, can help staff to come up with ideas about resources that can be provided to help engage him vicariously as well as actively. For example, as a retired plumber, a box of pieces of plastic pipe and fittings and other plumbing parts that he can repeatedly put together and take apart may engage him, particularly if it is readily available at times when care or meals are not scheduled. Additionally, he (and other residents) may be fond of music from the '50s, and staff could play CDs during unstructured times of the day. If he used to grow prized tomatoes, mounting an inexpensive poster at eye level that shows a plate of tomatoes can lead to conversations with other residents and staff about growing tomatoes, tomato sandwiches, and his mother canning tomatoes, as well as incorporate the image from the poster into conversations to cue upcoming activities such as meals or a horticulture program to be held on the patio.

Mr. Allen's ability to leave the group heading for the dining room or during activities, and then make his way out to the parking lot, suggests that taking him off the unit is teaching him how to leave. Setting up a small dining and activity area on the unit for residents like Mr. Allen who frequently exit or attempt to exit reduces the need to regularly take them off unit. Exit doors and frames could be painted the same color as the walls to make them harder for residents with dementia to detect.

There are several possible reasons Mr. Allen shows little interest in the after-lunch activities. Despite the efforts of activities staff, the programs may be too cognitively demanding for him, the room may get too noisy for him, or the activities may not be things he is interested in doing. Several changes may be helpful. Offering activities to a smaller group of residents with dementia would allow staff to more easily tailor programming to interests and abilities of residents with dementia and could help to limit noise and potential distractions associated with the number of people present. Offering it on-unit and in a quieter location would reduce noise and further limit potential distractions (from noise, views of outside, other residents, and staff) that may be present in the usual activity space. It also would have the advantage of not forcing a choice between limiting travel off-unit and participation in activities. Mr. Allen's wife could help staff to learn of his interests in order to offer activities that appeal to them.

In addition to increasing the availability of meaningful stimulation for Mr. Allen, the staff should look for ways to reduce sources of meaningless excessive stimulation. If a new wanderer alarm system that sends signals to pagers worn by staff is not affordable, they could investigate having the auditory alarm converted to a less aversive sound (e.g., play a distinctive song—one facility had their alarm play "I Am a Happy Wanderer") or use the system to send a different kind of signal (e.g., blinking lights). Use of overhead PA systems could be restricted to emergency announcements, volume of telephone and fax ringers lowered, acoustical paneling added to hallways to reduce how far sounds travel, and so forth. Poor lighting should be improved and glare and reflection reduced.

PRACTICE IMPLICATIONS

Suggestions for practical solutions that are either evidence-based or best practices have been provided throughout the chapter. There are, however, a few additional considerations that should be mentioned.

First and foremost, although the focus of this chapter was on physical environmental interventions to accommodate the person who wanders, the physical environment itself is only one facet of what must ultimately be a multifaceted approach. How caregivers understand and use environmental resources is equally, if not more, important. This is demonstrated by a post-occupancy evaluation of a dementia assisted living facility, where, after occupying the building for a year, researchers asked staff whether the residents used the color coding of the three wings to maintain orientation. Despite the fact that the color codes were linked to the theme of each wing and the smocks that staff wore, the staff were completely unaware of the color coding, and thus never pointed it out to the residents. Not surprisingly, staff did not think the color coding was effective for residents (Hoglund et al., 1994). This also illustrates the importance of familiarizing staff with environmental resources and how to incorporate them into caregiving.

Clearly, how staff use and reinforce the environmental cues that are available may be as important as their existence. Whether the goal is accommodating or preventing wandering, staff should view their role in the same light as the rest of their care-related interactions with residents. The goal is to support residents' abilities and autonomy to the greatest extent feasible. Repeatedly referring to highly visible cues to help a resident learn how to successfully navigate the unit and find their desired destinations is better than just taking the resident there.

A second important consideration is ensuring environmental interventions have adequate breadth and intensity. In addition to ensuring that the role of staff in residents' environmental use is understood and incorporated into care practices, it is critical to ensure that the right environmental changes and enough changes are made to achieve desired goals. In most cases, there are multiple interventions that can be expected to be helpful in addressing a specific problem. However, related interventions are often bundled in research studies, and it is not clear what the minimum set of components are to achieve minimal efficacy, for example, how many aversive noise sources have to be eliminated to avoid overstimulation, or how much painting, landmarking, and personalization is needed to be minimally effective in supporting independent wayfinding. Additionally, it is unknown which are the most critical changes and what the "value added" is for including additional components. If all you can afford to do is paint hallways and doors distinctive colors, is that enough to make a clinically significant improvement in problems residents experience in locating their rooms? The best answer at this time probably is, "it depends"—on how many residents are involved, how creative staff and families can be in finding ways to personalize room entries inexpensively, how much staff will compensate for inadequate directional and destination signage through verbal prompting, and so forth.

Finally, resident boredom is an important and correctable problem that has been associated with wandering (Kolanowski, Hurwitz, Taylor, Evans, & Strumpf, 1994; Perez et al., 2001). Lack of appropriate levels of engaging stimulation leads people with dementia to go in search of something more meaningful to them or more compatible with their tolerance for stimulation. Although formal, structured programming is critically important for residents with dementia in long-term care, ensuring appropriately engaging stimulation cannot be relegated solely to activities programming and activities staff. Access to secure outdoor space that is thoughtfully planned and landscaped can be enjoyed actively or vicariously, and raised planting beds that allow residents to "play in the dirt" alleviate boredom for some residents. For others, opportunities to listen to music, fold towels, and even tinker with an old car engage and stimulate. Importantly, these are activities that many residents are able to continue on their own once staff get them started. When the environment is structured so staff have a wealth of activity-based resources that appeal to different interests and different types and levels of preserved abilities, residents are more likely to be content and to spend less time walking around or attempting to leave the unit.

METHODOLOGICAL ISSUES

Sample Size and Study Design

Environmentally oriented wandering research has been plagued by the prevalence of small sample sizes, extensive reliance on case-study designs, and lack of comparison groups (Weisman, Calkins, & Sloane, 1994). For a number of reasons, wandering-oriented environmental research is usually conducted in field, not laboratory, settings. Sample size and study design problems are related to several realities of conducting environmental research in long-term care settings that are difficult to overcome.

The number of potentially eligible subjects at any single participating facility is usually limited. Increasing sample sizes typically involves participation of multiple facilities, which increases the cost and complexity of studies, and may introduce site level differences. In other types of applied geriatric research, site differences are usually accounted for by randomizing subjects at each site into intervention and control groups. However, environmental interventions are usually unit-level interventions. Thus, units, not individuals, need to be randomized, requiring a minimum of two study units at each site if randomization is to occur. Although most long-term care facilities have multiple units with long-stay residents with dementia who wander, these different units may vary in ways that impact the units' equivalency for purposes of randomization. For example, dementia special care units usually have fewer residents, are more self-contained, and may offer more activities programming for people with dementia than is the case for traditional units with mixed populations of residents with and without dementia. Some, but not all, provide a more supportive environment than do traditional units with mixed populations. Additionally, in most facilities, there are differences between residents with dementia residing in special care units and those residing in traditional units with mixed populations, and these differences may be important for some studies. For example, individuals with a history of exiting are not admitted to some facilities unless they can be placed on a unit with some type of exit control system. At these facilities, residents eligible for a study on environmental interventions to reduce exiting may all live on one unit.

Scope of Interventions

Some environmentally oriented wandering research has focused on single factor interventions or interventions with closely linked intervention components bundled together. Other environmentally oriented wandering research has occurred as part of research where the entire unit or building (accompanied by more staff, more staff training in dementia care, increased programming, etc.) is the intervention. The first approach has greater opportunity for scientific rigor and, potentially, unpacking the relative merits of intervention components, but the second, when done well, has greater ecological validity, recognizing the complex confluence of physical, social, and organizational factors that impact the setting and resident outcomes.

Difficulties of Evaluating Design Interventions

Evaluating design interventions pose challenges that are not common in studies evaluating other types of interventions in dementia care settings. Unlike research evaluating other types of interventions, for example training programs, when the study is over environmental interventions may remain whether or not successful or embraced by staff. If interventions are to be provided as part of research studies, some sponsors may question using research dollars to fund what they may see as capital improvements. Although "free" environmental modifications may be appealing to some administrators and staff, others may decline participation due to lack of facility control over a standardized research intervention. If researchers capitalize on "naturally occurring interventions" they may have concerns about their lack of control over the intervention and its implementation, including training care staff in intentions for its use with residents.

In multisite studies, it is difficult, if not impossible, to achieve fidelity of physical environment interventions across sites, particularly more complex, multicomponent interventions, because of differences in the overall design of different long-term care facilities and units. Conversely, if studies are done only at one site or at multiple sites with similar designs, results may not generalize well to sites with other designs.

Because staff play an important role in residents' use of environmental interventions and thus in assessing their effect on resident outcomes, researchers need to grapple with if or how staff roles will be dealt with as part of an intervention study. In general, the choices are for the research study to provide care related to the intervention or to train indigenous staff to fill this role. Providing care as part of the project can be costly, but indigenous staff may not consistently implement training in how to support residents' use of the interventions, likely weakening the intervention's effect.

Description of Interventions

Descriptions of interventions, and the larger context they are a part of, are often missing from research reports. Mixed and seemingly counter-intuitive results may be explained by missing details, such as fundamental differences in how interventions with the same name are designed, site differences that affect how standardized interventions are implemented across sites, and unmeasured differences in other environmental conditions. The availability of such descriptions would aid researchers in evaluating research findings and in replicating studies. They also would aid administrators and practitioners seeking to determine if proven solutions to wandering problems can be readily adopted at their facility.

GAPS IN RESEARCH

Most of what is advocated to address problems of wandering through environmental design comes more from thoughtful people who have seen a lot of what does not work and what does, than from research. At present, research that would be considered definitive by scientific standards has not been completed with regard to environmental design of long-term care settings and wandering. In many ways, the gaps in research have more to do with methodological issues than with topics yet to be addressed. However, there are some topics that have received limited attention and should be addressed in future research.

Environmental interventions to address wandering problems have been adapted by special care units and by traditional units whose residents include individuals with dementia, and in the context of new construction and renovation projects. Studies that compare the same intervention packages in these different applications would be particularly helpful to administrators and staff seeking to make decisions about the best interventions to target wandering in the context of their facilities.

Additionally, little is known about how interventions for wanderers impact other resident groups. There is reason to expect many environmental interventions that target problems experienced by residents who wander may also benefit residents with dementia who do not wander, as well as residents without dementia. For example, increasing the visual distinctiveness of decision points and destinations may also be helpful to residents with vision impairment, whether or not they have dementia.

SIDEBAR

- When doors and curtains were opened to allow in-room toilets to be seen from outside resident rooms, residents entered and used the toilets more often.
- How staff use and reinforce the wayfinding cues that are available may be as important as their existence. Repeatedly referring to highly visible cues to help a resident learn how to successfully navigate the unit and find their desired destinations is better than just taking the resident there.
- Ensuring appropriately engaging stimulation cannot be relegated solely to activities programming. When the environment is structured so staff have a wealth of activity-based resources that appeal to different interests and cognitive-function levels, residents are more likely to be content and not need to spend time walking around or attempting to leave.
- Although more extensive changes to address wandering problems are likely feasible in new long-term care facilities, existing facilities not planned for, but serving, people with dementia can incorporate numerous small scale design changes to enhance functioning and reduce environmental demands for residents with dementia.

CONCLUSION

Long-term care residents with dementia often experience excess disability as a result of the excessive environmental demands they experience in care settings not planned for their needs and abilities. With respect to wandering, environmental characteristics of long-term care settings not planned for residents with dementia often result in insufficient meaningful stimulation, excessive meaningless stimulation, inadequate visual access and cuing to locate and identify desired destinations, and too great an opportunity to leave the unit unobserved. There are a number of design approaches that are promising as a means to allow residents with dementia to use their preserved abilities to the fullest extent possible to remain engaged with the world around them, improve wayfinding, and reduce exiting, while helping staff to ensure their safety. These approaches have been evaluated through research and practice, and there are many that can be implemented as modifications to existing facilities as well as included in new construction.

Although more extensive changes to address wandering problems are likely feasible in new long-term care facilities, existing facilities not planned for, but serving, people with dementia can incorporate numerous small scale design changes to enhance functioning and reduce environmental demands for residents with dementia. Moreover, some design improvements can be addressed as part of routine maintenance, such as selecting paint colors that enhance the distinctiveness of resident room doors and reducing the distinctiveness of exits that residents who wander should not use without an escort. Other changes can be implemented through handyman type projects, such as changing the hinges so hall toilet room doors can be left open and visible to residents. Facilities can experiment with augmenting existing signage systems for residents with wayfinding problems by adding temporary signs produced on a color printer and placed where they are likely to be seen. Many proven techniques can be accomplished inexpensively or at no cost, such as by using large potted plants, or moving an existing distinctive piece of furniture to serve as landmarks.

Staff play a key role in helping residents to use supportive environments, thereby reducing wandering. How staff use and reinforce wayfinding cues in daily interactions with residents may be as important as the fact the cues are there. Resources that provide meaningful stimulation to residents during discretionary time will often go unused unless direct care staff provide an appropriate level of assistance to help residents access these resources.

Boredom has been associated with wandering, and residents need meaningful stimulation during discretionary time, which for people with dementia is anytime they are awake and not engaged in care or a structured activity designed for their preserved abilities. It is important to remember that what is meaningful to residents may differ from that thought to be meaningful to them by staff who do not know the residents well and by design professionals with a limited understanding of dementia. Although structured programs geared to the interests and abilities of residents with dementia are important, structured programming is unlikely to be available during all the times residents are awake but not engaged in care, meals, or planned activities. The availability of resources that offer meaningful stimulation during these times is critical as are efforts to reduce sources of stimulation that are meaningless to residents with dementia.

RESOURCES

Alzheimer's Association. (1997). *Key elements of dementia care.* Chicago, IL: Alzheimer's Association.

Brawley, E. (2005). *Design innovations for aging and Alzheimer's disease: Creating caring environments.* New York: John Wiley and Sons.

Calkins, M. (2001). *Creating successful dementia care settings* (Vols. 1–4). Baltimore, MD: Health Professions Press.

Cohen, U., & Weisman, J. (1991). *Holding on to home: Designing environments for people with dementia.* Baltimore, MD: Johns Hopkins University Press.

Silverstein, N. M., Flaherty, G., & Tobin, T. S. (2002). *Dementia and wandering behavior: Concern for the lost elder.* New York: Springer Publishing Co.

Warner, M. (2006). *In search of the Alzheimer's wandered: A workbook to protect your loved ones.* West Lafayette, IN: Purdue University Press.

REFERENCES

Algase, D. (1992). Cognitive discriminants of wandering among nursing home residents. *Nursing Research, 41*(2), 78–81.

Algase, D. L., Beck, C., Kolanowski, A., Whall, A., Berent, S., Richards, K., et al. (1996). Need-driven dementia-compromised behavior: An alternative view of disruptive behavior. *American Journal of Alzheimer's Disease, 11*(6), 10–19.

Algase, D. L., Kupferschmid, B., Beel-Bates, C. A., & Beattie, E.R.A. (1997). Estimates of stability of daily wandering behavior among cognitively impaired long-term care residents. *Nursing Research, 46*(3), 172–178.

Allen, G. L. (1999). Spatial abilities, cognitive maps, and wayfinding. Bases for individual differences in spatial cognition and behavior. In R.G. Gollege (Ed.), *Wayfinding behavior* (pp. 46–80). Baltimore, MD: Johns Hopkins University Press.

Ancoli-Israel, S., Klauber, M. R., Jones, D. W., Kripke, D. F., Martin, J., Mason, W., et al. (1997). Variations in circadian rhythms of activity, sleep, and light exposure related to dementia in nursing-home patients. *Sleep, 20*(1), 18–23.

Anthony, K., Proctor, A. W., Silverman, A. M., & Murphy, E. (1987). Mood and behaviour problems following the relocations of elderly patients with mental illness. *Age and Ageing, 16*(6), 355–365.

Arditi, A. (2005). Enhancing the visual environment for older and visually impaired persons. *Alzheimer's Care Quarterly,* 6(4), 294–299.

Baskaya, A., Wilson, C., & Ozcan, Y. Z. (2004). Wayfinding in an unfamiliar environment: Different spatial settings of two polyclinics. *Environment & Behavior, 36*(6), 839–867.

Bertram, M. (1989). The use of landmarks. *Journal of Gerontological Nursing, 14*(2), 6–8.

Brawley, E. (1997). *Designing for Alzheimer's disease: Strategies for better care environments.* New York: John Wiley and Sons.

Calkins, M. P. (1988). *Design for dementia: Planning environments for the elderly and the confused.* Owings Mills, MD: National Health Publishing.

Calkins, M. (2001). *Creating successful dementia care settings* (Vols. 1–4). Baltimore, MD: Health Professions Press.

Calkins, M. P. (2006). Personal Communication.

Chafetz, P. K. (1991). Behavioral and cognitive outcomes of SCU care. *Clinical Gerontologist, 11*(1), 19–38.

Cleary, T. A., Clamon, C., Price, M., & Shullaw, G. (1988). A reduced stimulus unit: Effects on patients with Alzheimer's disease and related disorders. *The Gerontologist, 28*(4), 511–514.

Cohen, U., & Weisman, J. (1991). *Holding on to home: Designing environments for people with dementia.* Baltimore, MD: Johns Hopkins University Press.

Cohen-Mansfield, J. (1986). Agitated behaviors in the elderly II. Preliminary results in the cognitively deteriorated. *Journal of the American Geriatrics Society, 24*(10), 722–727.

Cohen-Mansfield, J. (1991). The agitated nursing home resident. In M. S. Harper (Ed.), *Management and care of the elderly: Psychosocial perspectives* (pp. 89–103). Newbury Park, CA: Sage Publications.

Cohen-Mansfield, J., & Werner, P. (1998). The effects of an enhanced environment on nursing home residents who pace. *The Gerontologist, 38*(2), 199–208.

Connell, B. R. (1992). *'Elopement' opportunities among dementia patients in nursing homes: Architectural considerations.* Unpublished doctoral dissertation, Georgia Institute of Technology, Atlanta, GA.

Connell, B. R., & Calkins, M. (2004). Going outdoors is good for you: Research on the design of outdoor spaces for nursing homes and therapeutic benefits of their use by residents with dementia. In D. Miller & J. A. Wise (Eds.), *Proceedings of 35th Annual Conference of The Environmental Design Research Association,* 175.

Connell, B. R., & McConnell, E. S. (2000). Treating excess disability among cognitively impaired nursing home residents. *Journal of the American Geriatrics Society, 48*(4), 454–455.

Connell, B. R., McConnell, E. S., Mancil, G., & Coombs, T. (2001). Effect of vision status on behavior disturbance in NH residents with dementia. *The Gerontologist, 40*(S1), 379.

Connell, B. R., Sanford, J. A., Megrew, M. B., & Engel, P. A. (1997). Evaluation of environmental interventions for exiting behavior of dementia patients. *The Gerontologist, 37*(S1), 159.

Connell, B. R., Schuchard, R., & Griffiths, P. (2005). Wayfinding in nursing home residents. *The Gerontologist, 45*(S-II), 494.

Coons, D. (1988). Wandering. *The American Journal of Alzheimer's Care & Related Disorders and Research, 3*(1), 31–36.

Cronin-Golumb, A. (1995). Vision in Alzheimer's disease. *The Gerontologist, 35*(3), 370–376.

Dawson, P., Wells, D. L., & Kline, K. (1993). *Enhancing the abilities of persons with Alzheimer's and related dementias: A nursing perspective.* New York: Springer.

Day, K., & Calkins, M. P. (2002). Design and dementia. In R.B.A. Churchman (Ed.), *Handbook of environmental psychology.* New York: John Wiley & Sons.

Day, K., Carreon, D., & Stump, C. (2000). The therapeutic design of environments for people with dementia: a review of empirical research. *The Gerontologist. 40*(4), 397–416.

Dickinson, J. L., McLain-Kark, J., & Marshall-Baker, A. (1995). The effects of visual barriers on exiting behavior in a demented care unit. *The Gerontologist, 35*(1), 127–130.

Gilmore, G. C., & Whitehouse., P. J. (1995). Contrast sensitivity in Alzheimer's disease: A 1-year longitudinal analysis. *Optometry and Vision Science, 72*(2), 83–91.

Hall, G. R. (1999). When traditional care falls short. Caring for people with atypical presentation of dementia. *Journal of Gerontological Nursing, 25*(2), 22–32.

Hall, G. R., Kirschling, M. V., & Todd, S. (1986). Sheltered freedom—an Alzheimer's unit in an ICF. *Geriatric Nursing, 7*(3), 132–137.

Hanley, I. G. (1981). The use of signposts and active training to modify ward disorientation in elderly patients. *Journal of Behavioral Therapy and Experimental Psychiatry, 12*(3), 241–247.

Henderson, V. W., Mack, W., & Williams, B. W. (1989). Spatial disorientation in Alzheimer's disease. *Archives of Neurology, 46*(4), 391–394.

Hogan, M. J. (2003). Divided attention in older but not younger adults is impaired by anxiety. *Experimental Aging Research, 29*(2), 111–136.

Hoglund, J. D., Dimotta, S., Ledewitz, S., & Saxton, J. (1994). Long-term care design: Woodside Place—the role of environmental design in quality of life for residents with dementia. *Journal of Healthcare Design, 6,* 69–76.

Hussian, R. (1987). Wandering and disorientation. In L. Carstensen & B. Edelstein (Eds.), *Handbook of clinical gerontology* (pp. 177–189). New York: Pergamon Press.

Hussian, R., & Brown, D. (1987). Use of two-dimensional grid patterns to limit hazardous ambulation in demented patients. *Journal of Gerontology, 42(5)*, 558–560.

Hutton, J. T. (1985). Eye movements in Alzheimer's disease: Significance and relationship to visuospatial confusion. In J.T. Hutton & A. D. Kenny (Eds.), *Senile dementia of the Alzheimer type* (pp. 3–33). New York: Alan R. Liss.

Judd, S., Marshall, M., & Phippen, P. (1998). *Design for dementia.* London, England: Journal of Dementia Care, Hawker Publications Ltd.

Kirasic, K. C. (2000). Age differences in adults' spatial abilities, learning environmental layout, and wayfinding behavior. *Spatial Cognition and Computation, 2*(2), 117–134.

Kolanowski, A. M., Hurwitz, S., Taylor, L. A., Evans, L., & Strumpf, N. (1994). Contextual factors associated with disturbing behaviors in institutionalized elderly. *Nursing Research, 43*(2), 73–79.

Lawton, M. P. (1981). Sensory deprivation and the effect of the environment on management of the senile dementia patient. In N. Miller & G. Cohen (Eds.), *Clinical studies of Alzheimer's disease and senile dementia* (pp. 227–251). New York: Raven Press.

Lawton, M. P., Fulcomer, M., & Kleban, M. (1984). Architecture for the mentally impaired elderly. *Environment and Behavior, 16*(6), 730–757.

Lawton, M. P., & Nahemow, L. (1973). Ecology and the aging process. In C. Eisdorfer & M. P. Lawton (Eds.), *Psychology of adult development and aging* (pp. 619–674). Washington, D.C.: American Psychological Association.

Liu, L., Gauthier, L., & Gauthier, S. (1991). Spatial disorientation in persons with early senile dementia of the Alzheimer's type. *American Journal of Occupational Therapy, 45*(1), 67–74.

Martino-Saltzman, D., Blasch, B. B., Morris, R. D., & McNeal, L. W. (1991). Travel behavior of nursing home residents perceived as wanderers and nonwanderers. *The Gerontologist, 31*, 666–672.

Morgan, D. G., & Stewart, N. J. (1998). High versus low density special care units: Impact on the behavior of elderly residents with dementia. *Canadian Journal on Aging, 17*(2), 143–165.

Mosimann, U. P., Felblinger, J., Ballinari, P., Hess, C. W., & Muri, R. M. (2004). Visual exploration behavior during clock reading in Alzheimer's disease. *Brain, 127*(Pt 2), 431–438.

Namazi, K. H., & Johnson, B. D. (1991a). Environmental effects on incontinence problems in Alzheimer's disease patients. *The American Journal of Alzheimer's Care and Related Disorders & Research*, 6(6), 16–21.

Namazi, K. H., & Johnson, B. D. (1991b). Physical environmental cues to reduce the problems of incontinence in Alzheimer disease units. *The American Journal of Alzheimer's Care and Related Disorders & Research*, 6(6), 22–28.

Namazi, K. H., & Johnson, B. D. (1992). Pertinent autonomy for residents with dementias: Modification of the physical environment to enhance independence. *The American Journal of Alzheimer's Care and Related Disorders & Research, 7*(1), 16–21.

Namazi, K., Rosner, T., & Calkins, M. (1989). Visual barriers to prevent ambulatory Alzheimer's patients from exiting through an emergency door. *The Gerontologist, 29*(5), 699–702.

Namazi, K. H., Rosner, T. T., & Rechlin, L. R. (1991). Long-term memory cuing to reduce visuo-spatial disorientation in Alzheimer's disease patients is a special care unit. *The American Journal of Alzheimer's Care and Related Disorders & Research*, 6(6), 10–15.

Netten, A. (1989). The effect of design of residential homes in creating dependency among confused elderly residents: A study of elderly demented residents and their ability to find their way around homes for the elderly. *International Journal of Geriatric Psychiatry, 4*(3), 143–153.

Netten, A. (1993). *A positive environment? Physical and social influences on people with senile dementia in residential care.* Aldershot, England: Ashgate.

Nolan, B., Mathews, R., Truesdell-Todd, G., & VanDorp, A. (2002). Evaluation of the effect of orientation cues on wayfinding in persons with dementia. *Alzheimer's Care Quarterly, 3*(1), 46–49.

Norris-Baker, L., Weisman, G., Lawton, M. P., Sloane, P., & Kaup, M. (1999). Assessing special care units for dementia: The professional environmental assessment protocol. In E. Steinfeld & G. S. Danford (Eds.), *Enabling environments: Measuring the impact of environment on disability and rehabilitation* (pp. 165–182). New York: Plenum.

Passini, R., Rainville, C., Marchand, N., & Joanette, Y. (1995). Wayfinding in dementia of the Alzheimer's type: Planning abilities. *Journal of Clinical and Experimental Neuropsychology, 17*(6), 820–832.

Perez, K., Proffitt, M., & Calkins, M. (2001). *Minimizing disruptive behaviors* (Vol. 3). Baltimore, MD: Health Professions Press.

Ryan, J. P. McGowan, J., McCaffrey, N., Ryan, G. T., Zandi, T., & Brannigan, G. G. (1995). Graphomotor perseveration and wandering in Alzheimer's disease. *Journal of Geriatric Psychiatry and Neurology, 8*(4), 209–212.

Sanford, J., Fazenbaker, S., & Connell, B. R. (1992). Alarm system technology in elopement prevention. *Technology and Disability, 2*(1), 22–33.

Sloane, P. D., Mitchell, C. M., Weisman, G., Zimmerman, S. I., Long, K. M., Lynn, M., et al. (2002). The Therapeutic Environment Screening Scale for Nursing Homes (TESS-NH): An observational instrument for assessing institutional environments for persons with dementia. *Journal of Gerontology, 57B*(2), S69–S78.

Swanson, E. A., Maas, M. L., & Buckwalter, K. C. (1993). Catastrophic reactions and other behaviors of Alzheimer's residents: Special units compared with traditional units. *Archives of Psychiatric Nursing, 7*(5), 292–299.

Weisman, G., Calkins, M., & Sloane, P. (1994). The environmental context of special care. *Alzheimer's Disease and Associated Disorders, 8*(Supp. 1), S308–S320.

West, R. (1999). Visual distraction, working memory, and aging. *Memory and Cognition, 27*(6), 1064–1072.

Yao, L., & Algase, D. (2006). Environmental ambience as a new window on wandering. *Western Journal of Nursing Research, 28*(1), 89–94.

Zeisel, J., Hyde, J., & Levkoff, S. (1994). Best practices: An environment-behavior model for Alzheimer special care units. *The American Journal of Alzheimer's Care and Related Disorders & Research, 9*(2), 4–21.

CHAPTER SEVENTEEN

Evidence-Based Practice Protocols for Wandering

Elizabeth R. A. Beattie and Laura M. Struble

Those who are enamored of practice without science are like a pilot who goes into a ship without rudder or compass and never has any certainty where he is going. Practice should always be based upon sound knowledge of theory.

Leonardo da Vinci, Notebooks, 1508–1518

It has become a crucial mission in the core health care disciplines to make clinical decisions based on the best available scientific evidence. This follows a paradigm shift to evidence-based practice, beginning in medicine in the nineteenth century. Sackett and colleagues defined evidence-based medicine as the "conscientious, explicit, and judicious use of current best evidence in making decisions about the care of individual patients" (Sackett, Rosenberg, Gray, Haynes, & Richardson, 1996, p. 71). The best evidence must then be applied by a clinician with expertise in considering the unique values and needs of the person. The final aspect of the evidence-based practice process is evaluation of the "effectiveness of care and the continual improvement of the process" (DePalma, 2000). Thus, the goals of evidence-based practice are to deliver effective care based on the best research; resolve problems in the clinical setting; achieve excellence in care delivery, even exceeding quality assurance standards; and introduce innovation (Grinspun, Virani, & Bajnok, 2001/2002). Evidenced-based practice is supported by the Agency for Health Care Policy and Research (AHCPR) who support the use of clinical guidelines to reflect best practice in multiple disciplines.

The culture of evidence-based practice has deepened and extended over the last decade, making the expectation of best practice protocol development, and adherence to protocol, the norm for quality assurance within many health-related disciplines and care circumstances. Research from multiple disciplines confirms the outcomes of evidence-based practice as resulting in better patient care (Newhouse, 2006). For example, it has been reported that patients who receive research-based nursing care make "sizable gains" in behavioral knowledge and physiological and psychosocial outcome compared with those receiving routine nursing care (Heater, Becker, & Olson, 1988). The purpose of this chapter is to review the current status of evidence-based practice in wandering and identify challenges to the development of an evidence base for excellent clinical practice.

To develop and carry out evidence-based practice we must have sufficient theory-driven, empirically tested, published intervention research on wandering behavior and skill in accessing and critically analyzing research. The practice freedom and autonomy to implement changes in practice that are determined likely to produce better patient outcomes is also essential. Wandering behavior associated with dementia is an excellent target for evidence-based practice, because elements of the behavior are high risk and can result in injury or death. Wandering also occurs in multiple community contexts within and beyond the home, and in acute and long-term care settings. Thus, any evidence-based practice requires relevance to, and applicability in, multiple, complex settings. It is imperative to generate evidenced-based practice specific to wandering because, as with other complex behaviors, ineffective care may easily be delivered in response to the high risk aspects of the behavior while lower risk issues tend to be overlooked yet have insidious long-term impact. Traditionally wandering has been seen as one of a cluster of behavioral symptoms exhibited by persons with dementia. Thus, management strategies, in the absence of empirical evidence, have tended to target symptom clusters with arguably different, sometimes conflicting and overlapping, etiologies or root causes. Haphazard, often creative, problem solving has emerged from an intuitive practice base, but this does not necessarily improve the overall quality or process of care and patient outcomes and may result in increased caregiver burden (Miyamoto, Ito, Otsuka, & Kurita, 2002). Adopting traditional approaches to care with questionable validity can lead to the use of ineffective interventions and more importantly may cause harm to patients who wander if the person strays into unsafe territories. In addition, an intuition-based practice may be inconsistent with patient and family values. For example, physically retraining, restricting movement, or using loud alarms attached to patients are upsetting to patients and families.

CHALLENGES TO THE DEVELOPMENT OF EVIDENCE-BASED PRACTICE FOR WANDERING

Wandering as a "Problem" Behavior

An important issue for the science of wandering has been the idea that wandering is not a problematic behavior for persons with dementia. This issue has arisen from the notion that a wanderer is only suffering if their behavior is intrusive to others, or places them at high risk, and that, indeed wandering provides exercise benefits that outweigh the potentially detrimental aspects of the behavior. In the absence of definitive studies that reveal the subjective experience of wandering, the Need-Driven Dementia Compromised Behavior (NDB) model (described previously in Chapter 2) proffers a lens for considering the multiple facets of wandering as meeting extant need. Further, the impact of wandering on the performance of functional activities of daily living, while yet to be extensively explored by research, can be well-described by any first-line caregiver (see discussion in Chapter 6). When considering potential harm to the person with dementia it is useful to think of wandering behavior as occurring on a continuum of activity level, with some low frequency, duration, and intensity wandering causing minimal issues for the person with dementia or their caregiver (see Case Study #1). On the other end of the continuum wanderers who experience frequent, prolonged walking without rest or distraction, and whose wandering involves safety issues,

Case Study #1

It is still early morning in the assisted living facility (ALF), at least an hour until breakfast. Mr. Rich Styles, a 77-year-old retired accountant, walks quietly and slowly along the corridor past the closed bedroom doors of other residents. He has been a resident for about a year and has moderate-stage dementia. The night attendant, Trudy, smiles at him as he passes and asks him if he wants a drink. He shakes his head, smiles back and keeps walking. For the next half hour, as she completes her work, she sees him pass several times. His robe has come undone and his pajama pants are slipping. She gets him to pause while she pulls them up and ties his robe again, walking with him the 50 yards to the end of the long corridor. The morning clatter of breakfast and residents getting ready for the day has begun as she leaves at the end of her shift. By this time, Mr. Styles is asleep in a comfortable chair in the foyer near the fireplace. Tim, the nursing assistant, is calling his name for breakfast but gets no response.

such as poor navigation into walls or furniture, elopement attempts, and fatigue, elicit greater concern from caregivers (see Case Study #2). These examples illustrate differences in the temporal expression of wandering and thus in the level of concern caregivers express about it.

The Lack of a Universal Definition of Wandering

Evidence-based practice associated with management of wandering has been further hindered by the lack of a universal, widely utilized definition of the behavior (see also discussion in Chapter 1). Clinicians, researchers, and caregivers can speak to each other about the behavior with the comfort of recognition of the phenomenon; however the lack of adoption of a universal definition has slowed progress toward more precise, consistent understandings both within and across disciplines. One definition, developed within nursing science as a Nursing Diagnosis almost a decade ago, has yet to be routinely seen in published wandering literature (The North American Nursing Diagnosis Association [NANDA], 2001). The reasons for this lack of widespread utilization likely stem from the limited discourse in the literature about what constitutes wandering

Case Study #2

She pauses for a moment by the large windows with the view through the trees to the lake. The scene is peaceful and beautiful in the late fall afternoon, with sunlight falling on the colored leaves and glinting on the water. Then she is off again, passing others in the busy nursing home halls. Her stride is long, quick, and sure. She wears a jogging suit and white jogging shoes with one lace untied and trailing. She reaches a gaggle of residents and visitors congregated near the recreational room and pushes through the throng without stopping or looking. She heads through the recreation room, returning once again to the long enclosed porch, bumping into a parked wheelchair and almost stumbling. She steadies herself against a linen trolley and circles the porch perimeter again and again. The nurse comes to find her to give her routine medication but has to walk along side her as she continues to move. She can't persuade Ruth to stop, sit down, and rest. Ruth's lips are dry and cracked, she has a bleeding skin tear where she bumped into the wheelchair, and her pants look wet. Ruth's daughter Pearl arrives to help her with dinner, as she has three times a week for 4 years, and the nurse remarks to her, "She's not slowing down for anyone or anything today—wouldn't let us bathe her and hasn't eaten much"!

and a lack of exposure to, and use of, nursing diagnostic language in other health disciplines. A consensus approach to the use of a definition would assist the field in moving toward evidence-based practice, while simultaneously encouraging discourse about elements of the definition that may result in lack of commitment to its use.

Wandering Measurement

Where definition is an issue, measurement accuracy, quality, and consistency also become an issue. While there may be multiple theoretical perspectives on wandering, a universal definition creates a framework for measurement and supports the meaningful comparison of studies and samples and the replication that builds evidence that forms the foundations of evidence-based practice. Since the behavior is multifaceted, fundamental measurement strategies for determining frequency, duration, intensity, and temporal distribution as core features of wandering, as well as for wandering outcomes, are critical. Where strong measurement techniques have been employed there is the emergence of a growing body of empirical work that is replicable, and that underpins intervention development. For example, the use of rhythm theory to underpin ambulation measurement has given clear definition to the timing and coding of ambulation cycles and quantified temporal distribution of wandering (Algase, Kupferschmid, Beel-Bates, & Beattie, 1997). Until strong and consistent measurement techniques further penetrate the field of wandering science the quality of evidence from which to evolve evidence-based practice protocols will remain poor.

Wandering Etiology

Definition and measurement often can occur more quickly when the etiology of a disease or behavior is well understood. For example, in diabetes research and practice the etiology of diabetes is clear, and simple tests with unequivocal outcomes determine core treatment. Where complex human behavior intersects with treatment, such as adherence to a treatment regime, the association between etiology, the definition of nonadherence, and management strategies becomes less straightforward. However, in dementia, the etiology of wandering as a behavioral symptom remains unknown and may remain so for some time until there are more animal studies of wayfinding and studies involving brain morphology specific to wandering. In the absence of known etiology we are still charged with providing responsive, dignity-enhancing care for persons with dementia who wander. As the purview of wandering science expands to include not only persons with dementia, but persons whose wandering is associated with other functional brain diseases and traumatic brain injury, and persons whose wandering occurs while they are wheelchair bound versus ambulating, the matter of etiology becomes more pressing, because treatment may be different for wandering resulting from different types of disease. While understanding etiology itself is not essential to developing evidence-based practice, making the lack of knowledge of the etiology of wandering explicit serves to move this agenda forward as a research priority.

Conceptual Clarity About Wandering

The science of wandering has also be inhibited by the lack of clear delineation of wandering from other closely related phenomena seen in person with dementia, most importantly agitation, anxiety, and general restlessness (see also Chapter 2). The absence of well-conceived concept analyses in the literature perpetuates loose understandings of what *is* and *is not* wandering, resulting in poorly targeted interventions focused at symptom clusters rather than single behaviors. Further, the widespread use of pharmacological agents to mitigate behavioral symptoms in persons with dementias masks behavior and dampens the impression of the severity of wandering, making clear delineation more difficult (see also Chapter 12). While the judicious use of medication to manage behavioral symptoms is essential in some persons with dementia, nonpharmacological solutions with more idiosyncratic, person-centered goals will arguably be demonstrated to have greater efficacy in wandering as the science develops further (see also Chapter 12). Evidence available today shows early promise in our understandings of the personalities of wanderers and of the characteristics of the social and physical environments of long-term care in which they have traditionally been studied and may impact the development and nature of wandering (Song, 2003; Yao, 2004).

Wandering Study Designs and Study Environments

The standards for strength of evidence set in evidence-based practice are challenging for wandering research. Findings of research studies addressing wandering may be difficult to publish, because they often rely on small samples or use multiple case studies that are viewed as weak evidence. This situation is as much about a misunderstanding of the quality of evidence produced by rigorous multiple-case design studies as it is unfamiliarity with the complexities of wandering research itself. Traditionally, most studies have drawn samples from long-term care settings, and subjects have tended to be moderately to severely impaired, because these are the stages of the disease at which the behavior tends to become problematic for caregivers. Informed consent for participation has most often been given by legally designated representatives of these vulnerable, aged subjects. The numbers of persons with dementia who have to be systematically evaluated against rigorous inclusion criteria to yield a robust sample, or set of multiple cases, is frequently large and may involve the use of multiple complex settings unfamiliar with the research enterprise. This is an expensive investment in time and funds prior and during the conduct of the study, particularly because human subject requirements have become more stringent. Wanderers, by definition are considered an "at risk" population, prone to injury and behavioral issues while participating in a research study, so morbidity and mortality are a greater concern than in a younger population. Further, until the recent development of a proxy measure for wandering (Algase, Beattie, Bogue, & Yao, 2001), observational work with wanderers has relied upon the use of accelerometers and video cameras for capturing the behavior, approaches that are time and personnel expensive, even when well-tolerated by subjects (Algase, Beattie, Leitsch, & Beel-Bates, 2003). The utility and strength of single and multiple case designs, especially in pilot intervention work, should not be underestimated at this stage in the development of wandering science for its ability to build a body of knowledge.

As the science of wandering develops investigators are moving beyond traditional long-term care research settings into the home, community, and acute care, and to the use of existing extant datasets, such as the Minimum Data Set for long-term care to capture data on mobility and medical history data in large groups of patients, as well as the Safe Return® data from the American Alzheimer's Association (Rowe and Glover, 2001; see also Chapter 13). Persons with dementia who wander are beginning to be studied not only as individuals but as one member of a dyad involving both the wanderer and the caregiver. These settings and subject configurations impose new measurement and operational challenges. As technology improves, our ability to locate lost persons with dementia more readily has increased dramatically (see also Chapter 15). We are faced with new ethical dilemmas in wandering science that bring together important questions about risk benefit for the person with dementia, their caregivers, their families, and society at large. This transitional, developing nature of wandering science brings with it an imperative to continue to pursue evidence-based practice development even before the science is fully there to support it. This is demonstrated clearly in the single published evidence-based practice protocol, which, while laudable in intent, relied by necessity on evidence with minimal strength in the evidence hierarchy due to methodological weakness (Futrell & Melillo, 2002). Any evidence-based practice to be developed in the future will need to encompass new understandings of the multiple dimensions of wandering and the unique environmental features, physical, social, and emotional, that serve to mitigate or promote it.

A Critical Mass of Investigators

The development of a critical mass of well-educated investigators in any field of study is necessary to surface the persistent research questions that need to be answered and to establish strong records of scholarship that underpin funding. Until recently the small cohort of wandering researchers themselves had limited exposure to each other and to new ideas in the field except via the literature and regular generic geriatric meetings. The formation of the International Wandering Consortium in 2003 brought together a critical mass of American investigators with a commitment to the study of the phenomena. This pioneering group has links with investigators in other countries including the United Kingdom, Korea, and Australia. It can be argued that the recent emphasis on intervention studies, especially Stage III and IV controlled trials at the National Institute of Health (NIH), disadvantages science that is still predominantly at the descriptive level, as is the case with the science of wandering. The natural course and characteristics of wandering as it emerges in dementia, and evolves through the illness, has not been systematically studied, except in several small current pilots. A challenge to the new generation of investigators is to develop more robust, cost-efficient ways of obtaining necessary data and sharing data willingly for secondary analyses with appropriate safeguards for privacy in place. This will assist in the development of a critical mass of investigators with the credentials and research experience required to achieve the type of funding necessary to sustain a program of research in this area. Such investigators are also well-prepared to critique emerging work in the field, because of their familiarity with, and commitment to, the behavior.

A Model of Evidence-Based Practice to Evaluate the Development of Wandering

There are multiple models for research utilization in nursing and other health disciplines to support evidence-based practice. The models include: (1) the Conduct and Utilization of Research in Nursing (CURN) project (Haller, Reynolds, & Horsely, 1979); (2) the Stetler Model of Research Utilization (Stetler & Marram, 1976); and (3) the Iowa Model for Research in Practice (Titler et al., 1994). For the purposes of this chapter a recent framework for evidence-based practice, the ACE Star Model (Stevens, 2004), was selected as a useful organizing framework to evaluate the development of wandering evidence-based practice. The

ACE model depicts a circular model that is configured as a 5-point star, illustrating the five major, iterative states of knowledge transformation: (1) knowledge discovery (research), (2) evidence synthesis, (3) translation into practice recommendations, (4) integration into practice, and (5) evaluation (see Figure 17.1). The asterisks indicate the domains of evidence-based practice where wandering science has published evidence.

The first star point in the ACE model is Discovery, original research where new knowledge is uncovered through research and scientific inquiry. In the wandering literature, there is an increasing body of empirical work beginning with the scope of the problem. It is estimated in the United States that there are 125,000 reports of wanderers with dementia leaving the safety of their home and caregivers, unwilling or unable to return home. Sixty percent of people with Alzheimer's disease wander and attempt to leave home at least once during the course of their disease. Of the wanderers who succeed in elopement, 72 percent attempt to do so again (Warner, 2005). Recent work has begun to tease out the characteristics of the elopements of identified wanderers into unsafe situations, placing themselves at risk of injury and death (Aud, 2004; Rowe & Glover, 2001; Rowe & Bennett, 2003). The majority of other published wandering science is descriptive or exploratory at this time and is widely

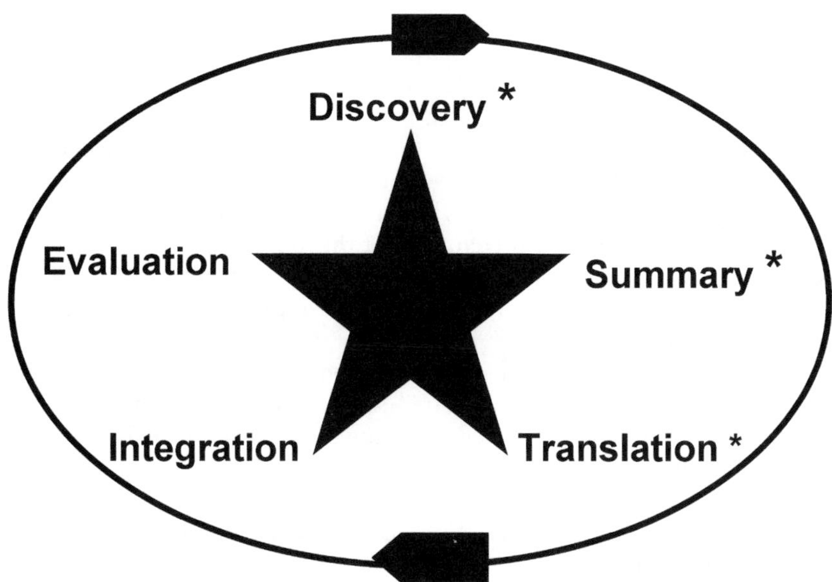

FIGURE 17.1 ACE star model of EBP: Knowledge transformation.
Source: Stevens (2004).

referenced in this book. The results of the first large, multisite explanatory study of identified wanderers conducted in long-term care by the Need-Driven, Dementia-Compromised Behavior Collaborative Research Group (NDB-CRG) will be available early in 2007 (see Chapter 2 for more information).

The second star point in the ACE model is Evidence Synthesis. At this time there are only five syntheses of wandering studies in the published literature (Algase, 1999; Siders et al., 2004; Price, Hermans, & Grimley Evans, 2002; Peatfield, Futrell, & Cox, 2002; Lai & Authur, 2003). These authors summarize the literature associated with wandering as a way to clarify what is known about a topic, as well as to identify gaps in science.

At the third ACE star point, Translation into Practice Recommendations, there are three protocols that focus on wandering (Algase, 1999; Algase & Struble, 1992; Beattie, 2004); each of these protocols focus on wandering assessment and a synthesis of these protocols can be found in Chapter 5. There is one evidence-based practice protocol for wandering (Futrell & Melillo, 2002) developed by the Gerontological Nursing Interventions Research Center (GNIRC) Research Translation and Dissemination Core at the University of Iowa College of Nursing and available for purchase at http://www.nursing.uiowa.edu/center/gnirc/protocols.htm. There is one assessment tool for wandering with solid psychometrics, titled the Algase Wandering Scale, which includes versions for use in community-based settings and another for long-term care settings (Algase et al., 2001) (see Appendix B). Several protocols that include wandering but are not specific to wandering are also available (Clarke, 2006; Doody et al., 2001; Zeisel, Hyde, & Levkoff, 1994). One evidence-based practice recommendation for wandering assessment that utilizes evidence supporting the Need-Driven Dementia Behavior Model is Beattie (2004). The Need-Driven Dementia Behavior Model was described previously in Chapter 2. At the time of preparation of this book there were very few evidence-based recommendations for wandering assessment or interventions to manage wandering and no published studies testing these recommendations.

A national call for "best practices" being used in the United States was sent out Spring 2006 and netted several clinical, educational, and policy innovations. We reviewed these submissions and have included a few in this chapter.

1. Staff at the Northport VA Medical Center developed a patient education brochure related to wandering, as well as a local policy they are willing to share (see Appendix C). For more information, contact Vivian E. Bugaoan, LCSW, Assistant Chief, Social Work Service (vivian.bugaoan@med.va.gov); you can view these

materials at http://www.visn8.med.va.gov/patientsafetycenter/wandering/.

2. VA Headquarters, under the leadership of the National Center for Patient Safety in Ann Arbor, issued a VA Directive that addresses how to prevent, detect, and respond to wandering behavior of VA patients (see Appendix C). For more information, you can view these materials at http://www.visn8.med.va.gov/patientsafetycenter/wandering/.
3. Staff at the Employee Education Center in the Veterans Health Administration have developed an electronic training program made available and required by all staff at all levels and disciplines as well as family members of high risk patients. The course link for "Missing Patient Directive" is http://vaww.sites.lrn.va.gov/mp/mpbegin.html. This was submitted by William W. Van Stone and can be found in Appendix C. The post-test exam requires logging into a Test System and may be restricted to VA employees. Instructions are available at this link: http://vaww.sites.lrn.va.gov/mp/teststatus.html. The link directly to the exam is: https://vaww.ees.aac.va.gov/.
4. A Patient Safety Officer at the VA in Reno, Judith O'Neal, RN, submitted a VHA Missing Patient Directive, two tools that have been incorporated into their electronic medical records: Wander Risk Assessment Tool and a Warning Flag for Wander Risk, as well as a slide presentation outlining a Missing Patient Process Improvement Program. These documents can be found in Appendix C. For more information, you can view these materials at http://www.visn8.med.va.gov/patientsafetycenter/wandering/, or contact Ms. O'Neal at (Judith.Oneal@va.gov).
5. At the Sepulveda and Greater LA VA Medical Centers, staff have developed an admission assessment form to screen for patients who may be at high risk for wandering. This screening tool, submitted by Fern Pietruszka (Fern.Pietruszka@va.gov), can be found in Appendix C, or you can view these materials at http://www.visn8.med.va.gov/patientsafetycenter/wandering/.
6. Kelly Fethelkheir RN (Kelly.Fethelkheir@va.gov) developed a Wandering Prevention Stop Sign used hospital-wide at the Bay Pines VA Medical Center in Florida. They have also developed an educational program, which is in Appendix C; for more information, you can view these materials at http://www.visn8.med.va.gov/patientsafetycenter/wandering/.

The state of published protocols and evidence-based practice recommendations in this area clearly does not reflect what is occurring in practice as clinicians adapt practice to keep wandering persons with dementia safe. However, there has been no systematic attempt to describe variation in practice or test standardized approaches.

Clinicians seeking evidence-based protocols for wandering currently have limited options, because evidence-based practice in wandering science is in its infancy. The resources in this book serve as a clinical guide to the scope of currently available wandering science at the time of publication. The necessary, pressing work of the cohort of wandering scientists is the amassing and synthesis of evidence and the further development of theory to support rigorous, targeted studies that minimize the risky elements of wandering. Meaningful translation of wandering study findings into clinical practice can begin to occur as the body of evidence becomes strong enough to support the infusion of useful changes or modifications into clinical practice and the systematic benchmarking of evidence-based practice outcomes. As we move forward in the development of the science of wandering it is imperative to emphasize that evidence-based practice involves not only the determination of research study quality, but the critique of existing management guidelines and systematic reviews. The finest clinical care generated from evidence-based practice evolves based on the hierarchy of evidence, and then relies on expert opinion when science is lacking.

REFERENCES

Algase, D. L. (1999). Wandering in dementia: State of the science. In J. J. Fitzpatrick (Ed.), *Annual review of nursing research*. New York: Springer.

Algase, D. L., Beattie, E.R.A., Bogue, E., & Yao, L. (2001). The Algase Wandering Scale: Initial psychometrics of a new caregiver reporting tool. *American Journal of Alzheimer's Disease and Other Dementias, 16*(3), 141–152.

Algase, D. L., Beattie, E.R.A., Leitsch, S. A., & Beel-Bates, C. A. (2003). Biomechanical activity devices to index wandering behavior. *American Journal of Alzheimer's Disease and Other Dementias, 18*(2), 85–92.

Algase, D., Kupferschmid, B., Beel-Bates, C., & Beattie, E. (1997). Estimates and stability of daily wandering behavior among cognitively impaired long-term care residents. *Nursing Research, 46*(3), 172–178.

Algase, D. L., & Struble, L. M. (1992). Wandering: What, why and how? *Geriatric Mental Health Nursing*. Thorofare, NJ: Slack, Inc.

Aud, M. (2004). Dangerous wandering: Elopements of older adults with dementia from long-term care facilities. *American Journal of Alzheimer's Disease and Other Dementias, 19*(6), 361–368.

Beattie, E.R.A. (2004). Nursing management of wandering behavior. In B. Keane (Ed.), *Practical nursing management for residential care*. Melbourne, Australia: AusMed Publications.

Clarke, C. (2006). Risk and ageing populations: Practice development research through an international research network (with members of the International Collaborative

Research Network on Risk and Ageing Populations). *International Journal of Older People Nursing, 1,* 169–176.

DePalma, J. (2000). Evidence-based clinical practice guidelines. *Seminars in Perioperative Nursing, 9*(3), 115–120.

Doody, R. S., Stevens, J. C., Beck, C., Dubinsky, R. M., Kaye, J. A., Gwyther, L., et al. (2001). Practice parameter: Management of dementia (an evidence-based review). Report of the Quality Standards Subcommittee of the American Academy of Neurology. *Neurology, 56,* 1154–1166.

Futrell, M., & Melillo, K. D. (2002). Evidence-based protocol. Wandering. *Journal of Gerontological Nursing, 28*(11), 14–22.

Grinspun, D., Virani, T., & Bajnok, I. (2001/2002). Nursing best practice guidelines: The RNAO project. *Hospital Quarterly,* 54–58.

Haller, K. B., Reynolds, M. A., & Horsley, J. A. (1979). Developing research-based innovation protocols: Process, criteria and issues. *Research in Nursing and Health, 2,* 45–51.

Heater, B. S., Becker, A. M., & Olson, R. (1988). Nursing interventions and patient outcomes. A meta-analysis of studies. *Nursing Research, 37,* 303–307.

Lai, C. K., & Arthur, D. G. (2003). Wandering behaviour in people with dementia. *Journal of Advanced Nursing, 44*(2), 173–82.

da Vinci, Leonardo. (n.d.). *Notebooks.* Brainy quote. Retrieved July 14, 2006, from http://www.brainyquote.com/quotes/quotes/l/leonardoda140595.html.

Miyamoto, Y., Ito, H., Otsuka, T., & Kurita, H. (2002). Caregiver burden in mobile and non-mobile demented patients: A comparative study. *International Journal of Geriatric Psychiatry, 17*(8), 765–773.

Newhouse, R. P. (2006). Evidence and the executive: Examining the support for evidence-based nursing practice. *Journal of Nursing Administration, 36,* 7–8.

North American Nursing Diagnosis Association (NANDA). (2001). *Nursing diagnosis: Definitions and classification, 2001–2002* (pp. 206–207). Philadelphia, PA: Author.

Peatfield, J. G., Futrell, M., & Cox, C. L. (2002). Wandering: An integrative review. *Journal of Gerontological Nursing, 28*(4), 44–50.

Price, J. D., Hermans, D. G., & Grimley Evans, J. (2002). Subjective barriers to prevent wandering of cognitively impaired people (Cochrane Review). In *The Cochrane Library, Issue 3.* Oxford: Update Software.

Rowe, M. A., & Bennett, V. (2003). A look at deaths occurring in persons with dementia lost in the community. *American Journal of Alzheimer's Disease and Other Dementias, 18*(6), 343–348.

Rowe, M., & Glover, J. (2001). Antecedents, descriptions and consequences of wandering in cognitively-impaired adults and the Safe Return (SR) program. *American Journal of Alzheimer's Disease and Other Dementias, 16*(6), 344–352.

Sackett, D. L., Rosenberg, W. N., Gray, J.A.M., Haynes, R. B., & Richardson, W. D. (1996). Evidence-based medicine: What it is and what it isn't. *British Medical Journal, 312,* 71–72.

Siders, C., Werner, D., Brown, L., Algase, D. L., Beattie, E.R.A., Schonfeld, L., et al. (2004). Evidence for implementing nonpharmacological interventions for wandering. *Rehabilitation Nursing, 29*(6), 195–206.

Song, J. A., (2003). Relationship of premorbid personality and behavioral responses to stress to wandering behavior of residents with dementia in long term care facilities (Doctoral dissertation, University of Michigan, 2003). *Proquest Dissertations and Theses 2003.* Section 0127, Part 0569, AAT 3096205, 209 pages.

Stetler, C. B., & Marram, G. (1976). Evaluating research findings for applicability in practice. *Nursing Outlook, 24*(9), 559–563.

Stevens, K. R. (2004). ACE Star Model of EBP: Knowledge Transformation. *Academic Center for Evidence-based Practice.* Retrieved May 16, 2005, from http://www.acestar.uthscsa.edu.

Titler, M. G., Kleiber, C., Steelman, V., Goode, C., Rakel, B., Barry-Walker, J., et al. (1994). Infusing research into practice to promote quality care. *Nursing Research, 43*(5), 307–313.

Warner, M. L. (2005, September). *In search of the Alzheimer's wanderer.* Purdue University Press. Retrieved August 18, 2006, from http://www.agelessdesign.com.

Yao, L., (2004). Locomoting responses to environment in elders with dementia: A model construction and preliminary testing (Doctoral dissertation, University of Michigan, 2004). *Proquest Dissertations and Theses 2004.* Section 0127, Part 0569, AAT 3137969, 151 pages.

Zeisel, J., Hyde, J., & Levkoff, S. (1994). Best practices: An Environment Behavior (E-B) model of physical design for special care units. *Journal of Alzheimer's Disease, 9*(2), 4–21.

PART V

Future Directions

CHAPTER EIGHTEEN

A Research Agenda to Build the Science Associated With Wandering

Audrey L. Nelson and Donna L. Algase

INTRODUCTION

While the number of studies related to wandering has increased in recent years, many gaps in science remain, limiting the empirical evidence on which to base important clinical decisions. These gaps in science contribute to significant variation in practice associated with assessment practices for wandering as well as interventions used to manage wandering. Indeed, fundamental questions on the potential harm versus the benefits of wandering behavior remain unresolved.

Despite these shortcomings, in the past decade, several important milestones have been reached to propel the science of wandering forward. The purpose of this chapter is to (1) describe the conceptual, methodological, and practical limitations that continue to thwart scientific progress, while highlighting milestones likely to propel the science forward; (2) present a research agenda to inform the directions and methods for future research related to wandering; and (3) project scientific and clinical breakthroughs expected over the next 5 years.

METHODOLOGICAL ISSUES AFFECTING WANDERING SCIENCE

Scientists face multiple challenges in designing and implementing wandering-related research. These challenges are organized as (1) conceptual, (2) methodological, and (3) practical; each will be briefly described.

Conceptual Issues

Conceptual clarity is needed to distinguish wandering from: (1) other symptoms of dementia (e.g., aggression, anxiety or agitation/general restlessness, pacing); (2) wandering outcomes (e.g., intrusion, elopement); (3) wandering correlates (e.g., packing to leave, door-testing, lingering near exits, shadowing); (4) wandering etiologies or contributing factors (e.g., impaired attention); and (5) other constructs related to navigation through space (wayfinding and spatial orientation). These terms are often used interchangeably, which can mask study results. To date published studies have suffered from the following conceptual issues: (1) inadequate conceptual and operational definition of wandering (described in Chapter 1), (2) inability to differentiate correlates of wandering from etiologies or contributing factors, and (3) use of atheoretical approaches.

As described in Chapter 17, there is a strong need for a standardized definition of wandering—for both clinicians, interested in evidence-based practice, as well as researchers, seeking robust research designs based on sound conceptual foundations. In the past 2 years, several new tools have been developed that should promote science in this area, including:

- Development of new and emerging conceptual models for explaining and predicting wandering (described previously in Chapter 2)
- Differentiation of wayfinding and wandering constructs
- Mechanisms underlying spatial disorientation in dementia (Duffy, 1999)
- Conceptualization of "wheelchair wandering" and beginning work to characterize the unique patterns and risks associated with this new concept
- Systematic compilation of Wandering-Related Terms and Definitions, toward standardization of definitions (Algase, Moore, Gavin-Dreschnack, & VandeWeerd, in press)
- Creation of a Conceptual Map of Wandering that explicates the four domains that circumscribe wandering behavior: locomotion, drive, space, and time (Algase, Moore, et al., in press)

Methodological Issues

Evolution of methodologies can be considered a marker for the maturity of a field of scientific inquiry; in the field of wandering studies, methodologies are in an early stage of advancement. Methodological issues in wandering science will be reviewed as they relate to research designs, research samples, observation, and measurement of the efficacy of wandering interventions.

Research Designs

To date, research in wandering reflects an overreliance on case studies and cross-sectional designs, with few prospective longitudinal designs or randomized controlled trials. Few studies have included control or comparison groups to remove potential confounds and very few have included random selection of subjects or random assignment of subjects to groups. Most studies related to wandering have relied on small sample size with insufficient power to detect effects even when differences exist. Rarely can a single study change practice; in order to increase the replicability of studies, the dependent variables and interventions need to be more clearly operationalized.

One explanation for the dearth of randomized controlled trials (RCT) to test wandering interventions is that randomization of individuals is costly and often impractical in nursing homes or other institutional settings, where the intervention is typically facility-wide (e.g., environmental modifications or use of wander alarm systems). Alternatives to RCTs include controlled trials and time series designs, which have been used. Studies using these designs have rarely addressed necessary design sensitivity concerns, such as (1) blinding observers to the nature of the intervention; (2) obscuring the presence of observers or monitoring equipment that might affect resident and caregiver behavior; (3) capturing resident, family, and caregiver responses to the intervention; (4) including rigorous inclusion/exclusion criteria to decrease the heterogeneity of the sample, which could confound the findings; and (5) monitoring the progression of dementia over time, which could mask important findings.

Research Samples

Historically, wandering studies have chiefly focused on nursing home residents or those in advanced stages of dementia and more severe levels of cognitive impairment and less on community-based persons with mild or moderately advanced stages of dementia and less severe levels of impairment. Consequently, little is known about the early onset of wandering, its emergence and earliest behavioral manifestations, nor about how such behaviors change and evolve in response to the progressive cognitive decline characteristic of Alzheimer's and related dementias. This knowledge gap has impaired the development of stage-specific wandering interventions in dementia care. Furthermore, the use of heterogeneous samples in some studies may mask the unique etiologies or treatment responses of subpopulations, for example, wheelchair wanderers or wanderers with non-Alzheimer's dementias.

Interventions

While the number of intervention studies reported in the literature is growing, the quality has been hampered by a lack of detail regarding the process of how the intervention was implemented. This missing or ambiguous information results in mixed or counterintuitive results that might have been explained through contextual factors or other missing details. This level of specificity in the intervention and process of implementation is needed to explain results, promote replication of studies, facilitate research translation to clinical practice, and help to build a business case. Advancements in the design and testing of interventions have been modest but do include the creation of a typology and index of wandering technologies (VISN 8 Patient Safety Center of Inquiry, 2005) as well as the cataloguing and critique of work completed to date through the design of evidence tables that catalog and critique interventions to manage wandering (Siders et al., 2004).

Outcome Measures

Scientific progress has been delayed as a result of narrowly defined outcomes, typically limited to the number of exits. This narrow focus largely ignores outcomes with the potential to guide clinical practice and build science, including exiting attempts, shadowing, lurking, and negative health consequences such as malnutrition, incontinence, and fatigue. Long-term outcomes, such as quality of life, have been summarily ignored in wandering research. One explanation is that researchers had limited access to valid and reliable measurement tools. Much progress has been made in the past 5 years in this area, which should contribute to stronger science. Advancements in the development and validation of measurement tools for wandering, include:

- Biomechanical Measures for Wandering, which include counting and timing both phases of all ambulation cycles occurring during observation (Algase, Beattie, Lietsch & Beel-Bates, 2003);

- Martino-Saltzman and colleague's typology for a coding scheme to characterize wandering behaviors (Martino-Saltzman, Blasch, Morris, & McNeal, 1991);
- Revised Algase Wandering Scale (Community Version and Long-Term Care Version) to assess and quantify wandering risk (Algase et al., 2004; see also Appendix B);
- Wayfinding Effectiveness Scale to determine the extent to which decrements in wayfinding ability are reflected in wandering behavior (Algase, Son, et al., in press).;
- Behavioral Response to Stress Scale to measure an individual's pattern of behavior in response to stressful situations, reflecting four behavioral domains commonly observed within this population: motor behaviors, verbal behaviors, aggressive behaviors, and passive behaviors (Gilley, Wilson, Bennett, Bernard, & Fox, 1991); and
- The use of Radio Frequency Identification Device (RFID) technology as a meta-technology to objectively test the effectiveness of simpler technologies available to home-based caregivers by actively monitoring the incidence of lingering near exits, shadowing other household residents, and detecting successful elopements.

Data Collection Intervals

More work is needed to refine the optimal intervals for data collection. Because wandering behaviors are rarely static and can be intermittent, positive results of intervention studies may be hidden, not because of a lack of intervention effectiveness, but rather, because the duration of the study may not be enough to detect a clinically meaningful change. In studies reported to date, most focused exclusively on immediate outcomes (days or a few weeks), ignoring intermediate (months) and long-term effects (years) of the interventions.

Practical Issues

Due to cost and convenience, most research on wandering has been conducted in nursing homes, largely ignoring home settings, assisted living facilities, or other settings where direct observation is costly, intrusive, and difficult. The numbers of subjects needed for statistical power is frequently large, and many subjects must be screened to achieve these numbers. This can be an expensive investment in time and funding. Typically, studies on wandering have relied on direct observation, which is quite time consuming and costly. Advancements in measurement, including new technology systems, should provide a solution to this problem. Another problem that arises is the ethical issues surrounding use of technology for clinical and research purposes (e.g., global tracking systems). Further, obtaining informed consent from persons with dementia is challenging, particularly when data is to be collected over time and the subject's condition is likely to deteriorate. Plans to obtain valid and reliable proxy measures can also be daunting.

RESEARCH AGENDA

After a careful review of the literature, consulting with experts of many disciplines, and discussions with caregivers of wandering individuals and clinicians who treat them, we have created a research agenda to guide the field over the next 5 years. The agenda is organized by study type: epidemiological, interventional, technology assessment, qualitative, and measurement/psychometrics.

Epidemiology Studies Needed

1. Prospectively examine the early trajectory of wandering, including the onset of wandering behaviors, by focusing on persons with mild dementia and following them over time as wandering behaviors emerge.
2. Determine variations in pattern, frequency, and duration of wandering behaviors in types of dementia (e.g., Alzheimer's disease, frontotemporal dementia, or vascular dementia).
3. Link competing biological etiologies associated with wandering behaviors identified in the literature to specific types of wandering (e.g., random, lapping, and pacing) and degrees of wandering intensity (e.g., frequency and duration).
4. Predict institutionalization, getting lost, injury, and death in wanderers based on patterns of wandering (e.g., random, lapping, and pacing), intensity of wandering (e.g., frequency and duration), and level of cognitive impairment.
5. Identify the profiles of wandering responsive to pharmacological interventions.
6. Characterize wheelchair wandering behaviors and compare with ambulatory wandering.
7. Examine the epidemiology (incidence, prevalence, caregiver and care recipient characteristics, and consequences) of getting lost behaviors.
8. Test new and emerging conceptual models on wandering for predicting adverse events associated with wandering.

Intervention Studies Needed

1. Test wandering interventions targeting specific diagnoses, impairments, and clinical settings, targeting understudied populations with unique wandering risk factors, such as non-Alzheimer's type dementia, persons with TBI, those with psychiatric diagnoses without dementia, and wheelchair wanderers.
2. Develop and test setting-specific protocols for fast recovery of wanderers who get lost.
3. Develop and test strategies to train caregivers in long-term care settings on effective strategies to mitigate the negative consequences of wandering behaviors.
4. Examine cost effectiveness of training programs to safely manage wandering behavior in nursing homes, assisted living facilities, continuing care retirement communities, acute care, and home care settings.
5. Test predictive models of potentially hazardous, high-risk wandering and the impact on patient and caregiver outcomes.
6. Develop and test interventions linked to contributing factors (or risk assessment) to mitigate potentially hazardous, high-risk wandering.
7. Evaluate the effectiveness of interventions for specific types of wandering (e.g., random, lapping, and pacing), intensity of wandering (e.g., frequency and duration), and care settings (acute care, LTC, and community-based).
8. Develop community-based prevention and intervention programs to mitigate risky wandering.
9. Prospectively evaluate the cost effectiveness of the Safe Return® project on a national sample of veterans with dementia.
10. Examine the effectiveness of search protocols for wanderers in institutions versus home-based settings.
11. Extend wandering research conducted primarily in nursing homes to community-based settings using robust research designs.

Technology Assessment Studies Needed

1. Examine the cost-effectiveness and acceptance of wandering technologies such as visual barriers, camouflage, and alarm systems used in home settings.
2. Examine research applications of technologies (unobtrusive measures for quantifying exit attempts or lurking by doors) and rehabilitation interventions for preventing elopement, and protection when elopement occurs, as well as minimizing injuries associated with wandering behaviors, such as falls or malnutrition.

3. Conduct head-to-head evaluations of the 80+ commercially available products associated with management of wandering, to develop practical knowledge for providers for prescribing and use in institutional settings.
4. Compare the effectiveness of subjective barriers (e.g., contrasting tape (grid or stripes) applied to door or floor, mirrors, cloth panels (to conceal door or doorknob), or murals to disguise the door) to prevent wandering in cognitively impaired people.
5. Conduct technology assessments for low-cost, noninvasive locator systems, targeting specific settings (e.g., home-based, acute care, and long-term care).
6. Conduct technology assessments for low-cost technologies (e.g., visual barriers, verbal warning systems, ambient conditions such as lighting), targeting specific types of wandering patterns (e.g., random, lapping, and pacing).
7. Test the use of Global Positioning Systems (GPS) in high-risk wanderers for preventing injuries and death associated with getting lost.
8. Evaluate the effectiveness of wandering technologies for specific types of wandering (e.g., random, lapping, and pacing), degrees of wandering (e.g., frequency and duration), and care settings (acute care, LTC, and community-based).
9. Test the effectiveness of personalized robotic devices to cue appropriate behavior, reorient, and reduce agitation in the lost wanderer.

Qualitative Research Studies Needed

1. Examine the meaning and potential health benefits of wandering behaviors from the perspective of the patient.
2. Discover effective caregiver strategies used to reduce the degrees of wandering (e.g., frequency and duration) and risks associated with wandering behavior.
3. Describe cross-cultural differences in wandering behaviors and interventions used to control and manage wandering, including cognitive restructuring and patient and caregiver responses to interventions.

Psychometric Studies Needed

1. Establish construct validity of wandering and convergence validity of various measurement approaches, including rating scales, observation tools, and technology measures (e.g., RFID).

ANTICIPATED SCIENTIFIC BREAKTHROUGHS

As mentioned previously, the science associated with wandering is emerging. In the past 5 years, several scientific milestones have been achieved to propel the science forward, including defining more clearly the construct of wandering, development of valid and reliable measures, and an explosion of technologies available. Within the next 3–5 years, we project the following scientific breakthroughs will occur in this research area:

1. Based on research in progress at the Tampa VA Patient Safety Center of Inquiry and University of South Florida, within the next 2–5 years Radio Frequency Identification Devices (RFID) will replace costly observational methods in institutions and extend capacity for understanding wandering behaviors in the home for detecting and measuring specific wandering behaviors (e.g., exiting attempts, lurking by exits, shadowing, or persistence). This will also improve outcome measurement of targeted interventions across settings. RFID applications will be expanded beyond observational and measurement techniques to include product and research development for tracking the locomotion of individuals who wander in group settings.
2. In the next 5 years, at least two large-scale studies will be completed to capture the onset of wandering behaviors prospectively following a large cohort of persons newly diagnosed with dementia (Tampa VA Patient Safety Center of Inquiry and University of Michigan).
3. Given several new and emerging conceptual models available to guide research questions, we would expect explanations and predictions of wandering to become more focused.
4. Planned research at the Tampa VA Patient Safety Center of Inquiry includes use of sociotechnical probabilistic risk modeling (STPR) to provide a better understanding of conditions precipitating the occurrence of rare but serious adverse events associated with wandering in long-term care settings.
5. Research at the Tampa VA Patient Safety Center of Inquiry is currently in progress to determine the efficacy of visual barriers as deterrents for exiting and exit-seeking behaviors in the home setting.
6. Pilot work has been initiated to extend valid measurement of wandering behaviors to a new population of wheelchair wanderers. We expect that in the next 3–5 years, we will be able to characterize this as a new population of "at-risk" veterans.

ANTICIPATED CLINICAL CONTRIBUTIONS

The lag between research findings and clinical application is unfortunately significant. Despite this, we are optimistic that given existing research achievements and projected research planned over the next few years, the following clinical achievements are possible, for a subset of highly motivated "early adopters":

1. Reduce variation in practice through use of standardized definitions, assessment tools, and outcome measures specific to care settings (acute care, long-term care, and community-based).
2. Standardize quality improvement approaches for tracking adverse events, examining root causes, implementing system changes, mitigating adverse events associated with wandering, and evaluating outcomes over time.
3. Promote culturally competent care for persons who wander and their caregivers.
4. Develop a business case for implementing wandering interventions and technologies in institutional and community-based settings.

CONCLUSION

Building a new science base is painstaking work, requiring a core group of committed individuals with necessary expertise and resources. The International Consortium of Research in Wandering, formed in 2003, is committed to this goal. To assure efficiency and effectiveness of efforts to build science and impact clinical practice, we have developed this research agenda. Clinicians and researchers interested in participating or monitoring our progress can access the following Web page: http://www.visn8.med.va.gov/patientsafetycenter/wandering/

Together, we can make a difference in improving the safety and quality of life for persons who wander and the caregivers to whom their care is entrusted.

REFERENCES

Algase, D. L., Beattie, E.R.A., Lietsch, S. A., & Beel-Bates, C. A. (2003). Biomechanical activity devices to index wandering behavior. *American Journal of Alzheimer's Disease and Other Dementias, 18*(2), 85–92.

Algase, D. L., Moore, D. H., Gavin-Dreschnack, D., & VandeWeerd, C. (in press). Wandering definitions and terms. In A. Nelson (Ed.), *Evidence-based protocols for safety managing wandering behaviors.* New York: Springer Publishing.

Algase, D. L., Son, G. R., Beattie, E., Song, J., Leitsch, S., & Yao, L. (2004). The interrelatedness of wandering and wayfinding in a community sample of persons with dementia. *Dementia and Geriatric Cognitive Disorders, 17*(3), 231–239.

Algase, D. L., Son, G-R., Beel-Bates, C., Song, J., Yao, L., Beattie, E.R.A., et al. (in press). Initial psychometric evaluation of the wayfinding effectiveness scale. *Western Journal of Nursing Research.*

Duffy, C. J. (1999). Visual loss and Alzheimer's disease: Out of sight, out of mind. *Neurology, 52*(5), 10–11.

Gilley, D. W., Wilson, R. S., Bennett, D. A., Bernard, B. A., & Fox, J. H. (1991). Predictors of behavioral disturbance in Alzheimer's disease. *Journal of Gerontology, 46,* 362–371.

Martino-Saltzman, D., Blasch, B., Morris, R., & McNeal, L. (1991). Travel behavior of nursing home residents perceived as wanderers and non-wanderers. *Gerontologist, 11,* 666–672.

Siders, C., Nelson, A. L., Brown, L. M., Joseph, I., Algase, D., Beattie, E., et al. (2004). Evidence for implementing non-pharmacological interventions for wandering. *Rehab Nursing, 29,* 195–206.

VISN 8 Patient Safety Center of Inquiry (2005). *Wandering technology resource guide.* Retrieved September 20, 2006, from http://www.visn8.med.va.gov/visn8/patientsafetycenter/wandering.

APPENDIX A

Compendium of Wandering-Related Terms and Definitions

TERMS AND DEFINITIONS

Term	Map term or group	Type of Definition*	Definition	Citation
Definitions From Scientific Literature				
Abscond	Abscond	O	Being absent from the ward, w/o permission, for at least 1 hour	Bowers, Alexander, & Gaskell (2003)
		O	Leaving (hospital) grounds without permission	Muller (1962); Antebi (1967); Bowers, Jarrett, Clark, Kiyimba, & McFarlane (1999)
		O	Absent w/o permission and cause for serious concern	Falkowski, Watts, Falkowski, & Dean (1990)
		O	Absence of a patient sufficient to cause concern on part of trained nursing staff	Tomison (1989)

(Continued)

TERMS AND DEFINITIONS (Continued)

Term	Map term or group	Type of Definition*	Definition	Citation
		O	Missing from ward w/o permission for more than 24 hours	John, Gangadhar, & Channabasavanna (1980)
		O	Any unauthorized absence necessitating staff intervention	Meyer Martin, & Lange (1967)
		O	Any unauthorized departure of a patient from hospital grounds	(1) Molnar, Keitner, & Swindall (1985); (2) Bowers et al. (1999)
		O	Leaving the ward without consent	Sommer (1974)
Active wandering	Inappropriate to circumstance	C	Determined wanderer appears to be searching for something or attempting to keep busy	Hirst & Metcalf (1989)
Agenda behavior	Inappropriate to circumstance	C	Planning and behavior that cognitively impaired use in attempt to meet their felt social, emotional, or physical needs at a given time	Rader (1987)
Aimless walking	Aimless	O	Subject walks around (either inside or outside) w/o any evidence of purpose. Not used if there appears to be a purpose, however bizarre, or if walking meets criteria for checking, trailing, or pottering	Hope & Fairburn (1990)

(Continued)

TERMS AND DEFINITIONS (Continued)

Term	Map term or group	Type of Definition*	Definition	Citation
Aimless wanderer	Aimless	C	Confused about where he is, but nurse is not. Moves about purposelessly, looking for some unknown location, thinking he is in his previous home, or entering other patient's rooms and exploring their belongings.	Butler & Barnett (1991)
Aimless wander-ing	Aimless	C	Outdated way of thinking—assumes purposelessness ... usually a reason for the behavior	Mather (2001)
		C	Stems from loneli-ness and separation	Algase & Struble (1992)
		C	Complex human activity, generally involving walking-type movements that may take on various forms over time and place in the same person and between differ-ent people	Dewing (2005)
		C	Searching for "miss-ing" or unattainable people or places	Dewing (2005)
Akathesi-acs	Aimless	C	Restless, aimless movers who pace or fidget, whose wandering is often secondary to prolonged use of psychotropic drugs	Rader (1987)

(Continued)

TERMS AND DEFINITIONS (Continued)

Term	Map term or group	Type of Definition*	Definition	Citation
Attempts to leave home	Exit seeking	O	Subject makes attempts to leave his residence, but is prevented by CG. Purpose of this term is to include those whose behavior might fall into one of the other categories if their movements were not restricted. In most cases CG restricts subject's movements or previous wandering problems	Hope & Fairburn (1990)
AWOL	AWOL	O	Patients who's absent without leave	Bowers et al. (1999)
Being lost	Solitary	C	Having destination, but losing direction	Wolanin & Phillips (1981)
Checking	Checking	O	Person repeatedly seeks whereabouts of carer or occasionally another person	Hope & Fairburn (1990)
Continuous wanderer	Continuous	O	Defined as ambulating more than 50% of wakeful time	Thomas (1995)
Critical wanderer	Boundary transgression	C	(1) Strays from nursing unit, but does not understand implications of his wandering. Becomes critical when he leaves premises unattended. Most dangerous, linked to out-of-facility deaths. (2) Anyone with dementia who has wandered away (disappeared of their own free will) from their caregiver	(1) Butler & Barnett (1991); (2) Koester & Stooksbury (1992)

(Continued)

TERMS AND DEFINITIONS (Continued)

Term	Map term or group	Type of Definition*	Definition	Citation
Direct	Direct	O	Walking directly from point A to point B without deviations, hesitations, or direct changes	Martino-Salzman Blasch, Morris, & McNeal (1991); Algase, Beattie, Bogue, &Yao (2001)
Direct toward appropriate purpose	Repetitive	O	Walking toward an appropriate purpose, but is repeated with inappropriate frequency	Hope & Fairburn (1990); Futrell & Melillo (2002)
Direct toward inappropriate purpose	Inappropriate to circumstance	C	Walking appears to be directed toward a purpose, but that purpose is inappropriate	Hope & Fairburn (1990); Futrell & Melillo (2002)
Direct travel	Direct	O	Travel from one location to another w/o diversion	Martino-Salzman et al. (1991)
		O	Straightforward movement to a destination	Martino-Salzman et al. (1991)
Door testing	Exit seeking	O	Any behavior with the primary goal of opening the locked doors on a special care unit. Includes but not limited to pulling, pushing, ramming, kicking, and knocking or pounding on door.	Kinkaid & Peacock (2003)
Elope	Boundary transgression	C&O	Run away	Zencius & Wesolowski (1990)
Elopement	Elopement	C	Getting lost from one's own dwelling (which may put demented individual at risk)	Lai & Arthur (2003)

(Continued)

TERMS AND DEFINITIONS (Continued)

Term	Map term or group	Type of Definition*	Definition	Citation
		C	Boundary transgressions	Lai & Arthur (2003)
		C	Puts the wanderer's safety at risk	Lai & Arthur (2003)
		C&O	(C) Running or walking away from a caregiver without consent; (O) Any movement away from the therapist more than 1.5 m without permission	Tarbox, Wallace, & Williams (2003)
		C&O	Dangerous wandering, passing beyond the safe environment's boundaries, the act of wandering away from a safe residence	Aud (2004)
		C&O	Unescorted exiting	Connell (2003)
Entry into restricted area	Boundary transgression	O	Adult day care participant crosses a piece of masking tape 0.6 m in front of threshold of office door	Feliciano, Vore, LeBlanc, Baker (2004)
		C&O	When wandering around becomes wandering away	Aud (2004)
Exit seeking and trespassing; exit seeking and inappropriate entry	Exit seeking, boundary transgression	O	(2) attempting to leave a protective environment and entering into the nursing station unprompted	(1) Cohen-Mansfield & Werner (1998); (2) Hussian (1988)

(Continued)

TERMS AND DEFINITIONS (Continued)

Term	Map term or group	Type of Definition*	Definition	Citation
Exit attempts, exiting behavior	Exit seeking	O	(1) Resident pressed panic bar on locked NH exit door; (2) Resident approached point two meters in front of observed NH exit door; (3) leaving the NH unit through an emergency exit door equipped with an alarm; (4) resident opening either of two NH exit doors equipped with a buzzer; (5) NH exit door contacts	(1) Dickenson, McLain-Kark, Marshall-Baker (1995); (2) Mayer & Darby (1991); (3) Namazi, Rosner, & Calkins (1989); (4) Chafetz (1990); (5) Hewawasam (1996)
Escapist wanderer	Escapist	C	Patient knows where he is (or at least where he is not) and can slip away from facility undetected. Nurse does not know his location. His wandering represents concerted attempt to get somewhere. If restrained, often becomes angry or fearful; gentle assurances do not deter him	Butler & Barnett (1991)
Excessive activity	Persistent	O	Person is on the move for an abnormally large proportion of the time while awake. In extreme form, person does not sit for more than a few minutes at a time.	Hope & Fairburn (1990)

(Continued)

TERMS AND DEFINITIONS (Continued)

Term	Map term or group	Type of Definition*	Definition	Citation
Exit seekers	Exit seeking	O	Newly admitted residents who try to open locked exit doors	Hussian & Davis (1983)
Exit-door contact	Exit seeking	O	Touching or opening exit door; exiting ward	Mayer & Darby (1991)
External wandering	Boundary transgression	C	Wandering external to care settings	Miskelly (2004)
Getting lost behavior (GLB), Getting lost	Disoriented	O	(1) Getting lost in familiar and unfamiliar interior and exterior environments; (2) difficulty in finding the way about the home and/or around the neighborhood; (3) the number of times patient at home brought back to the house by caregiver; (4) Differentiates wandering and becoming lost	(1) Chiu, Algase, Liang, Liu, & Lin (2005); (2) Ballard, Mohan, & Patel (1991); (3) McShane et al. (1998) (4) Rowe (2003)
High energy level/goal directed	Exit seeking	C	Wants to go home	
Hyperactivity	Repetitive	C&O	Central increased drive to walk interacting with cognitive impairment; the patient walks around the house or garden carrying out meaningful tasks but inappropriately often	Hope et al. (2001)

(Continued)

TERMS AND DEFINITIONS (Continued)

Term	Map term or group	Type of Definition*	Definition	Citation
Invasion	Invasion	C	Entering other people's rooms	Lai & Arthur (2003)
Lapping	Lapping	O	Walking in a looping repetitive path having at least three legs	Algase, Beattie, Bogue, & Yao (2001); Martino-Salzman et al. (1991)
		O	Circuitous movement revisiting points sequentially along a path or track	Lai & Arthur (2003)
		O	Repetitive travel characterized by circling large areas	Futrell & Melillo (2002)
Modelers	Modeling	O	People who tag onto or "shadow" other pacers	Hussian & Davis (1983)
Modeling	Modeling	C	Following others around	Rader (1987)
Needs to be brought back home		O	Subject has been brought back to residence on at least one occasion. Maybe subject was unable to get home w/o help, but not necessarily so. Often not possible to know whether or not subject could have returned unaided.	Hope & Fairburn (1990)
Nocturnal wandering	Nocturnal	O	Walks around inappropriately at night; term is not used if subject gets up only to go to toilet	Hope & Fairburn (1990)

(Continued)

TERMS AND DEFINITIONS (Continued)

Term	Map term or group	Type of Definition*	Definition	Citation
		O	Associated with onset of darkness and related to person's loss of spatial relationships in the dark	Matteson & Linton (1996)
		C	Often most troublesome type of wandering—can be passive or active	Hirst & Metcalf (1989)
Overtly goal-directed/ searching behavior	Inappropriate to circumstance	O	Constantly searching for something that is often unattainable (mother, home, abstract objects, etc.) often associated with calling out repeatedly or approaching one person after another in pursuit of this goal	Snyder, Rupprecht, Pyrek, Brekhus, & Moss (1978)
Overtly goal-directed/industrious behavior	Inappropriate to circumstance	O	Characterized by a seemingly inexhaustible drive to do things or remain busy; often commenting on need to perform a stated task or gesturing as if working	Snyder et al. (1978)
Overtly non–goal-directed behavior	Aimless	O	Aimlessly drawn to one stimulus after another, momentarily attentive then diverted again; often stating a question or apparent goal, but rarely following through	Snyder et al. (1978)

(Continued)

TERMS AND DEFINITIONS (Continued)

Term	Map term or group	Type of Definition*	Definition	Citation
		C	Newly admitted residents who try to open locked exit doors	Lai & Arthur (2003)
Pacing	Pacing	O	Walking back and forth between two points	Martino-Salzman et al. (1991) Algase, Beattie, Bogue, & Yao (2001)
		O	Repetitive back and forth movement within a limited area	Futrell & Melillo (2002)
		C	Fretful locomotion	Dewing (2005)
Passive wandering	Aimless	C	Wandering appears to be aimless; such wanderers are easily distracted and thus potentially easier to manage	Hirst & Metcalf (1989)
Pottering	Pottering	O	Partial attempts to carry out household tasks, that with further cognitive decline, becomes less and less meaningful	Hope et al. (2001)
Problem behavior	Inappropriate to circumstance	O	Defined by the level of aggression, frequency of behavior, and level of inappropriateness by social standards	Banazak (1996)
		O	Person walks around house or garden apparently trying, but ineffectively, to carry out task of own accord	Hope & Fairburn (1990)

(Continued)

TERMS AND DEFINITIONS (Continued)

Term	Map term or group	Type of Definition*	Definition	Citation
Purposeful wanderer	Direct	C	Resident walks around in his room, along corridors, or elsewhere with apparent intent; patient knows where he is and nurse knows his location	Butler & Barnett (1991)
Random walking	Random	O	Walking in haphazard fashion using multiple changes in direction, and no obvious route to the eventual stopping point	Martino-Salzman et al. (1991) Algase, Beattie, Bogue, & Yao (2001)
		C	Haphazard movement without repeating points in sequence	Lai & Arthur (2003)
Random travel	Random	O	Roundabout or haphazard travel to many locations within an area w/o repetition, no obvious route to stopping point	Martino-Salzman et al. (1991)
		O	Inefficient, frequent direction changes and hesitations	Algase, Beattie, & Therrien (2001)
Risky wandering/safe wandering	Problematic	C	Depends on the person doing the wandering, the knowledge and skills of caregivers and clinicians, the context or setting of care, and the workplace culture	Dewing (2005)

(Continued)

TERMS AND DEFINITIONS (Continued)

Term	Map term or group	Type of Definition*	Definition	Citation
Self stimulators	Aimless	C	Those wanderers whose purpose is to provide stimulation rather than to exit	Rader (1987)
	Exit seeking	C	Those who perform other self-stimulating activities, such as turning doorknobs, in addition to continuous pacing	Hussian & Davis (1983)
Shadowing	Shadowing	C	Following behind a caregiver	Dewing (2005); Algase et al. (2004)
Sporadic wanderer	Sporadic	O	Moves about less than half of their wakeful time	Thomas (1995)
Tag	Tagging		Shadowing another pacer	Hussian & Davis (1983)
Trailing	Trailing	O	Follows right behind care provider	Hope & Fairburn (1990); Hope et al. (2001)
		C	Extreme form of checking where person follows CG or other around excessively, and very closely behind	Futrell & Melillo (2002)
Trespassing	Trespassing	C	(1) Locomotion into unauthorized spaces; (2) Inappropriate entry	Dewing (2005)
Unattended wandering	Boundary transgression	C	Forays into the community without the supervision of caregiver	Rowe & Glover (2001)

(Continued)

TERMS AND DEFINITIONS (Continued)

Term	Map term or group	Type of Definition*	Definition	Citation
Unpurposeful wandering	Perseverative	O	Neuroleptic-induced pacing and restlessness	Hussian & Davis (1983)
Wandering behavior	Wandering	O	Observed agitation or restlessness, walking, standing, and pacing	Linton, Matteson, & Byers (1997)
Wanderers/Nonwanderers	Wandering	C&O	Wanderers: Diagnosis of some form of chronic dementia; middle or late stage dementia; physically capable of walking or moving independently; frequent ambulation defined as at lest 30% of wakeful time; nonuse of psychotropic drugs. Nonwanderers: Diagnosis of some form of chronic dementia; middle or late stage dementia; not previously defined as a wanderer; physically capable of walking or moving about independently; ambulation not exceeding 12% of wakeful time; nonuse of psychotropic drugs.	Thomas (1995)
Definitions From Policy/Regulatory Literature				
High risk patient	Problematic	O	(1) Are legally committed; or (2) Have a court-appointed legal guardian; (3) Are a danger to self or others;	James A. Haley Veterans' Hospital, Tampa, FL. Hospital Policy Memorandum No 00- 16, 9/2003

(Continued)

TERMS AND DEFINITIONS (Continued)

Term	Map term or group	Type of Definition*	Definition	Citation
			(4) Lack cognitive ability to make relevant decisions; (5) Have physical or mental impairments that increase their risk of harm to self or others	
Wandering patient	Escapist	O	A high-risk patient who has shown a propensity to stray beyond the view or control of employees, thereby requiring a high degree of monitoring and protection to ensure the patient's safety	
Missing patient	Boundary transgression	O	A high-risk patient who disappears from an inpatient or outpatient treatment area, or during transport, while under supervision by hospital staff	
Absent patient	Boundary transgression	O	A patient who leaves the treatment area without knowledge or permission of staff but who does not meet high-risk criteria	
Wandering	Wandering	C	• Locomotion with no discernible, rational purpose. A wandering resident may be oblivious to his	Centers for Medicare & Medicaid Services (CMS) Revised Long-Term Care Resident Assessment

(Continued)

TERMS AND DEFINITIONS (Continued)

Term	Map term or group	Type of Definition*	Definition	Citation
			or her physical or safety needs • Wandering behavior should be differentiated from purposeful movement (e.g., a hungry person moving about the unit in search of food). • Wandering may be manifested by walking or by wheelchair. • Do not include pacing as wandering behavior. Pacing back and forth is not considered wandering, and if it occurs, it should be documented in Item E1n, "Repetitive physical movements."	Instrument User's Manual, version 2.0, December 2002
Elopement	Boundary transgression	C	A patient that is aware that he/she is not permitted to leave, but does so with intent	VHA National Center for Patient Safety Escape and Elopement Management (2001) vaww.ncps.med.va.gov
Escape	Boundary transgression		Act of becoming free from surroundings, to avoid a threat, perceived or real	
Pacing	Pacing		Walking back and forth with no apparent destination	

(Continued)

TERMS AND DEFINITIONS (Continued)

Term	Map term or group	Type of Definition*	Definition	Citation
Purposeful wandering	Inappropriate to circumstance		Roaming with a desired location in mind, even if not in reality	
Unpurposeful wandering	Aimless		To roam about without a fixed course, aim, or goal	

* C = Conceptual, O = Operational

REFERENCES

Algase, D. L., Beattie, E. R., Bogue, E. L., & Yao, L. (2001). The Algase wandering scale: Initial psychometrics of a new caregiver reporting tool. *American Journal of Alzheimer's Disease and Other Dementias, 16*(3), 141–151.

Algase, D. L., Beattie, E. R., & Therrien, B. (2001). Impact of cognitive impairment on wandering behavior. *Western Journal of Nursing Research, 23*(3), 283–295.

Algase, D. L., & Struble, L. M. (1992). Wandering behavior: What, why, and how? Geropsychiatry. In K. Buckwalter (Ed.), *Geriatric mental health nursing: Current and future challenges* (pp. 61–74). Thorofare, NJ: Slack.

Algase, D. L., Son, G. R., Beattie, E., Song, J. A., Leitsch, S., & Yao, L. (2004). The interrelatedness of wandering and wayfinding in a community sample of persons with dementia. *Dementia and Geriatric Cognitive Disorders, 17*(3), 231–239.

Antebi, R. (1967). Some characteristics of mental hospital absconders. *British Journal of Psychiatry, 113*(503), 1087–1090.

Aud, M. A. (2004). Dangerous wandering: elopements of older adults with dementia from long-term care facilities. *American Journal of Alzheimer's Disease and Other Dementias, 19*(6), 361–368.

Ballard, C. G., Mohan, R. N. C., Bannister, C., Handy, S., & Patel, A. (1987). Wandering in dementia sufferers. *International Journal of Geriatric Psychiatry,* 6(8), 611–614.

Banazak, D. A. (1996). Difficult dementia: six steps to control problem behaviors. *Geriatrics, 51*(2), 36–42.

Bowers, L., Alexander, J., & Gaskell, C. (2003). A Trial of an anti-absconding intervention in acute psychiatric wards. *Journal of Psychiatric and Mental Health Nursing, 10,* 410–416.

Bowers, L., Jarrett, M., Clark, N., Kiyimba, F., & McFarlane, L. (1999). Absconding: Outcome and risk. *Journal of Psychiatric and Mental Health Nursing,* 6(3), 213–218.

Butler, J. P., & Barnett, C. A. (1991). Window of wandering. *Geriatric Nursing, 12*(5), 226–227.

Chafetz, P. K. (1990). Two-dimensional grid is ineffective against demented patients' exiting through glass doors. *Psychology of Aging, 5*(1), 146–147.

Chiu, Y. C., Algase, D., Liang, J., Liu, H. C., & Lin, K. N. (2005). Conceptualization and measurement of getting lost behavior in persons with early dementia. *International Journal of Geriatric Psychiatry, 20*(8), 760–768.

Cohen-Mansfield, J., Werner, P., Marx, M. S., Freedman, L. (1991). Two studies of pacing in the nursing home. *Journal of Gerontology, 46*(3), M77–M83.

Connell, B. R. (2003). Why residents wander—and what you can do about it. *Nursing Homes: Long Term Care Management.* Retrieved May 10, 2007, from http://www.nursinghomesmagazine.com/Past_Issues.htm?ID=1315.

Department of Veterans Affairs (2001). *Escape and elopement management.* Retrieved August 23, 2006, from http://www.va.gov/ncps/CogAids/EscapeElope/index.html.

Dewing, J. (2005). Screening for wandering among older persons with dementia. *Nursing Older People, 17*(3), 20–22, 24.

Dickinson, J. I., McLain-Kark, J., & Marshall-Baker, A. (1995). The effects of visual barriers on exiting behavior in a dementia care unit. *Gerontologist, 35*(1), 127–130.

Falkowski, J., Watts, V., Falkowski, W., & Dean, T. (1990). Patients leaving hospital without the knowledge or permission of staff: Absconding. *British Journal of Psychiatry, 156,* 488–490.

Feliciano, L., Vore, J., LeBlanc, L. A., & Baker, J. C. (2004). Decreasing entry into a restricted area using a visual barrier. *Journal of Applied Behavior Analysis, 37*(1), 107–110.

Futrell, M., & Melillo, K. D. (2002). Evidence-based protocol wandering. *Journal of Gerontological Nursing, 28*(11), 14–22.

Hewawasam, L. (1996).The use of two-dimensional grid patterns to limit hazardous ambulation in elderly patients with Alzheimer's disease. *Nursing Times Research, 92*(22):41–44.

Hirst, S. T., & Metcalf, B. J. (1989). Whys and whats of wandering. *Geriatric Nursing, 10*(5), 237–238.

Hope, T., & Fairburn, C. (1990). The nature of wandering in dementia: A community-based study. *International Journal of Geriatric Psychiatry, 14*(5), 239–245.

Hope, T., Keene, J., McShane, R. H., Fairburn, C. G., Gedling, K., & Jacoby, R. (2001). Wandering in dementia: A longitudinal study. *International Psychogeriatrics, 13*(2), 137–147.

Hussian, R.A. (1988). Modification of behaviors in dementia via stimulus manipulation. *Clinical Gerontologist, 8*(1), 37–43.

Hussian, R. A., & Davis, R. (1983). *Analysis of wandering behavior in institutionalized geriatric patients.* Presented at meeting of the Association for Behavioral Analysis, Milwaukee, WI, 1983.

John, C. J., Gangadhar, B. N., & Channabasavanna, S. N. (1980). Phenomenology of 'escape' from a mental hospital in India. *Indian Journal of Psychiatry, 22*(2), 247–250.

Kincaid, C. Peacock, J. R. (2003). Effect of a wall mat on decreasing four types of door-testing behaviors. *Journal of Applied Gerontology, 22*(1), 76–88.

Koester, R. J., & Stooksbury D. E. (1992). Lost Alzheimer's subjects-profiles and statistics. *Response, 11*(4), 20–26.

Lai, C. K., & Arthur, D. G. (2003). Wandering behaviour in people with dementia. *Journal of Advanced Nursing, 44*(2),173–182.

Linton, A. D., Matteson, M. A., & Byers, V. (1997). The relationship between premorbid life-style and wandering behaviors in institutionalized people with dementia. *Aging Clinical and Experimental Research, 9*(6), 415–418.

Martino-Salzman, D., Blasch, B. B., Morris, R. D., & McNeal, L. W., (1991). Travel behavior of nursing home residents perceived as wanderers and non-wanderers. *Gerontologist, 31,* 666–672.

Mather, L. A. (2001). Wandering: Repaving the way you think. *Contemporary Long Term Care, 24*(12), 8–13.

Matteson, M. A., & Linton, A. (1996). Wandering behaviors. *Journal of Gerontological Nursing, 22*(9), 39–46.

Mayer, R., & Darby, S. J. (1991). Does a mirror detect wandering in demented older people? *International Journal of Geriatric Psychiatry, 6,* 607–609.

McShane, R., Gedling, K., Keene, J., Fairburn, C., Jacoby, R., & Hope, T. (1998). Getting lost in dementia: a longitudinal study of a behavioral symptom. *International Psychogeriatrics, 10*(3), 253–260.

Meyer, G. G., Martin, M. B., & Lange, P. (1967). Elopement from the open psychiatric unit: A two year study. *Journal of Nervous and Mental Disease, 144,* 297–304.

Miskelly, F. (2004). A novel system of electronic tagging in patients with dementia and wandering. *Age Ageing, 33*(3), 304–306.

Molnar, G., Keitner, L., & Swindall, L. (1985). Medicolegal problems of elopement from psychiatric units. *Journal of Forensic Sciences, 30*(1), 44–49.

Muller, D. J. (1962). The 'missing' patient. *British Medical Journal 1,* 177–179.

Namazi, K. H., Rosner, T. T., & Calkins, M. P. (1989).Visual barriers to prevent ambulatory Alzheimer's patients from exiting through an emergency door. *Gerontologist, 29*(5), 699–702.

Rader, J. (1987). A comprehensive staff approach to problem wandering. *The Gerontological Society of America, 27*(6), 756–760.

Rowe, M. (2003). People with dementia who become lost. *American Journal of Nursing, 103*(7), 32–39; quiz 40.

Rowe, M. A. & Glover, J.C. (2001). Antecedents, descriptions and consequences of wandering in cognitively-impaired adults and the Safe Return (SR) program. *American Journal of Alzheimer's Disease and Other Dementias, 16*(6), 344–352.

Snyder, L. H., Rupprecht, P., Pyrek, J., Brekhus, S., & Moss, T. (1978). Wandering. *The Gerontologist, 18*(3), 272–280.

Sommer, G. (1974). A short term study of elopement from a state mental hospital. *Journal of Community Psychology, 2,* 60–62.

Tarbox, R. S., Wallace, M. D., & Williams, L. (2003). Assessment and treatment of elopement: A replication and extension. *Journal of Applied Behavior Analysis, 36*(2), 239–244.

Thomas, D. W. (1995). Wandering: A proposed definition. *Journal of Gerontological Nursing, 21*(9), 35–41.

Tomison, A. R. (1989). Characteristics of psychiatric hospital absconders. *British Journal of Psychiatry, 154,* 368–371.

Wolanin, M. O., & Phillips, L.R.F. (1981). *Confusion: Prevention and care.* St. Louis: C.V. Mosby.

Zencius, A. H., Wesolowski, M. D., & Burke, W. H. (1990). A comparison of four memory strategies with brain-injured adults. *Brain Injury, 4*(1), 33–38.

APPENDIX B

Measurement Tools for Wandering

REVISED ALGASE WANDERING SCALE: COMMUNITY VERSION (RAWS-CV)

Directions for Administration

To prepare the instrument for use, put items in numerical order and omit subscale headings. Reproduce the form in large print (no smaller than 12 point) and use a high-quality printer to enhance readability of the instrument by respondents.

Respondents can complete the instrument independently or by having it read to them. Survey, face-to-face, telephone, or Web-based formats are all suitable, but choice of format should be based on characteristics of the target audience.

Respondents should be caregivers who live with, provide care to, or are in direct contact with the person with dementia for a minimum of 8 hours per week. This criterion is to assure that they have sufficient opportunity to observe or gain direct knowledge of the behavior that is being rated.

In completing the instrument, respondents should be directed to think of the person with dementia as they are in the present and to reflect on the immediately preceding week to inform their response.

Directions for Scoring

Items constituting each subscale are listed in the table below.

At least 75 percent of the items in a subscale require a valid rating in order to compute a useable score. When there are missing items, reduce the denominator in the computing equation to equal the number of valid ratings for that subscale. This same computation rule applies to the overall RAWS-CV scale score as well.

Revised Algase Wandering Scale (RAWS): Community Version

Please circle the number beside the statement that best describes your family member's current ability or behavior. Use the following scale: 1 = never or unable; 2 = seldom; 3 = sometimes; 4 = usually; 5 = always.

TABLE B.1. Subscales and Related Items for the Revised Algase Wandering Scale—Long-term Care Version

Subscale	No. of items	Item numbers
Persistent walking (PW)	12	1, 5, 6, 9, 23, 25, 26, 28, 29, 32, 33, 34
Repetitive walking (RW)	7	2, 3, 10, 12, 17, 20, 37
Eloping behaviors (EB)	6	8, 14, 16, 27, 30, 36
Spatial disorientation	4	18, 22, 24, 35
Negative outcomes	4	11, 19, 21, 31

TABLE B.2 Revised Algase Wandering Scale—Community Version

	1 never/ unable	2 seldom	3 sometimes	4 usually	5 always
A. Persistent Walking (PW)					
1. He/she does a lot of spontaneous walking.	1	2	3	4	5
5. He/she goes to many different places while walking.	1	2	3	4	5
6. He/she gets up and walks during the night.	1	2	3	4	5
7. He/she walks around restlessly.	1	2	3	4	5
9. He/she walks around between awakening and breakfast.	1	2	3	4	5
13. He/she walks about aimlessly.	1	2	3	4	5
23. He/she travels many different routes while walking.	1	2	3	4	5
25. He/she walks around between lunch and dinner.	1	2	3	4	5
26. He/she often changes direction or course while walking.	1	2	3	4	5
28. He/she walks around between breakfast and lunch.	1	2	3	4	5
29. He/she walks for an odd or inappropriate reason.	1	2	3	4	5
32. He/she walks around between dinner and bedtime.	1	2	3	4	5
33. He/she walks without an apparent destination.	1	2	3	4	5
34. He/she walks during inappropriate times.	1	2	3	4	5

(Continued)

	1 never/ unable	2 seldom	3 sometimes	4 usually	5 always
B. Repetitive walking (RW)					
2. He/she walks intensely between two places.	1	2	3	4	5
3. He/she paces up and down.	1	2	3	4	5
10. He/she walks back and forth between two places in a repetitive way.	1	2	3	4	5
12. He/she walks in one continuous direction.	1	2	3	4	5
17. He/she goes repeatedly to the same location(s) while walking.	1	2	3	4	5
20. He/she repeatedly travels the same route while walking.	1	2	3	4	5
37. He/she walks in a continuous route, as if on a track.	1	2	3	4	5
C. Eloping Behavior (EB)					
8. He/she runs off.	1	2	3	4	5
14. While walking alone, he/she walks beyond intended destination.	1	2	3	4	5
16. He/she attempts to get outside.	1	2	3	4	5
27. He/she stands at the outdoor wanting to go out.	1	2	3	4	5
30. He/she attempts to find or go to familiar locations, even unrealistic ones.	1	2	3	4	5
36. He/she attempts to leave his/her own area.	1	2	3	4	5

38. He/she gets lost outside the house.	1	2	3	4	5
39. He/she enters private or unauthorized areas.	1	2	3	4	5
D. Spatial Disorientation (SD)					
18. He/she cannot locate own room without help.	1	2	3	4	5
22. He/she cannot locate bathroom without help.	1	2	3	4	5
24. He/she gets lost inside the house.	1	2	3	4	5
35. He/she cannot locate dining room without help.	1	2	3	4	5
E. Negative outcome (NO)					
11. While walking alone, he/she has fallen down.	1	2	3	4	5
19. He/she has been found with some major injury.	1	2	3	4	5
21. He/she has been found with some minor injury.	1	2	3	4	5
31. While walking alone, he/she bumps into obstacles or other people.	1	2	3	4	5
F. Mealtime impulsivity (MI)					
4. He/she walks off during meals.	1	2	3	4	5
15. During meals, he/she tries to leave the table or walks away.	1	2	3	4	5

REVISED ALGASE WANDERING SCALE—LONG-TERM CARE VERSION (19 ITEMS)

Administration and Scoring Instructions

Purpose

The Revised Algase Wandering Scale for Long-Term Care (RAWS-LTC) was developed for estimating the degree of wandering behavior in residents of long-term care settings. The LTC version was derived from earlier and longer versions of the Algase Wandering Scale and contains three subscales consistently validated across earlier versions: persistent walking, spatial disorientation, and eloping behavior. The RAWS-LTC has 19 items and can be administered in 10 minutes.

Publications relating to earlier versions of the AWS are found in:

Algase, D. L., Beattie, E.R.A., Bogue, E., & Yao, L. (2001). The Algase Wandering Scale: Initial psychometrics of a new caregiver reporting tool. *American Journal of Alzheimer's Disease and Other Dementias, 16*(3), 141–152.

Algase, D. L., Beattie, E.R.A., Song, J., Milke, D., Duffield, C., & Cowan, B. (2004). Validation of the Algase Wandering Scale (Version 2) in a cross cultural sample. *Aging & Mental Health, 8*(2), 133–142.

Song, J., Algase, D. L., Beattie, E.R.A., Milke, D. L., Duffield, C., & Cowan, B. (2003). Comparison of U.S., Canadian and Australian participants' performance on the Algase Wandering Scale–Version 2 (AWS-V2). *Research & Theory for Nursing Practice: An International Journal, 17*(3), 241–256.

Administration

The AWS is completed by nursing staff as it applies to the behavior of a particular resident. Respondents should have provided care to the person

TABLE B.3 Subscales and Related Items for the Revised Algase Wandering Scale—Long-term Care Version

Subscale	No. of items	Item numbers
Persistent walking (PW)	9	1, 3, 9, 10, 12, 13, 4, 16, 19
Eloping behaviors (EB)	4	4, 7, 8, 15
Spatial disorientation (SD)	6	2, 5, 6, 9, 17, 18

Scores are computed by averaging the ratings for all items within the subscale or for the instrument overall. For example, if items on the SD subscale are scored as follows, #18 = 2, #22 = 3, #24 = 3, and #35 = 2, the subscale score would be (2 + 3 + 3 + 2)/4 or 2.5. Computing scores as item means allows for comparison of subscales scores of unequal length.

with dementia over several recent shifts. This criterion is to assure that they have sufficient opportunity to observe or gain direct knowledge of the behavior that is being rated. In completing the instrument, respondents should be directed to think of the person with dementia as they are in the present and to reflect on the immediately preceding week to inform their response. Staff may complete the instrument unaided, or it may be read to them by another individual.

To prepare the instrument for use, put items in numerical order and omit subscale headings. Reproduce the form in large print (no smaller than 12 point) and use a high quality printer to enhance readability of the instrument by respondents. Survey, face-to-face, telephone, or Web-based formats are all suitable, but choice of format should be based on characteristics of the target audience.

Scoring

Items 1 through 23 constitute the RAWS-LTC; items in each subscale are listed in the following table.

Items 20 through 24 are used for reliability and validity estimation. These items may be deleted if these estimates are not desired.

Values for items range from 1 through 4, with the value 1 assigned to the first response listed for each item.

Scores are computed by averaging the ratings for all items within the subscale or for the instrument overall. For example, if items on the subscale are #4 = 3, #5 = 3, #16 = 3, and #18 = 2, the subscale score would be (3 + 3 + 3 + 2)/4 or 2.75. Scores computed as item averages allow for comparison of subscales scores of unequal length. A valid rating is needed on 75 percent of items to compute a useable score. When there are missing items, reduce the denominator in the computing equation to equal the number of valid ratings for that subscale. This same computation rule applies to the overall RAWS—LTC scale score as well.

Revised Algase Wandering Scale—LTC (19 items)

University of Michigan, School of Nursing
Wandering Research Project

TABLE B.4 Revised Algase Wandering Scale— Long-term Care Version

Subject ID ____________ Facility ____________

Please put a check beside the statement that best describes this resident.

PERSISTENT WALKING

1. Resident has a reduced amount of spontaneous walking.	___	walks the same or more as others of same age and ability
	___	walks less than others of same age, ability
	___	walks only minimally, e.g., to go to bathroom
	___	does not walk spontaneously unless prompted
19. Resident has an increased amount of spontaneous walking.	___	walks about the same as others of same age and ability
	___	walks distinctly more than average, but will sit for periods
	___	walks distinctly more than average, rarely sits
	___	walks distinctly more than average, never sits
3. Resident walks about on own.	___	only if prompted
	___	occasionally during the day
	___	frequently during the day
	___	almost constantly during the day
9. Resident walks around restlessly.	___	never
	___	on a few occasions
	___	regularly but not daily
	___	on a daily basis
10. Resident paces up and down.	___	never
	___	on a few occasions
	___	regularly but not daily
	___	on a daily basis

16. Resident walks around after awakening but before breakfast.	___	never
	___	less than others of same age and ability
	___	the same as others of the same age and ability
	___	more than others of same age and ability
12. Resident walks around between breakfast and lunch.	___	never
	___	less than others of same age and ability
	___	the same as others of the same age and ability
	___	more than others of same age and ability
13. Resident walks around between lunch and dinner.	___	never
	___	less than others of same age and ability
	___	the same as others of the same age and ability
	___	more than others of same age and ability
14. Resident walks around after dinner but before bedtime.	___	never
	___	less than others of same age and ability
	___	the same as others of the same age and ability
	___	more than others of same age and ability
ELOPING BEHAVIOR		
4. Resident attempts to leave their authorized area.	___	never
	___	on a few occasions
	___	regularly but not daily
	___	on a daily basis
7. Resident runs off.	___	never
	___	on a few occasions
	___	regularly but not daily
	___	on a daily basis

(Continued)

Subject ID ____________________ Facility ____________________

8. Resident enters unauthorized areas.	___	never
	___	on a few occasions
	___	regularly but not daily
	___	on a daily basis
15. Resident was returned to authorized area after leaving unnoticed.	___	never
	___	only once
	___	more than once, but not often
	___	often

SPATIAL DISORIENTATION

2. Resident gets lost.	___	never
	___	on a few occasions
	___	regularly but not daily
	___	on a daily basis
5. Resident cannot locate bathroom without help.	___	requires no help
	___	sometimes requires help
	___	usually requires help
	___	always requires help
6. Resident cannot locate dining room without help.	___	requires no help
	___	sometimes requires help
	___	usually requires help
	___	always requires help

9. Resident cannot locate own room without help.	___	requires no help
	___	sometimes requires help
	___	usually requires help
	___	always requires help
17. Resident walks about aimlessly.	___	always has an identifiable destination/goal
	___	usually has an identifiable destination/goal
	___	sometimes has an identifiable destination/goal
	___	never has an identifiable destination/goal
18. While walking alone, resident bumps into obstacles or other people.	___	never
	___	on a few occasions
	___	regularly but not daily
	___	on a daily basis
VALIDATION ITEMS		
20. Resident is a wanderer.	___	definitely not
	___	at times
	___	yes, but it is not a problem
	___	yes, and it is a problem

(Continued)

Subject ID ____________		Facility ____________
21. I am	___	a nurse aid
	___	a licensed practical nurse
	___	a registered nurse
	___	a social worker
	___	a dietitian or dietary aid
	___	a physical therapist
	___	an occupational therapist
	___	an activity therapist
	___	a unit clerk
	___	other
22. I have worked with this resident.	___	only today
	___	today and once before
	___	several times
	___	many times
23. I have attended classes on dementia.	___	never
	___	once
	___	several times
	___	often
24. I consider myself	___	inexperienced with dementia
	___	a beginner in caring for persons with dementia
	___	experienced in dementia care
	___	an expert in dementia care

Are there any comments you would like to make, either about this resident or about our research?

Wandering Research Project, University of Michigan, 400 N. Ingalls, Ann Arbor MI 48109-0499

APPENDIX C

Wandering Resources

- Sample Policies/Directives/Templates
  - Management of Wandering and Missing Patient Events Directive
  - Management of Cognitively Impaired, Wander Risk Veterans in Medical Center Outpatient Clinics (sample)
  - Sample Respite Admission Questionnaire
- Resources
  - The National Center for Patient Safety (www.patientsafety.gov)
  - The Missing Patient Directive Web Course
- Training Courses (from slide presentations)
  - Bay Pines VAMC Geriatric Psychiatry Unit "Don't Get Lost" Inpatient and Day Treatment Programs Wandering Prevention Training Course
  - Missing Patient Process Improvement Presentation
- Family/Caregiver Educational Materials
  - Family/Caregiver Brochure

SAMPLE POLICIES/DIRECTIVES/TEMPLATES

Management of Wandering and Missing Patient Events Directive

This is a VA Directive that addresses how to prevent, detect, and respond to wandering behavior of VA patients. It is accompanied by an Employee Education Service electronic training program made available and required by all staff at all levels and disciplines as well as family members of high risk patients.

Department of Veterans Affairs
Veterans Health Administration
Washington, D.C. 20420

VHA DIRECTIVE 2002–013

March 4, 2002

Management of Wandering and Missing Patient Events

1. PURPOSE: This Veterans Health Administration (VHA) Directive establishes policy to ensure that each Department of Veterans Affairs (VA) medical facility has an effective and reliable plan to prevent and effectively manage wandering and missing patient events that place patients at risk for harm.
2. BACKGROUND
   A. In VHA facilities, patients straying beyond the normal view or control of employees may be at risk for injury or death. Although VA has responsibility for all patients under its care, physically or mentally impaired patients require a distinctly higher degree of monitoring and protection.
   B. To prevent accidental deaths and injuries, VHA must:
      (1) Recognize, specify, and maintain appropriate staff responsibility for the whereabouts of patients;
      (2) Systematically assess all patients to determine the risk potential for those who may wander or become missing from a treatment setting;
      (3) Detect missing patients early; and
      (4) Initiate prompt search procedures.
   C. Definitions
      (1) *High-risk Patient.* A high-risk patient is one who is incapacitated because of frailty, or physical or mental impairment. Patients are considered incapacitated if, at a minimum, they:
         (a) Are legally committed;
         (b) Have a court appointed legal guardian;
         (c) Are considered dangerous to self or others;
         (d) Lack cognitive ability (either permanently or temporarily) to make relevant decisions; or
         (e) Have physical or mental impairments that increase their risk of harm to self or others.
      (2) *Wandering Patient.* A wandering patient is a high-risk patient who has shown a propensity to stray beyond

the view or control of employees, thereby requiring a high degree of monitoring and protection to ensure the patient's safety.

(3) *Missing Patient.* A missing patient is a high-risk patient who disappears from an inpatient or outpatient treatment area or while under control of VA, such as during transport. Examples of situations when patients who meet the above criteria should be considered missing include, *but are not limited* to, the following:
   (a) Inpatient or day treatment high-risk patient not present to receive a scheduled medication, treatment, meal, or appointment, and whose whereabouts are unknown.
   (b) A high-risk patient checked in for an outpatient clinic appointment who is not present for the appointment when called, and whose whereabouts are unknown.
   (c) High-risk outpatients from a community facility who do not return to their community facility following the appointment, whose whereabouts are unknown.
   (d) A high-risk patient who is using VA-sponsored transportation (Disabled American Veterans vans, VA drivers, VA shuttles) who does not report to that transportation for the return trip.
   (e) High-risk patients who do not return from pass as scheduled and whose whereabouts are unknown.

(4) *Absent Patient.*
   (a) An absent patient is one who leaves a treatment area without knowledge or permission of staff, but who *does not meet* the high-risk criteria outlined for a missing patient and is *not* considered incapacitated.
   (b) An otherwise absent patient should be classified as a missing patient when one or a combination of additional environmental or clinical factors may, in the judgment of the responsible clinician, increase the patient's vulnerability and risk. Conditions that might lead to this decision may include, but are not limited to, the following:
      i. Weather conditions, i.e., the patient has inappropriate dress, the patient's safety is compromised;

ii. Construction sites or other dangerous conditions exist nearby;

iii. Recent trauma, unexpected bad news, or abrupt change in clinical status;

iv. Local geographic conditions increase risk; or

v. Homelessness, in combination with other factors that create risk.

(5) *Assessment.* An assessment is a clinical evaluation of patients with regard to their capacity to make decisions relative to their immediate physical safety or well being. Past history may be a guide, as well as information obtained by friends, relatives, or caregivers. Patients whose mental status may change rapidly, such as those suffering from post-surgical delirium or drug-induced psychosis, may require repeated assessments during the day. An assessment is a clinical event and should be recorded in the medical record, whether paper-based or electronic. Staff may be alerted to patients at special risk through electronic "flags" or reminders.

D. Preliminary Search. As soon as it is determined that a high-risk patient is missing, a preliminary search must be initiated to include nearby ward or clinic areas, offices and adjacent areas such as lobbies, stairwells, elevators, etc., and will be coordinated by locally designated staff in each clinical area.

E. Full Search. If a missing patient is not located during the preliminary search and the clinical assessment indicates the patient is at high-risk, a full search is authorized by the medical center Director, or designee.

(1) VA Police, Security Service, and appropriate medical center staff on duty participate in the search to include all areas of the facility in addition to those covered by the preliminary search, such as:

(a) All grounds areas, parking lots, ball fields, tennis courts, outdoor seating and picnic areas, woods, and areas off, but contiguous to, the property (e.g., local neighborhood attractions, with specific instructions as to what action(s) to initiate if the patient is found since there *is no legal authority,* lacking an extreme exigency, for patients to be physically detained against their will off facility property) as appropriate; and

(b) All other buildings, elevators, designated smoking areas, accessible areas for outpatient clinics, construction sites, and other structures.

(2) When appropriate during or following the full search, VA Police and Security Service must contact the appropriate outside law enforcement agencies to file a missing persons report providing all the needed data so as to ensure that the patient is entered into the National Crime Information Computer (NCIC) system. These agencies must also be informed in a timely manner to cancel this alert when a missing patient is recovered. This policy should not preclude those Police and Security Services units from entering this data themselves provided they have the capability to do so.

3. POLICY: It is VHA policy for all facilities to maintain:
   A. A system of identifying high-risk patients needing a higher degree of monitoring and protection.
   B. A detailed plan for assessment, identification, and prevention of wandering.
   C. A detailed plan for searching and locating of missing patients. *NOTE:* This policy is applicable to all sites and levels of care such as: hospital, domiciliary, and nursing care facilities; residential bed care facilities (psychiatric residential rehabilitation and treatment programs); VA-owned or leased, off-ground health care facilities; day centers, day hospitals, and day treatment centers; and Community Based Outpatient Clinics (CBOCs), or independent clinics.
4. ACTION
   A. Responsibilities
      (1) *Network Directors.* Network Directors are responsible for ensuring that each medical center within their respective Veterans Integrated Service Network (VISN) has local policy that meets the guidelines established in this directive.
      (2) *Medical Center Directors.* Medical center Directors are responsible for:
         (a) Developing local policies that require:
            i. Timely assessments of patients and documentation of such assessments;
            ii. Early intervention to minimize wandering risks;
            iii. Clear designation of responsibility for security of construction and other environmental hazards to minimize risks of inappropriate or unauthorized access to unsafe areas;

iv. Timely and thorough search procedures;
v. Staff competency with ongoing education and training in the care of wandering or missing patients;
vi. Missing patient events to be referred for Root Cause Analysis (RCA) or Aggregated Review consistent with VA's National Center for Patient Safety (NCPS) procedures described in the Patient Safety Improvement Handbook; and
vii. Continuous learning through the integration of lessons learned from drills, close calls, or actual missing patient events.

(b) Each medical center must establish and publish a local plan (policy) that reflects the full scope of services to be provided and designates all sites of care to be involved, in order for the effective prevention and management of wandering patients and of missing patient events to be achieved. This plan must define preparation for and responses to missing patient events; it needs to include, but is not limited to:
i. Designation of persons who can perform a clinical review of patients when they have "disappeared" to determine if they are either "missing" or "absent," and designation of persons who will follow up with the patient, family, or extended family regarding those patients considered "absent" to assure their safety. *NOTE:* If there are concerns regarding an absent patient, it is recommended that a telephone call be placed to the next of kin or other designated individual, to ascertain the patient's whereabouts in lieu of a search, i.e., to validate the patient's safety.
ii. Designation of who may declare a patient "missing" and under what circumstances as well as who will determine the level of search required for each category of patient.
iii. Command responsibilities and procedures both during administrative hours and nonadministrative hours, including designation of a Search Command Post and Search Coordinator.
iv. Time frames, based on local circumstances, for initiating preliminary and full searches,

for notifying relatives (next of kin), and for determining when the full search for an incapacitated missing patient is considered to be unsuccessful.

v. Designation of persons who will communicate with relatives, guardians, other responsible persons, and nearby treatment facilities, as appropriate, until a missing patient is found.

vi. Specific staff assigned to given areas to ensure that all areas are searched and to avoid random or uncoordinated searches. Use of a grid search is recommended (see Att. A).

vii. Immediate notification of VA Police in the event that a missing patient is found to be deceased on VA property. The Federal Bureau of Investigation (FBI), State and local police, the Office of the Medical Examiner, and local management officials are to be notified. The police will establish and maintain the area as a possible crime scene, ensuring that the body and premises are not disturbed until instructions and the proper authorization have been received. After positive identification is confirmed, notification of next of kin is accomplished in accordance with local policy. *NOTE:* Local law enforcement agencies and officials should be oriented and become involved with the search activities of the VA medical center by being invited to policy and operational planning sessions.

viii. Designation of responsibility to maintain the Missing Patient Register, i.e., entering the names of missing patients as soon as the full local search has failed to locate them, and removing their name from the Register as soon as they are located. *NOTE:* This process will aid in flagging patients who may present to other VA facilities and will allow analysis of national patterns.

(c) Ensuring that the prevention or management of wandering patients and the management and reporting of actual missing patient events is integrated into initial orientation, annual, and other ongoing education and training of staff, especially within those special units or sites designated for the care of high-risk patients.

(d) Ensuring that the comprehensive review and assessment of each facility's processes and any aggregated data on actual missing patient events or close calls are incorporated into the appropriate committee activity at each facility to continuously and systemically enhance environmental safety.

(3) *Employees.* All employees, including both clinical and nonclinical staff, are responsible for assessing, reviewing, and developing processes to enhance patient safety associated with wandering or missing patient events within the scope of their job, as well as intervening when appropriate.

(4) *NCPS.* NCPS is responsible for reviewing RCAs and Aggregate Reviews involving missing patients that are submitted to NCPS. NCPS is responsible for disseminating and making relevant information from the RCAs and Aggregate Reviews available to VHA facilities to foster the reduction and elimination of risks. This information may be communicated in numerous ways, including advisories, alerts, newsletters, and national calls.

(5) *Employee Education Service (EES).* EES will support the establishment of a national training program on wandering and missing patients to be made available at all VA facilities to assure minimum uniform training standards by October 1, 2002. This program should be directed toward relevant staff at all levels and disciplines as well as family members of high-risk patients. The program should include information from the NCPS on the requirements and basic procedures for addressing missing patients as described in the VHA Handbook 1050.1, Patient Safety Improvement Handbook.

B. Prevention and Management. The prevention and effective management of wandering and missing patient events is based on clinical assessment of cognitive ability for each patient and the associated safety risks. Each facility must determine the frequency for assessing the cognitive ability of patients with regard to their safety and developing safety measures, as appropriate for the patient's condition.

(1) *Assessment of Cognitive Impairment.* At a minimum, the clinical assessment of cognitive impairment must be recorded in the patient's record:

(a) At the time of inpatient admission, discharge, or transfer between units or care setting;
(b) As a component of each initial and annual outpatient evaluation;
(c) When there is a reported change in mental status for any reason; and
(d) In absentia, i.e., when they have disappeared from a clinical setting.

NOTE: If the patient is at high-risk, then assessment and the safety measures appropriate for the patient need to be part of the treatment plan, which must be discussed among the patient's health care providers. In addition, that assessment and the safety measures need to be included in the alert that comes to the attention of all applicable health care providers when the patient's record is accessed. The assessment must occur. The assessment and related safety measures must be discussed by the patient's treatment team and documented as being discussed.

(2) *Minimizing Risks.* Because of the documented risks inherent in the aging veteran population, VHA aims to be as proactive as possible in minimizing risks for patients under its care. As a result, the following processes must be integrated into each facility's policy for the prevention or effective management of wandering and missing patient events:
(a) Policies on patient privileging, requirements for patient supervision and surveillance, and search procedures with regard to early identification of missing patients;
(b) Each facility must consider actual or close call missing patient events in accordance with NCPS guidelines and VHA Handbook 1050.1 and integrate the resulting information into education and training of staff and improving existing processes to enhance patient safety;
(c) Initial and annual training of all relevant staff regarding policy and search policies and procedures for identifying, assessing, and finding missing patients;
(d) Missing Patient Drills that integrate findings from environmental rounds or other patient safety processes (such as aggregated RCAs), must be conducted at each medical center or site of jurisdiction, including CBOCs. Once staff have received initial training, additional drills must be conducted

at least annually (or more frequently, if judged prudent due to local circumstances) to effectively evaluate known areas of vulnerability throughout and surrounding the facility. Once staff are fully trained, an actual search during which the search plan is fully implemented and a critique is completed may take the place of the drill for the shift involved in the actual search. It is recommended that the sites for missing patient drills be prioritized based on known areas of vulnerability and lessons learned from RCAs and other risk management or performance improvement processes; and

(e) The systematic and comprehensive monitoring and assessment of hazardous areas and construction sites must be an integral part of this process. It is essential to plan appropriate security measures, including method for promptly discovering breaches and response to such a discovery, for areas of the medical center that contain hazards such as: construction sites, staging areas, areas involved in maintenance procedures, mechanical spaces, utility areas, crawl spaces, electrical vaults and closets, shops, utility plants, storage areas, water towers, lakes, ponds, rivers, streams, laboratories, research space, and morgues. (*NOTE:* Essentially any area that when entered by an untrained individual could reasonably be considered to hold potential danger must be integrated into local processes.) Any portion of the security plan where failure is not immediately obvious (such as fire or motion alarms) must be periodically checked for proper function.

C. High-Risk Patients

(1) *Electronic Technology.* The use of electronic technology for those patients considered to be high-risk may be used *only* as one tool to enhance and augment other processes for minimizing the risk of patients wandering away from a designated area or site of care. This use must not be considered as a substitute for professional vigilance and systematic verification of patient location such as during change of shift rounds for inpatient and other supervised settings. When electronic technology is in use:

(a) There must be systematic and frequent checks of all critical components of the system with clear designation of responsibility for monitoring and maintaining that system. A basic check of the system in high-risk areas is encouraged at a minimum of every 24 hours to assure proper functioning as intended to minimize risk. Maintenance of the system must be consistent with manufacturer's guidelines; however, a complete systems check must be performed at least annually. A proactive assessment of potential vulnerabilities of the system and its use (e.g., failure Modes Effects Analysis) should be performed to guide the appropriate use of the system (see VHA Handbook 1050.1, sub par. 5d).

(b) Electronic devices or systems must be re-evaluated at the time of each wandering or missing patient event to assess possible contributing factors.

(2) *Activities.* A comprehensive review and assessment of locations for activities away from the facility must be conducted and integrated in the planning of recreational activities to facilitate safety, especially for those patients known to be high-risk. Supervision of patients must be consistent with review findings.

(3) *Identification.* Each facility must establish processes to assure the availability of pictures and physical descriptions for all high-risk patients in the event that they are suspected to be missing as a means to enhance the effectiveness of search procedures. Patient Identification System photographs may be used where available.

(4) *Transport.* Each facility must take special precautions during the transport of known high-risk patients or those reported to have a change in mental status, in the absence of clinical assessment.

5. REFERENCES
   A. M-1, Part I, Chapter 13.
   B. M-2, Part I, Chapter 35.
   C. DM&S Supplement MP-I, Part I, Change 42.
   D. Vet. Affairs Opinion Gen. Counsel Prec 37–91 (1991).
   E. National Center for Patient Safety (NCPS) guidelines.
   F. VHA Handbook 1050.1, Patient Safety Improvement Handbook.
6. FOLLOW-UP RESPONSIBILITY: Mental Health Strategic Health Care Group (116) is responsible for the content of this Directive. Questions may be referred to 202-273-8435.
7. RESCISSIONS: VHA Directive 96–029 is rescinded. This VHA directive expires March 31, 2007.

S/Tom Sanders for
Frances M. Murphy, M.D., M.P.H.
Acting Under Secretary for Health

Attachment

DISTRIBUTION: CO: E-mailed 3/5/2002
FLD: VISN, MA, DO, OC, OCRO, and 200—E-mailed 3/5/2002

ATTACHMENT A

Patient Searches Using Grid Sectors

1. Work with facility engineering staff to obtain a site plot of the facility and surrounding areas. Superimpose a grid map to delineate the grid sectors.
2. One individual is to be responsible to gather all pertinent information concerning the grid search. This needs to include:
   a. Search grid sector assignments;
   b. Times and by whom grid sectors are searched;
   c. Times and by whom each building is searched;
   d. Times and to whom notifications and requests are made; and
   e. Result of search.
3. The indoor search needs to include all buildings within the assigned search area to include any unsecured: stairwells, closets, attics, crawl spaces, equipment rooms, all smoking shelters, indoor construction areas, bathrooms, vending areas, and all other areas large enough for the subject to hide.
4. The outdoor search needs to include brush and open areas, all parking areas, all government and nongovernment vehicles, all courtyard areas, all shrubbery around buildings, all construction areas, all outlying structures on grounds not assigned to interior search personnel, and any other area where a subject could have wandered.
5. The outdoor search is to be a methodical and complete visual inspection of open terrain for a lost or injured person, or for indications and marks of a person's movement. Larger areas are to be divided into smaller, more manageable grids. Each grid is approximately 500 by 500 feet and is designated with coordinates as illustrated on the search grid maps.
6. Each search team is assigned to a grid or number of grids. Each grid is to be searched from south to north by a search team in sweeps by lines of team members spaced abreast. Several sweeps

may be necessary to completely cover assigned grids. A leader directs the search team.

7. The leader is responsible for the safety of team members and to make sure the search of assigned grids is complete. Failure to check one small area may result in search failure.
8. If the subject is found, the search team will render first aid if needed and notify command post of the location and, if needed request that medical personnel be sent. If the subject is unharmed, the search team will transport the subject back to the appropriate treatment area.
9. If the subject is found deceased, the subject and area surrounding the subject will be cordoned off and preserved as a possible crime scene until instructions and the proper authorization have been received.

Management of Cognitively Impaired, Wander Risk Veterans in Medical Center Outpatient Clinics (Sample)

(Provided by Vivian E. Bugaoan, LCSW, Northport VA Medical Center, Northport, NY)

Department of Veterans Affairs Center Memorandum 122–13
Northport, New York 11768

Subj. Management of Cognitively Impaired, Wander Risk

Veterans in Medical Center Outpatient Clinics

1. PURPOSE AND SCOPE: To establish policy and procedures for the identification, assessment, and management of cognitively impaired veterans who attend medical center outpatient clinics and are at risk to wander.
2. POLICY: Outpatient veterans identified as a wander risk will be escorted during clinic appointments by a competent family member/significant other or VA escort. It is the policy of the Medical Center to:
   A. Assess the wander risk potential of outpatient veterans who have a DSM IV dementia diagnosis.
   B. Develop an individualized plan to provide for the escort/accompaniment of wander [risk veterans.]
   C. Instruct wander risk outpatient veterans and their families/caregivers regarding safety precautions to be taken in the community and outpatient clinic.
   D. Evaluate the biopsychosocial environment of cognitively impaired wander risk veterans to determine the need for

community psychosocial support services to enhance/sustain community living.

E. Take appropriate action to locate a wander risk veteran and ensure their safety should they become missing during an outpatient clinic visit.

3. DEFINITIONS:

A. *Wander Risk:* A veteran with a dementia diagnosis whose degree of cognitive impairment is such that clinical staff assess that veteran is unable to reliably get from one place to another in a clinic setting without being accompanied/escorted is considered to present a wander risk.

B. *Outpatient Clinic[s]:* This includes the clinical pavilion in Building 200, other areas of Building 200 where ambulatory services are provided to outpatient veterans, and [Mental Health Clinic / Bldg. 64].

C. *Missing:* A cognitively impaired outpatient veteran who has been assessed as a wander risk will be considered missing if:

1) Veteran is transported to the Medical Center, but does not appear for scheduled clinic appointment.

2) Veteran presents for outpatient clinic appointment, but leaves prior to completion of treatment.

3) Veteran does not appear at designated area for transportation home by DAV.

4. PROCEDURES:

A. The identification of wander risk in a cognitively impaired veteran attending an outpatient clinic will occur during scheduled clinic appointments.

B. An outpatient veteran with a dementia diagnosis will be [assessed by their primary care provider for wander risk and document the assessment in the medical record].

C. A veteran with a dementia diagnosis who is not assessed as a wander risk will be reassessed by their primary care provider when the provider identifies a significant change in the veteran's mental status during a subsequent clinic visit.

D. The *primary care provider* who determines that veteran is a wander risk will:

1) [Immediately] advise the veteran/family/caregiver, as appropriate, of the provider's assessment of wander risk and the need for the veteran to be escorted/accompanied during all clinic visits. [The primary provider will document this discussion in the veteran's medical record.]

2) Provide veteran/family with initial education to outline precautions that family members and caregivers can take

in the home and community setting when caring for a veteran at risk for wandering.

3) The clinician will ensure that the veteran has been issued a color photo Veteran Identification Card (VIC) as this VIC photo is available under the VISTA Image Display in CPRS. If an ID card was issued from another facility, the admissions supervisor should be contacted to gain access. If the veteran does not have a new color photo VIC card, the veteran should be escorted to Central Intake to have a picture taken.
4) Immediately refer the veteran and family/significant other to the outpatient clinic social worker.
5) Document these actions in a progress note.

E. The clinic Social Worker will:
   1) Meet with the veteran/family/significant other, as appropriate, to provide further education regarding the assessment of wander risk and the precautions that family members and caregivers can take in the clinic and community to ensure the veteran's safety. [The social worker will give the veteran/family/significant other the Medical Center Brochure: "Protecting a Person Who Wanders."]
   2) Provide a biopsychosocial assessment to include:
      (a) Evaluation of veteran's safety in his home environment and ability of caregiver to meet veteran's needs.
      (b) Evaluation of community support services that would enhance/sustain veteran's ability to remain in a community setting.
      (c) Evaluation of [veteran's] need for alternate level of care.
      (d) Plan of psychosocial intervention to assure veteran safety in the community, address veteran psychosocial needs, and provide caregiver support.
   3.) Develop with the veteran/family/significant other an individualized plan to provide for the escort/accompaniment of the veteran in clinic settings.

F. Specific measures to escort/accompany veterans to clinic appointments will be initiated by the interdisciplinary team as follows and will [involve] the veteran's community residence and the psychosocial support services available to the veteran.
   1) For veterans residing independently in the community or with a family member:
      (a) Veteran's family member/significant other will be instructed by the primary care provider to accompany veteran to all clinic appointments. If veteran

utilizes DAV transportation, the [clinic social worker] will provide a letter for DAV, stating that the veteran requires accompaniment by the family member/significant other.

(b) For those veterans whose family members are unable to accompany them and who utilize DAV transportation, the family member will contact the ER [Nurse Manager] (extension 2380) when scheduling DAV transportation and arrange for veteran to be met at the DAV drop off location by an assigned VA escort. The escort will accompany the veteran to his clinic, return veteran to the DAV pick-up point, and wait with the veteran until the DAV van arrives and veteran is placed on the van. The family member will advise DAV when scheduling transportation that veteran will be met by VA escort.

2) For veterans residing in Contract Nursing Homes:

(a) The VA Contract Nursing Home (CNH) Coordinator or VA Public Health Nursing (PHN) Coordinator will notify the Contract Nursing Home Director of Nursing that the veteran is a wander risk and develop a plan with the CNH to ensure that veteran is accompanied to all clinic appointments by VA Escort Services.

(b) The CNH Coordinator or PHN Coordinator will notify the following VA staff of veteran's status as a wander risk:

i. CNH Coordinator
ii. Public Health Nurse Coordinators
iii. ER Nurse Manager

(c) Escort Procedure for Scheduled Clinic Appointments:

i. The Contract Nursing Home will notify the PHN Coordinator of the date and time of clinic appointments
ii. Transport of CNH veterans to the medical center is scheduled by the VA travel coordinator. The VA travel coordinator will e-mail the CNH Coordinator and PNH Coordinator at least 24 hours in advance of scheduled appointment that travel has been arranged.
iii. The PHN Coordinator will coordinate with VA Escort and VA travel to ensure that veteran is dropped off and picked up at the VA Escort

office by VA travel and a VA escort is assigned to accompany the veteran during the visit to the Medical Center.

(d) Escort Procedures for Unscheduled Clinic Appointments:

i. The CNH will inform the ER Nurse Manager that the veteran is a wander risk and needs VA Escort.

ii. The ER Nurse Manager will assign VA Escort or ER staff during off tours to remain with and supervise the veteran.

(e) Other Escort Procedures:

i. A small number of CNHs routinely provide escort for veterans on contract. Since this service is not included in the contracted per diem rate, this option can only be utilized with the CNH's agreement.

3) For veterans residing in Community Residential Care Program [Adult] Homes:

(a) The CRC Social worker will advise the CRC home that veteran is considered a wander risk and develop a plan with the home [to ensure veteran's accompanied to VA appointments].

(b) Options include:

i. The CRC home assigns a member of their staff [or another responsible resident] to [accompany] the veteran to clinic and provide escort to clinic appointments. Since such escort services are not part of the monthly rate paid by the veteran to the home, an additional special rate may be negotiated by CRC for this service.

ii. If veteran travels to clinic by DAV, the CRC home will contact the ER Nurse Manager (extension 2380) after scheduling DAV transportation and arrange for veteran to be met at the DAV drop-off location by an assigned VA escort person. The VA escort will accompany veteran to his clinic, return the veteran to the DAV pick-up point and wait with the veteran until the DAV van arrives and veteran is placed on the van. The home will advise DAV when scheduling the transportation that the veteran will be met by a VA escort.

G. Search Procedures: In the event that a wander risk veteran is found to be missing, the following actions will be initiated:
   1) The veteran will be overhead paged in the clinical pavilion and in Building 200.
   2) The clinic staff will conduct a preliminary search of the clinic area, nearby offices and adjacent areas such as bathrooms, the smoking shelter, the DAV van pick up, and HART bus pick up.
   3) A clinical practitioner will contact veteran's residence to ensure that veteran has not returned home on his own.
   4) The VA Police should be contacted if the above efforts do not result in finding the missing veteran. Police should be provided with a description of the veteran, to include clothing and other identifying features. The VA Police will conduct a preliminary search of the medical center grounds.
   5) If these efforts to find the veteran fail, and if the treating physician assesses that the veteran is a danger to himself/herself or others, the treating physician will contact the Medical Center Director, Associate Director or Chief of Staff requesting authorization for a full search (Code Green). If a full search is authorized, procedures outlined in CM 07B-05 shall be followed.

5. REFERENCES: Center Memorandum 07B-05, "Search for Missing Patients Plan," dated [April 15, 2005]
6. RESCISSION: Center Memorandum 122–13, dated [April 11, 2003]
7. Attachments:
   A. Brochure: Protecting a Person Who Wanders

[ROBERT S. SCHUSTER, MHCA]
[Director]
Dist. A

Sample Respite Admission Questionnaire

(Provided by Fern Pietruszka, Greater Los Angeles VA)

Respite Care Screening. The following questionnaire is used as part of the screening process for respite admissions to the Nursing Home Care Unit (NHCU). Each veteran and a caregiver/spouse is interviewed in person to determine if the NHCU can provide a safe respite admission for the veteran. This set of questions is for the caregiver. In conjunction with this subjective set of questions, we look at the veteran's cognition, transfer, and ambulation ability as well as the veteran's ability to sit through the full respite screening interview process. This helps to identify those veterans who may need one-to-one supervision and those who may also need additional evaluation of their cognitive status or medication needs prior to admission for respite.

Wander Risk Assessment

1.	Does the veteran walk around his usual environment aimlessly?	Yes	No
2.	Does the veteran get easily agitated with doing simple tasks such as dressing?	Yes	No
3.	Does the veteran frequently ask where he is?	Yes	No
4.	Does the veteran ask the same question(s) often throughout the day?	Yes	No
5.	Does the veteran get confused with any change in his routine?	Yes	No
6.	Does the veteran get confused with any change in his location?	Yes	No
7.	Has the veteran ever gotten lost?	Yes	No
8.	Has the veteran needed to be frequently re-directed in a task?	Yes	No
9.	Does the veteran have a conservator or DPA for Health Care?	Yes	No
10.	Can the veteran walk more than 200 yards?	Yes	No
11.	Can the veteran walk up stairs?	Yes	No
12.	Have you ever been told that the veteran has dementia or mental health illness?	Yes	No

RESOURCES

The National Center for Patient Safety (www.patientsafety.gov)

- TIPS Newsletter Nov/Dec 2005: Analyzing Missing Patient Events at the VA by Joseph M. DeRosier, PE, CSP, NCPS program manager and Lesley Taylor, BS, NCPS program analyst, http://www.patientsafety.gov/TIPS/tips.html

The Missing Patient Directive Web Course

For VA Employees only: http://vaww.sites.lrn.va.gov/mp/mpbegin.html

The Missing Patient Directive Web site was developed by The Employee Education System for the VHA Central Office.

The Management of Wandering and Missing Patient Events is a national initiative, created by a large multidisciplinary group chaired by William Van Stone of the Mental Health Strategic Health Care Group in VA Central Office.

Missing Patient Directive Committee Biographical Information (alphabetical)

Ron Alford

Joseph Derosier

Noel Eldrige

Linda M. Flynn

Gary Gillitzer

Lynn Litwa

Kimberly Radant

For non-VA Employees, following is the text of the Missing Patient Directive Presentation and Test that you can adapt for your own facility's use.

Missing Patient Directive Glossary, Presentation, and Text (adapt for your own facility's needs).

GLOSSARY

Absent Patient

A VA patient who leaves a treatment area without knowledge or permission of staff, but who does not meet the high-risk criteria outlined for a missing patient and is not considered incapacitated.

Assessment

A clinical evaluation by a mental health professional of the mental ability of a patient to care for him- or herself.

CBOC

Community Based Outpatient Clinics. VA clinics located some distance from a VA medical center.

Clinical Status

The assessment of a combination of illnesses or physical disabilities that may put a patient at risk.

Cognitive Ability

The ability of a person to remember, think, reason, and use judgment.

Contiguous

Contiguous to the property. Nearby to VA property.

Drills, Missing Patient

Regularly scheduled drills that imitate preliminary and full searches as they might occur at your own facility.

Electronic Technology

Electronic devices physically attached to a high-risk patient that ring an alarm at the nursing station when a high-risk patient nears an exit.

Extreme Exigency

An emergency situation involving patients.

Full Search

A full search includes all areas of the facility in addition to those covered by the preliminary search.

High-Risk Patient

A high-risk patient is one who is incapacitated because of frailty or physical or mental impairment.

Incapacitated Patient

A patient who is injured or debilitated physically or mentally to the extent that he or she is unable to function adequately.

Legally Committed

A legal process that varies state by state whereby a judge decides that a person must receive psychiatric treatment because of severe mental illness. While usually treatment must occur in a hospital, a number of states also have outpatient commitment.

Mental Status

A part of a psychiatric or mental examination that describes how well a patient's mind is functioning.

Missing Patient

A missing patient is a high-risk patient who leaves a treatment area without knowledge or permission of staff.

Missing Patient Register

The Missing Patient Register is a national computer system that has recently been replaced by a new Web-Based Missing Patient Register (WBMPR).

NCIC

National Crime Information Computer. A national system used by police that includes a list of persons who are reported missing.

NCPS

National Center for Patient Safety.

Preliminary Search

A preliminary search includes nearby ward or clinic areas, offices, and adjacent areas such as lobbies, stairwells, elevators.

Root Cause Analysis

A system for looking at problems and incidents that involve the safety of patients.

Wandering Patient

A high-risk patient who tends to stray beyond the view or control of clinical staff.

WBMPR

The Web-Based Missing Patient Registry is a national electronic program available at all VA facilities that lists the names of high risk patients who are missing along with the date and name of the facility where they were last seen.

Chapter 1: New Definitions

What is a High-Risk Patient?

A high-risk patient is one who is incapacitated because of frailty or physical or mental impairment. Patients are considered incapacitated if, at a minimum, they:

- Are legally committed;
- Have a court-appointed legal guardian;
- Are considered dangerous to self or others;

- Lack cognitive ability (either permanently or temporarily) to make relevant decisions;
- Have physical or mental impairments that increase their risk of harm to self or others.

In addition, patients whose mental status may change rapidly, such as those suffering from post-surgical delirium or drug-induced psychosis, become at risk. When there is a reported change in mental status for any reason, patients may require repeated assessments during the day to determine if they are at high risk.

What is Meant by an Assessment?

An assessment is a clinical evaluation of patients with regard to their capacity to make decisions relative to their immediate physical safety or well-being. Past history may be a guide, as well as information obtained by friends, relatives, or caregivers. Each facility must determine the frequency for assessing the cognitive ability of patients with regard to their safety and developing safety measures, as appropriate for the patient's condition.

Timing of Assessments

- Patients whose mental status may change rapidly, such as those suffering from post-surgical delirium or drug-induced psychosis, may require repeated assessments during the day. An assessment is a clinical event and should be recorded in the medical record, whether paper-based or electronic. An assessment may be recorded as part of the routine mental status during a physical or mental health examination or listed separately in the progress note. At a minimum, the clinical assessment of cognitive impairment must be recorded in the patient's record:
    - at the time of inpatient admission, discharge, or transfer between units or care setting;
    - as a component of each initial and annual outpatient evaluation;
    - when there is a reported change in mental status for any reason; and
    - in absentia, i.e., when they have disappeared from a clinical setting.

Staff may be alerted to patients at special risk through electronic "flags" or reminders.

Wandering Patient

What is a wandering patient? A wandering patient is a high-risk patient who has shown a propensity to stray beyond the view or control of employees, thereby requiring a high degree of monitoring and protection to ensure the patient's safety.

Missing Patient

A missing patient is a high-risk patient who disappears from an inpatient or outpatient treatment area or while under control of VA, such as during transport. Situations when patients meet the high-risk patient criteria and should be considered missing include, but are not limited to, the following:

- An inpatient or day treatment high-risk patient who is not present to receive a scheduled medication, treatment, meal, or appointment, and whose whereabouts are unknown.
- A high-risk patient who does not return from pass as scheduled and whose whereabouts are unknown. Of course, staff must determine the circumstances under which a high-risk patient may be given a pass and the safeguards established at the time.
- A high-risk patient who checked in for an outpatient clinic appointment but is not present for the appointment when called, and whose whereabouts are unknown. If someone accompanied the patient, that person should be located immediately if possible.
- A high-risk outpatient from a community facility who does not return to his or her community facility following the appointment and whose whereabouts are unknown.
- A high-risk patient who is using VA-sponsored transportation (Disabled American Veterans (DAV) vans, VA drivers, VA shuttles) who does not report to that transportation for the return trip.

Missing Patient Versus Absent Patient

How can you tell the difference between a missing patient and one who is just absent? An "absent patient" is one who leaves a treatment area without knowledge or permission of staff, but who does not meet the high-risk criteria outlined for a "missing patient" and is not considered incapacitated. The great majority of the patients we see are not at high-risk. Under some circumstances a patient whose whereabouts are unknown, and who usually would not be considered incapacitated or at high risk, may be in potential danger and should be considered missing. Those circumstances should be noted in the clinical record by a responsible clinician.

An otherwise "absent patient" should be classified as a "missing patient" when one or a combination of additional environmental and clinical factors may, in the judgment of the responsible clinician, increase the patient's vulnerability and risk. Conditions that might lead to this decision may include, but are not be limited to, the following:

- Weather conditions, i.e., the patient has inappropriate dress, and the patient's safety is compromised;
- Construction sites or other dangerous conditions exist nearby;
- There has been recent trauma, unexpected bad news, or an abrupt change in clinical status;
- There are local geographic conditions that increase risk; or
- Homelessness, in combination with other factors that create risk.

Chapter 2: The Search for Missing Patients

Preliminary Versus Full Search

Preliminary search definition: A preliminary search must be initiated as soon as it is determined that a high-risk patient is missing. A preliminary search includes nearby ward or clinic areas, offices, and adjacent areas such as lobbies, stairwells, elevators, and so forth. A preliminary search will be initiated and coordinated by locally designated staff in each clinical area as defined in your local facility's Missing Patient Plan.

Full search definition: A full search is authorized by the medical center Director, or designee, if the missing patient is not located during the preliminary search and a review of the clinical assessment confirms that the patient is at high-risk. VA Police and Security Service and appropriate medical center staff on duty participate in the search.

What Areas Must Be Searched Under a Full Search?

A full search includes all areas of the facility in addition to those covered by the preliminary search, such as:

- All buildings, elevators, designated smoking areas, accessible areas for outpatient clinics, construction sites, and other structures.
- All grounds areas, parking lots, ball fields, tennis courts, outdoor seating and picnic areas, woods, and areas off, but contiguous to, the property (e.g., local neighborhood attractions). See "Grid Search" below for details of planning, organizing, and per-

forming a systematic search of VA property. *NOTE:* The facility Missing Patient Plan must include specific instructions as to what action(s) to initiate if the patient is found off the grounds, because there is no legal authority, lacking an extreme exigency, for patients to be physically detained against their will off facility property.

Grid Search (Patient Searches Using Grid Sectors)

1. Work with facility engineering staff to obtain a site plot of the facility and surrounding areas. Superimpose a grid map to delineate the grid sectors.
2. One individual is to be responsible to gather all pertinent information concerning the grid search. This needs to include:
   a. Search grid sector assignments;
   b. Times and by whom grid sectors are searched;
   c. Times and by whom each building is searched;
   d. Times and to whom notifications and requests are made; and
   e. Result of search.
3. The indoor search needs to include all buildings within the assigned search area to include any unsecured: stairwells, closets, attics, crawl spaces, equipment rooms, all smoking shelters, indoor construction areas, bathrooms, vending areas, and all other areas large enough for the subject to hide.
4. The outdoor search needs to include: brush and open areas, all parking areas, all government and nongovernment vehicles, all courtyard areas, all shrubbery around buildings, all construction areas, all outlying structures on grounds not assigned to interior search personnel, and any other area where a subject could have wandered.
5. The outdoor search is to be a methodical and complete visual inspection of open terrain for a lost or injured person, or for indications and marks of a person's movement. Larger areas are to be divided into smaller, more manageable grids. Each grid is approximately 500 by 500 feet and is designated with coordinates as illustrated on the search grid maps.
6. Each search team is assigned to a grid or number of grids. Each grid is to be searched from south to north by a search team in sweeps by lines of team members spaced abreast. Several sweeps may be necessary to completely cover assigned grids. A leader directs the search team.

7. The leader is responsible for the safety of team members and to make sure the search of assigned grids is complete. Failure to check one small area may result in search failure.
8. If the subject is found, the search team will render first aid if needed and notify command post of the location and, if needed request that medical personnel be sent. If the subject is unharmed, the search team will transport the subject back to the appropriate treatment area.
9. If the subject is found deceased, the subject and area surrounding the subject will be cordoned off and preserved as a possible crime scene until instructions and the proper authorization have been received.

In What Ways Are VA Police Involved in a Search?

- VA Police and Security Service participate with appropriate medical center staff on duty in every full search.
- When appropriate during or following the full search, VA Police and Security Service must contact the appropriate outside law enforcement agencies to file a missing persons report providing all the needed data so as to ensure that the patient is entered into the National Crime Information Computer (NCIC) system.
- VA Police are to be notified immediately in the event that a missing patient is found to be deceased on VA property. The Federal Bureau of Investigation (FBI), State and local police, the Office of the Medical Examiner, and local management officials are to be notified as designated by your facility's Missing Patient Plan.

What Are Missing Patient Drills?

Every VA medical center and clinic, including CBOCs, must conduct Missing Patient Drills that replicate preliminary and full searches as they might occur at your own facility. Once staff have received initial training, additional drills must be conducted at least annually (or more frequently if judged prudent due to local circumstances) to effectively evaluate known areas of vulnerability throughout and surrounding the facility. Clinical settings that provide 24-hour care must train staff on all shifts initially and subsequently at least on an annual basis for each shift.

Missing Patient Drills that integrate findings from environmental rounds or other patient safety processes (such as aggregated RCAs), must be conducted at each medical center or site of jurisdiction, including CBOCs. Once staff have received initial training, additional drills must be conducted at least annually (or more frequently, if judged prudent due to local circumstances) to effectively evaluate known areas of vulnerability throughout and surrounding the facility. Once staff are fully trained, an actual search during which the search plan is fully implemented and a critique is completed may take the place of the drill for the shift involved in the actual search. It is recommended that the sites for missing patient drills be prioritized based on known areas of vulnerability and lessons learned from RCAs and other risk management or performance improvement processes.

How Can You Tell if a Missing Patient Might Be at Another VA Facility?

The new Web-Based Missing Patient Registry (WBMPR) is a software application available at all VA facilities that contains information on high-risk patients who are missing. It replaces a previous non-Web version. Each facility's Missing Patient Plan needs to designate at least one person who can access the WBMPR. The WBMPR user(s) will be given a user ID and password. Anyone with a user ID and password can access the WBMPR.

When a full search has failed to locate a missing patient, a WBMPR user should enter the name of that patient in the WBMPR. When the facility reports a patient as missing, the WBMPR will send an e-mail to selected officials at the reporting facility to inform them of the missing patient event, so each facility will need to maintain, in the WBMPR, a list containing the officials who should be notified by the WBMPR. A special feature of the WBMPR is that it will also automatically contact the officials on that e-mail list when their missing patient presents for care at another VA facility. In addition, the MPWBR will send an e-mail with pertinent information about the formerly missing patient to the officials on the MBMPR e-mail list that is maintained at the facility where that patient has presented for care.

Chapter 3: Prevention: Everyone's Responsibility

What Do I Have to Do With Missing Patient Events?

All employees, including both clinical and nonclinical staff, are responsible for assessing, reviewing, and developing processes to enhance patient safety associated with wandering or missing patient events within the scope of their job, as well as intervening when appropriate. The prevention and effective management of wandering and missing patient events is based on clinical assessment of cognitive ability for each patient and the associated safety risks.

Assessment

An assessment is a clinical evaluation of patients with regard to their capacity to make decisions relative to their immediate physical safety or well being. Past history may be a guide, as well as information obtained by friends, relatives, or caregivers. Patients whose mental status may change rapidly, such as those suffering from post-surgical delirium or drug-induced psychosis, may require repeated assessments during the day. An assessment is a clinical event and should be recorded in the medical record, whether paper-based or electronic. Staff may be alerted to patients at special risk through electronic "flags" or reminders.

To prevent accidental deaths and injuries, VHA must: (1) Recognize, specify, and maintain appropriate staff responsibility for the whereabouts of patients; (2) Systematically assess all patients to determine the risk potential for those who may wander or become missing from a treatment setting; (3) Detect missing patients early; and (4) Initiate prompt search procedures.

NOTE: If the patient is at high-risk, then assessment and the safety measures appropriate for the patient need to be part of the treatment plan, which must be discussed among the patient's health care providers. In addition, that assessment and the safety measures need to be included in the alert that comes to the attention of all applicable health care providers when the patient's record is accessed. The assessment must occur. The assessment and related safety measures must be discussed by each patient's treatment team and documented as being discussed.

What Do I Look at to See Where My Group Can Minimize Risks?

Because of the documented risks inherent in the aging veteran population, VHA aims to be as proactive as possible in minimizing risks for patients under its care. As a result, the following processes must be integrated into each facility's Missing Patients Plan and become part of the daily operation of the facility:

- Policies on patient privileging, requirements for patient supervision and surveillance, and search procedures with regard to early identification of missing patients.
- Initial and annual training of all relevant staff regarding policy and search policies and procedures for identifying, assessing, and finding missing patients.
- The systematic and comprehensive monitoring and assessment of hazardous areas and construction sites must be an integral part of this process.

- A comprehensive review and assessment of locations for activities away from the facility must be conducted and integrated in the planning of recreational activities to facilitate safety, especially for those patients known to be high-risk.
- Each facility must take special precautions during the transport of known high-risk patients and those reported to have a change in mental status, in the absence of clinical assessment.
- Each facility must establish processes to assure the availability of pictures and physical descriptions for all high-risk patients in the event that they are suspected to be missing as a means to enhance the effectiveness of search procedures. Patient Identification System photographs may be used where available.
- Missing Patient Drills that integrate findings from environmental rounds or other patient safety processes (such as aggregated Root Cause Analysis) must be conducted at each medical center or site of jurisdiction, including CBOCs. Aggregated Review should be done in response to one or more adverse events or close calls involving missing patients. It is recommended that the sites for missing patient drills be prioritized based on known areas of vulnerability and lessons learned from RCAs and other risk management or performance improvement processes.
- Each facility must consider actual or close call missing patient events in accordance with NCPS guidelines and VHA Handbook 1050.1, and integrate the resulting information into education and training of staff and improving existing processes to enhance patient safety.

How Does Root Cause Analysis Help Prevent Missing Patient Events?

VA considers reducing and preventing missing patient events an important part of improving patient safety. The VA National Center for Patient Safety (NCPS) has developed a system for looking at problems and incidents that involve the safety of patients called Root Cause Analysis (RCA). The RCA process is used to study selected incidents, including both actual events where a patient was harmed and close calls where an event almost occurred but was averted. VA NCPS emphasizes that we can learn as much from close calls as from actual events and that learning from close calls can help us to prevent adverse events, including missing patient events, before they happen. Your Patient Safety Manager is the person that you should contact after a missing patient event or close call has occurred. Using tools developed by NCPS your Patient Safety Manager will determine if an RCA should be performed.

Does Technology Help Us to Prevent High-Risk Patients From Leaving Without Permission?

Electronic devices physically attached to a high-risk patient that ring an alarm at the nursing station when a high-risk patient nears an exit have been in use for some time. The use of electronic technology for those patients considered to be high-risk may be used only as one tool to enhance and augment other processes for minimizing the risk of patients wandering away from a designated area or site of care. This use must not be considered as a substitute for professional vigilance and systematic verification of patient location, such as during change of shift rounds for inpatient and other supervised settings. Electronic devices and systems must be re-evaluated at the time of each wandering or missing patient event to assess possible contributing factors.

Electronic Devices

The use of electronic technology for those patients considered to be high-risk may be used only as one tool to enhance and augment other processes for minimizing the risk of patients wandering away from a designated area or site of care. This use must not be considered as a substitute for professional vigilance and systematic verification of patient location such as during change of shift rounds for inpatient and other supervised settings. When electronic technology is in use: (a) There must be systematic and frequent checks of all critical components of the system with clear designation of responsibility for monitoring and maintaining that system. A basic check of the system in high-risk areas is encouraged at a minimum every 24 hours to assure proper functioning as intended to minimize risk. Maintenance of the system must be consistent with manufacturer's guidelines; however, a complete systems check must be performed at least annually. A proactive assessment of potential vulnerabilities of the system and its use (e.g., failure Modes Effects Analysis) should be performed to guide the appropriate use of the system (see VHA Handbook 1050.1, sub par. 5d). (b) Electronic devices and systems must be re-evaluated at the time of each wandering or missing patient event to assess possible contributing factors.

TRAINING COURSES (FROM SLIDE PRESENTATIONS)

Bay Pines VAMC Geriatric Psychiatry Unit "Don't Get Lost" Inpatient and Day Treatment Programs Wandering Prevention Training Course

Gail Vaillancourt RN, Kelly Fethelkheir RN

The following information is from a slide presentation used during this training course.

Overview of Programs—Inpatient Program

- Treatment of acute mental and behavioral conditions
- Geared for diagnoses of dementia and depression and other psychiatric diagnoses
- 10-bed locked unit
- Specially trained staff
- Interdisciplinary Team consisting of Geriatric psychiatrist, Nurse Practitioner, Social Worker, Pharmacist, Dietician, Nursing, PT, OT, and KT.
- Daily case review

Overview of Programs—Outpatient Day Treatment Program

- Locked Unit
- Geared for dementia, depression, and other psychiatric diagnoses
- 25 patients attend daily from 9 A.M. to 2 P.M.
- Daily structure, support, and socialization
- Recreation, crafts, field trips, music, reminiscing, health education
- Lunch provided daily along with nutritious snacks
- Nursing intervention for psychiatric and medical problems
- Respite for caregivers

Philosophy

- Structure and routine
- Limit Goals
- Look at patients in a holistic way
- Patient and Caregiver are main focus
- "No-Fail Environment" for dementia patients*

* Stewart, J.T. (1995). Management of behavior problems in the demented patient. *American Family Physician, 52,* 2311–2322.

Goals of the Unit

- Provide comprehensive biopsychosocial care to veterans with age-related psychological and behavior problems
- Maximize their functional capacity and maintain the highest level of independence in the least restrictive environment
- Prevent relapse

No-Fail Environment

- Based on validation therapy
- Customer is always right
- Can prevent catastrophic reactions that can trigger a wandering event
- The most useful intervention that prevents agitation and behavioral problems
- Anosognosia—fail to recognize one's own deficits
- Support and educate staff and family
- Provide reassurance

Definition of Wandering

"aimless or purposeful motor activity that causes a social problem such as getting lost, leaving a safe environment or intruding in inappropriate places." (www.alz.org)

Types of Wandering

Random Wandering

- No apparent goal
- Aimless
- Random occurrence
- Passive in nature

Goal Directed

- Searching for something
- Purposeful
- Exit seekers

Wandering Statistics

- Time of year—Warmer season
- Time of day—6 A.M. to 12 midnight
- Usually found within one mile of point last seen
- Wander in straight lines until they encounter resistance
- Two-thirds of all dementia patients wander
- 7 of every 10 people diagnosed with dementia will wander and become lost
- It is the MOST frequent and challenging problem for caregivers

Critical Wanderers

- Definition: any person with dementia that wanders away from supervised care, a controlled environment, or cannot be located
- Each year over 125,000 people become critical wanderers
- *Survivability*—Only 50 percent of critical wanderers that require greater than 24 hours to locate will survive

Wandering Triggers

- Unfamiliar Environment
- Argumentative Situation
- Change in Schedule / Routine
- Medications
- Left alone in car
- Day care
- Unfamiliar sights or sounds
- Restlessness due to lack of physical activity
- Searching for food, drink, bathroom, or companion
- Trying to complete former tasks (work, etc.)

Geropsychiatry Inpatient Unit Wandering Prevention

- Identification of patients at risk for wandering
- Low patient to staff ratio
- Locked Unit
- ESO (Enhanced Safety Observation) for patients at risk for wandering. Staff visualizes patients on ESO at all times.
- Staff escorts ESO patients to ALL appointments
- Education of nonclinical personnel and volunteers

Geropsychiatry Day Treatment Wandering Prevention

- Locked Unit
- Identification of patients and use of Special ID badge for patients at risk for wandering
- Numerous roll calls by seasoned staff
- Escorted to and from unit and to all appointments by staff/trained volunteers
- Low patient to staff ratio
- Use of cell phones and walkie-talkies

- Educate staff, volunteers, and nonclinical staff about at-risk patients and those patients permitted to leave unit
- Medic-Alert Bracelets provided
- Continuous patient reassessments

*Missing Patient Protocol—High Risk Patient (*VA Center Memorandum 516–00–00–24)*

- Preliminary and immediate search of area by staff
- Notify VA police and provide description
- Notify Nursing Supervisor, Admitting Officer of the Day (AOD), and Physician
- Complete Report of Unauthorized Absence
- Notify family
- Critique of record of recovery goes to Quality Systems and a Root Cause Analysis is completed

REMEMBER...

Missing Patient Process Improvement Presentation

VA Sierra Nevada Health Care System (654), Reno, NV
Judith O'Neal, RN, Patient Safety Officer

Why?

- Prevent a catastrophic event due to patient elopement from facility
- Decrease risk of patient abuse/exploitation by preventing unauthorized persons from having access to the patients

Reno Presents Unique Problems

- 24-hour town
  - Transient
  - Gambling
  - Drinking
- Recent elopements have been patients leaving on unauthorized passes for "recreation"
- Due to clinician concerns, patient is bumped up to "missing" rather than "absent"

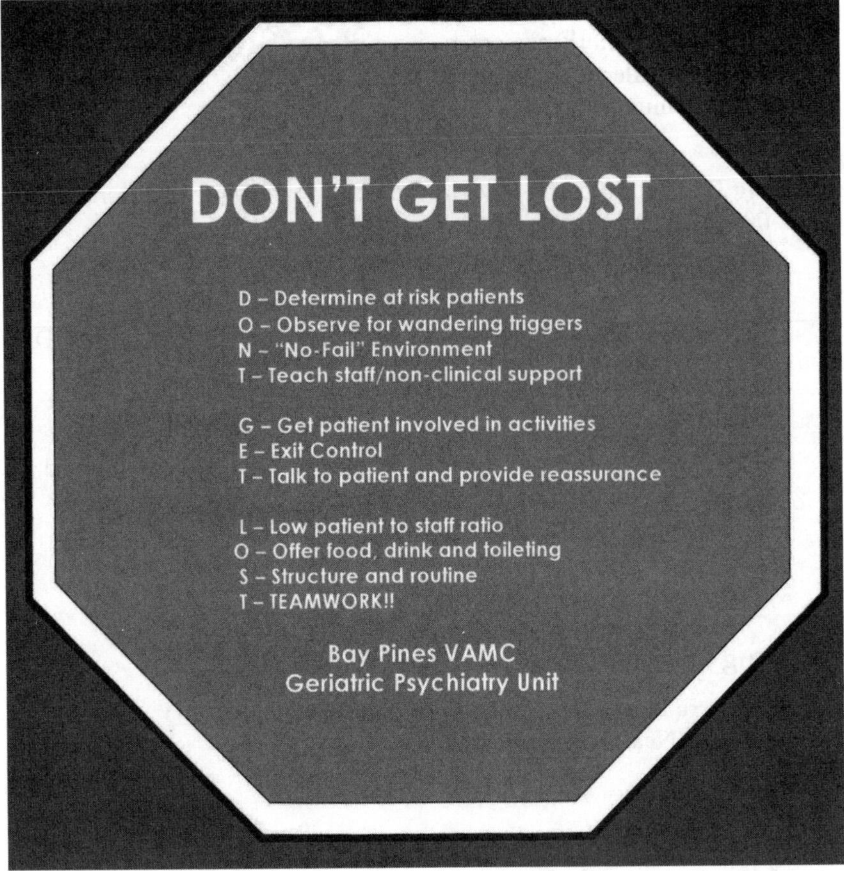

FIGURE C.1

Environmental

- Reduced the number of available TCU exits from 6 to 1
  - Locked four north doors and one east door of the TCU
  - Allows patient free access to court yard and entire unit
  - Doors automatically unlock in the advent of fire
  - Requires 1:1 monitoring of high-risk patients during fire
- This left only one exit resulting in faster staff response to code-alert alarm at main entrance.

Staff Education

- Clinician education "missing" vs. "absent"
- Missing Patient Directive revised with user-friendly checklist
- Missing patient and code alert included in mandatories

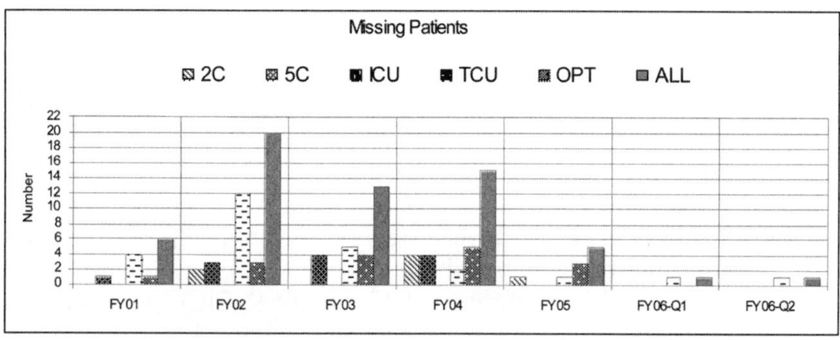

FIGURE C.2

- Missing patient education completed when new problems are identified by root cause analysis
    - Additional abuse/exploitation education for TCU staff (also in mandatories for all nursing personnel)
    - VA Police standby while secure door unlocked until relocked

Identify Wanderers

- Wander risk-assessment alert developed
- Chart is flagged
- Place code-alert on "high-risk" patient
- Place orange armband on "high-risk" patient
- TCU orange nameplates indicate "high risk" for wandering

Supportive Processes

- TCU pass procedure
    - sign out log
    - tracking tool

Table C.1 Missing Patient Process Improvement by FY

	2CMed/ Surg	5C Psych	ICU	TCU Transitional Care	Outpatient	All
FY01		1		4	1	6
FY02	2	3		12	3	20
FY03		4		5	4	13
FY04	4	4		2	5	15
FY05	1			1	3	5
FY06 Q1				1		1
FY06 Q2				1		1

- improved pass order
- templates

- Compressed guardianship process for high-risk patients
- Wander risk alert displays at check-in, PSAs assure 1:1 and document in record
- 1:1 suicidal patient in Triage
- Direct admits from Mental Health to inpatient Psych
- Involved local bus drivers—report patients in PJs and orange armbands trying to board
- National Crime Information Computer (NCIC) installed, VA Police trained, enter missing patients

Code "66"

- Overhead announcement "Code 66" summons the personnel pool similar to facility disaster plan
- All available staff respond
- VA police use facility map to make assignments
- Staff report back after search and are asked for recommendations for improvement next time
  - Send staff with radios to the outside areas
  - Purchase more radios
  - Critique is submitted with missing patient police report to Patient Safety Officer who forwards recommendations to responsible parties
- Frequent drills—initially

Staffing

- We wanted to place a staff person at the main entrance of the TCU with
  - Pictures of the high-risk patients
  - List of approved visitors
  - Monitor patient passes
- We did not have the resources to staff this low level position (we were already having difficulty filling patient transport positions)

FAMILY/CAREGIVER EDUCATIONAL MATERIALS

Family/Caregiver Brochure

(Provided by Vivian E. Bugaoan, LCSW, Northport VA Medical Center, Northport, NY)

FIGURE C.3

Taking calmly and in a reassuring voice can prevent the person from struggling and resisting your effects to re-direct him.

10. Involve Your Neighbors
Inform your neighbors of the person's condition and keep a list of their names and telephone numbers handy.
Ask your neighbors to call you or the police, if you cannot be reached, if they see the person walking alone in the neighborhood.

11. Be Aware of Hazards.
Places that appear safe to you can be dangerous for the person who wanders. Check around your home for possible hazards such as swimming pools, dense bushes, bus stops, tunnels and busy roadways.

12. Use Signs.
A confused person may start to wander looking for the bathroom at home. A sign on the bathroom door may help.

13. Consult Your Doctor.
Certain medications may make the confused person less restless. Other drugs can cause restlessness.
All medications, whether prescribed by the doctor or purchased over the counter, must be closely supervised by a doctor.

14. Enroll the Person in "Safe Return."
The Alzheimer Associate's Safe Return Program provides I.D. products, registration in a National Information/Photo Database, a 24-hour toll-free crisis line and a nationwide fax alert system.

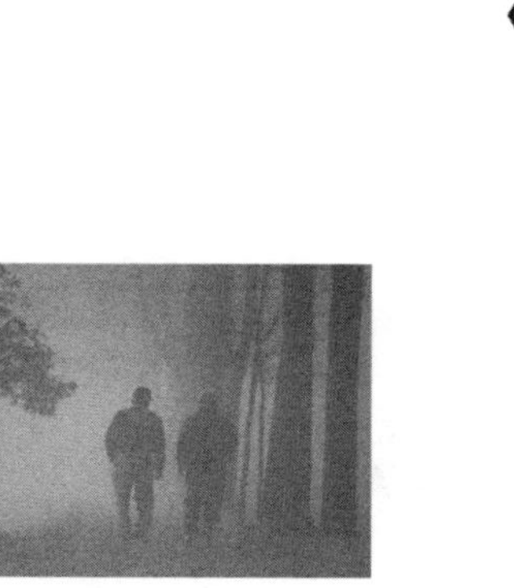

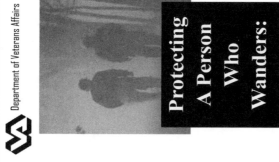

For further assistance in managing the needs of a person who wanders, please contact the clinic social worker or call Social Work Service, 516-261-4400 extension 7030.

Department of Veterans Affairs

Protecting A Person Who Wanders:

Helpful Hints and Safety Precautions

VA Medical Center
79 Middleville Rd.
Northport, NY 11768

Index